The GIANT BOOK of Women's Health Secrets

The GIANT BOOK of
Women's Health Secrets

By Kerri Bodmer
and Nan Kathryn Fuchs, PhD

Soundview Publications
Atlanta, Georgia

ISBN 1-885385-00-5

Cover design by Elizabeth Bame

Additional copies of this book may be purchased from Soundview Publications. Please call for more information. Soundview Publications also publishes Kerri Bodmer's monthly medical newsletter, *Women's Health Letter*. To subscribe, please call or write:

Soundview Publications, Inc.
Post Office Box 467939
Atlanta, Georgia 31146-7939
800-728-2288 or 770-399-5617

Table of Contents

Health Secrets From Jeanne Calment

This book is dedicated to the memory of Jeanne Calment, whose claim to fame was her longevity.

She was born February 21, 1875, in Arles, France, and died there, too, in 1997 at the age of 122 years, 5 months, and 2 weeks. She had held the record as the oldest living person in the world whose age had been verified by official documents.

How did she manage to live so long?

The French boast that it wasn't for a lack of bad habits, since she ate two pounds of chocolate a week and didn't give up smoking until she was 117.

But a closer look at this remarkable woman's life reveals some powerful health and longevity secrets that you can use, too.

As a young girl, Jeanne played in the same countrysides, and slept under the same starry-night skies, that inspired artist Vincent Van Gogh to create some of today's most-treasured paintings. She even met Van Gogh in the late 1880s.

At the age of 21, in 1896, she married a successful businessman. While he ran the store, she studied the piano, attended the opera, rode in hunting parties, played tennis, swam, and bicycled. (Therein lies Secret #1: interests and exercise — just two brisk 30-minute walks a week was recently shown to reduce the overall death rate by 44 percent!)

Although longevity ran in her family, with her mother living to age 86 and her father to age 93, her biographer Jean-Marie Robine believed Jeanne Calment's greatest strength was her unflappability. "I think she ... was immune to stress." She also quoted Jeanne as once saying, "If you can't do anything about it, don't worry about it." (That's Secret #2: good stress-management skills.)

This unflappability may have helped her better overcome grief in her life, as well. Her only child, a daughter, died young of pneumonia in 1934 and left her an eight-year-old grandson to raise. Her husband died of food poisoning in 1942, and her grandson died in an auto accident in 1960.

Nevertheless, Jeanne Calment bubbled with activity, enthusiasm, and humor, right up to the end.

She bicycled to her 100th birthday party. Then later, walked all over Arles thanking those who'd helped her celebrate. (There's Secret #3: good relationships.)

When her memory began to fail, she quipped to an interviewer, "When you're 117, see if you remember everything!"

When another visitor, upon leaving, said "until next year, perhaps," she retorted, "I don't see why not! You don't look so bad."

But perhaps her most famous one-liner was about her face which she treated with olive oil. She said, "I've never had but one wrinkle, and I'm sitting on it." (These are examples of Secret #4: humor.)

If you're smiling right now, note also how you feel. Good feelings pack a lot of health and healing power — and likely went a long way toward helping Jeanne Calment live so long.

But my main purpose in sharing Jeanne Calment's health and longevity secrets is to let you know that being healthier and living longer may be much easier than you may have imagined, as the pages of this book, *The Giant Book of Women's Health Secrets*, will also reveal.

Be happy, be healthy,
Kerri Bodmer

Is Stress Killing You Slowly?

Cultural anthropologists tell us that in present-day tribal societies, such as those found mainly in Africa and parts of Asia, people tend to work an average of about four hours a day. In addition, these societies are usually headed up by women and organized cooperatively, in which all major tasks such as growing food, cooking, washing, making clothes, and even child rearing, are shared group activities. Although such a lifestyle may sound strange to us, it spans 97 percent of human history.

In contrast, modern-day Western cultures feature 40-hour work weeks and single family units; living in single family dwellings, and relying on one or two adults in the household to be the sole providers of food, shelter, clothing, and a vast array of modern-day extras. If we want to have it all, we must do it all. This often doesn't even leave us enough time to get a good night's sleep, much less the opportunity to simply relax.

As a result, mental stress is now the #1 cause of life-threatening disease, according to many well-respected experts. The role it plays in the development of many serious diseases is well documented. Just last year, the *Journal of the American Medical Association* published the results of a Duke University five-year study that concluded mental stress is more dangerous to the heart than physical stress.

The study also indicated that the way we respond to mental stress is a strong predictor of whether or not we are vulnerable to heart attacks, even death. Since heart disease is the leading cause of death, ultimately claiming one of every two female lives, the single most significant thing every one of us can do to protect our health may very well be to reduce stress.

For many of us, stress is a vague concept. So let's start by defining it as clearly as possible.

Physical stress occurs when your body is over-burdened physically. Examples of physical stress include lack of sleep, poor nutrition, allergies, tobacco and other substance abuse, smog and other pollutants, extreme heat or cold, lack of water, overexertion, major and long-term illness, and acute trauma such as a broken bone. The common denominator of physical stress is that your body must spend extra energy, nutrients, and other resources to overcome it. This can lead to a deterioration of overall health. Examples include frostbite and smoking-related diseases, respectively.

Emotional stress manifests itself physically through our nervous system. When you are startled and your heart starts racing, that's emotional stress in its purest form. This is your fight-or-flight response. It prompts you to flee immediately, without thinking when you're facing a life-or-death situation. Imagine your car stranded on the tracks of an oncoming train. Your brain responds by automatically releasing stress hormones, which shift you into high gear:

● Your pupils dilate for sharper vision.

● Your bronchial tubes expand and breathing accelerates to increase oxygen intake.

● Your heart rate and blood pressure soar to speed this extra oxygen to muscles for extra energy.

● Your liver releases extra glucose and fatty acids for even more energy.

This type of stress is functional and it can literally save your life.

Modern life, however, is rife with situations that are not life-threatening, but can trigger milder versions of mental stress. You can be certain you are experiencing this when you have the above stress reactions in response to a non-life-threatening event. Many modern-day stressors, however, are often more subtle and difficult to recognize. Still, just about everyone experiences them, some of us more than others.

Instead of the classic fight-or-flight responses, these stressors can produce irritability, anxiety, tension, edginess, restlessness, and feeling overwhelmed. These types of stress, when experienced chronically or for extended periods of time, also put an extra physical burden on your body, which can cause your health to deteriorate and even kill you.

The physical burden comes into play because your body releases stress hormones, such as adrenaline and cortisol, in response to mental stress. The release of these hormones preempts and disrupts the normal flow of other hormones and thus the execution of certain normal bodily functions, as vital energy and other resources are diverted elsewhere. This is why a lack of emotional calm disrupts the progress of women in labor.

More commonly, both physical and mental stress can cause menstrual cycle irregularity.

These types of stress responses are our bodies' way of telling you it needs more tranquillity for optimum performance. Over extended periods of time, especially, failing to heed our bodies' calls for less stress can result in adverse effects on our health. To avoid these, we need to become better at avoiding, reducing, and managing stress, both physical and mental. Keep in mind that the lower our physical stress levels, the better we're able to handle mental stress.

Because of the effects of stress on our lives, the first chapter of this book deals with it and many of the other toxic emotions that inhibit our ability to fight disease. Until we conquer these negative influences, we can't move on to conquer the many health problems we may face. But once we've dealt with them, we can then employ the many other health secrets contained in this book.

Chapter 1

Replace Toxic Emotions With Healing Emotions

Have you ever been upset with a doctor who told you, "There's nothing wrong with you. It's all in your head," when you knew you weren't feeling well physically?

Whether you've ever had difficulty getting a specific diagnosis or not, your past or present illnesses probably got started or were helped along by toxic emotions. Most people don't realize that chronic and severe illnesses usually have an emotional component.

Toxic emotions make you feel tired, depressed, listless, and upset. They lower your immune system and help cause bothersome and serious illnesses. Most of all, they waste your time. They waste your life.

Anger, resentment, hate, bitterness, impatience, unkindness, negative thinking, and vindictiveness are all toxic emotions. When you hold on to them and live with them day in and day out, they create a great deal of stress. This constant stress lowers your immune system, contributing to illness.

Positive emotions, like love, enthusiasm, and happiness, cleanse your system and give you energy. They heal your body, mind, and spirit. They are responsible for serious illnesses going into remission and for your body's ability to heal itself more quickly.

Where It Begins

Our illnesses are rarely all physical or all emotional in origin. We've known this since the 1950's when Dr. Hans Selye, a biochemist, began writing about the effects of stress hormone activity and illness in his classic book, *The Stress of Life*. And in 1977, Kenneth Pelletier wrote *Mind as Healer, Mind as Slayer*, in which he described some of the diseases caused by stress: from heart disease and cancer to migraines and arthritis.

Today, the mind-body connection is accepted by more physicians, psychotherapists, and other health care professionals. Decades of scientific studies have shown that our minds do, indeed, control our bodies' chemistry, and that negative thoughts produce destructive chemicals that can harm us. It's time to take a closer look at your toxic emotions and your health, because the thoughts you think and the feelings you have can either help you become and stay healthy or can literally kill you.

We don't want you to assume that all you need to do to be healthy is to eliminate your toxic emotions and take a positive attitude toward life. Although that approach certainly has its merits. First, get a diagnosis of any physical symptoms you are experiencing from one or more doctors, so you know what you're dealing with. Then look at some of the emotional aspects of your problem and address it.

Psychological and Physiological Aspects of Stress

Just saying that emotions are toxic is not enough. We need to understand their physiological consequences. Toxic emotions lead to prolonged mental stress — and stress can kill us.

As far back as the 1930s, Harvard physiologist Walter Cannon believed our bodies regulated themselves according to our needs. This balance, or homeostasis, was affected by our blood pressure, body temperature, heart rate, blood sugar — and by stress. Cannon saw that when we were in particularly stressful conditions, our bodies adapted by working overtime to try to restore us to balance. He called this the "fight-or-flight" response. What this means is that when we're surprised by a bear in the woods we're either going to fight it, or run like crazy. This fight-or-flight response is affected by chemicals secreted in the brain that send a signal to the adrenal glands (glands that produce hormones like cortisol and adrenaline).

The adrenal hormones affect your nervous system and muscles. They are responsible for the shakiness you feel when you barely avoid an accident or are suddenly surprised by someone sneaking up on you. They give you superhuman strength to lift something far heavier than you could ordinarily to save someone from being crushed, and they give you the energy you need to run faster than you thought possible when you feel you're in danger.

This stress response was, most likely, the way many of our ancestors survived difficult situations, and in itself is not necessarily toxic. But we encounter stressors much more often in our daily lives, and although they may not be life-threatening, they overwork our glands, organs, nervous system, and brain. Our bodies can deal with a little stress. High levels of stress over prolonged periods of time, however, can be toxic — more than our bodies can handle.

Decades after Walter Cannon's work, Dr. George F. Solomon, a psychiatrist at Stanford University, decided that stress and emotions not only set off our fight-or-flight response, they also affected our immune systems. He began to experiment with the hypothalamus, a tiny part of the brain where hormone secretions associated with stress responses begin. Solomon, and an immunologist, Alfred Amkraut, found that when the hypothalamus in rats was damaged, their immunity decreased. This was the

---

Stress and Surgery

The thought of surgery is stressful, and stress has a direct impact on our health. Now, a study is showing that when a woman hears stress-reducing messages when she's under anesthesia, her recovery time is shortened.

Nearly 40 women who had hysterectomies (a procedure we discourage since 90 percent are estimated to be unnecessary and actually more harmful than beneficial), were separated into two groups. One group listened to a blank tape during the operation; the other group heard a tape with nine minutes of suggestions that they would not feel pain afterward, would not be sick, and the more they relaxed the better they would feel. The women who heard these suggestions improved greatly over those who heard nothing.

If you're undergoing surgery, consider finding or making a tape with these kinds of suggestions on it. Or bring a tape of your favorite inspirational music to be played. Often, surgeons talk about sports, failed operations, and other negative things. You have a right to ask your surgeon and the attending nurses to keep the talk positive and encouraging. By doing so, you may even surprise them in your recovery.

Anderson, Robert A., MD. "Surgical recovery and intraoperative suggestion," *The Townsend Letter*, June 1997.

beginning of the scientific study of the mind/body connection — and examination of the effects of toxic emotions.

What Happens When You're Under Stress

There are two areas in your body that are activated by stress. These are the autonomic nervous system, which is involuntary, and the endocrine system. The autonomic nervous system has two components, which are called the sympathetic and the parasympathetic nervous systems. The sympathetic system causes your involuntary muscles to tense up, and it activates your endocrine system. The parasympathetic system dilates your smooth muscles, causing you to relax.

When you're under stress, your sympathetic nervous system is activated; blood leaves your hands, feet, and stomach and starts to go to

Stress Slows Healing

We already know that emotional stress can adversely affect our physical health. Short-term stress can increase our susceptibility to catching a cold. And long-term stress can wear down our immune system until we become more susceptible to more serious conditions, including cancer. New research now suggests that stress can also impair our ability to heal. A study of 26 women who had breast biopsies timed the recovery periods of the women. Thirteen of them who were under the stress of caring for someone with Alzheimer's disease took an average of nine days longer to heal than the 13 women who weren't experiencing constant stress. If you are trying to heal from a surgery (or maybe another health problem), minimizing stress will help speed your recovery.

In addition, remember that all kinds of stressors add stress to your body — such as lack of sleep or a poor diet. When your body is on the mend, you need to take the best possible care of yourself on all fronts. This includes getting plenty of sleep and eating the best foods you can find. Keep your sugars and fats low, eat lightly, chew your food well, and eat plenty of whole grains, veggies, and fruit.

Lancet, November 4, 1995.

your head and torso. You get cold hands, chills, a knot in your stomach. Your muscles get tight — shoulders, neck, throat. You are feeling the effects of the fight-or-flight response.

The sympathetic nervous system works with your endocrine system when you're under stress. Your endocrine system — pituitary glands, thyroid, parathyroids, islets of Langerhans in your pancreas, and adrenal glands — become activated and secrete hormones inappropriately. Two of the most important ones in the stress response are ACTH (adrenocorticotrophic hormone) and TTH (thyrotrophic hormone), both released by the pituitary gland, which cause you to sweat, feel nervous and shaky, have a rapid heartbeat, and feel exhausted. These are the same kinds of feelings you would get from food poisoning. It's just a different kind of toxic reaction.

The sympathetic system also stimulates your adrenal glands to make adrenaline, and you may feel an adrenaline "rush." Adrenaline also sends a message to your liver to release glucose (sugar) for quick energy. It causes you to burn carbohydrates faster, opens up the arteries to your heart so you breathe faster, and raises your temperature. If your fight-or-flight response occurs only when you're facing a bear in the woods or escape an accident, your immune system won't suffer. That's what it's for. But if you are under stress constantly, your immune system may lose its ability to protect you from microorganisms and disease.

Stress and Immunity

Joseph Pizzorno, ND, founding president of Bastyr University, the first accredited university of natural medicine in the country, and author of *Total Wellness* (Prima Publishing, 1966) says, "In general, the degree of immunosuppression is proportional to the level of stress." So the more stress you're under, the weaker your immune system is likely to be.

Stress overactivates the sympathetic nervous system. Your immune system works best when the para-sympathetic nervous system is up and running and when the sympathetic system is not stimulating the production of adrenal hormones. These hormones have a toxic response in your body by lowering your white blood cells — your body's defense system — and they actually shrink your thymus gland. Your thymus is the gland that rules and supports your entire immune system.

Heart Disease and the Type A Personality

Back in the early 1970s, two researchers, Friedman and Rosenman, found that more men had heart disease than women, and not because of any dietary or hormonal differences. They discovered that their personalities were quite different. More men had what they called Type A personalities: They were excessively competitive and felt like they had to continually meet deadlines. Women, who were more likely to possess Type B personalities, were more relaxed, made time for leisure activities, and worked more for personal satisfaction than for money.

The Type A personality is toxic — always striving for the external, the material; the Type B personality takes better care of itself and is healing. In the two decades following this research on Type A and Type B personalities, women have achieved more in the workplace. And, as a result, there are now more women who have taken on the toxic Type A personality — along with all the harmful effects it produces.

Climbing the corporate ladder, however, needn't result in toxic emotions. Many high-achieving women benefit health-wise from higher levels of personal satisfaction and self-esteem.

In addition, the feelings of frustration and powerlessness that are common among pink-collar workers, as well as many homemakers and mothers, are toxic and have been linked to higher rates of heart disease.

Heart disease is now as prevalent among women as men. In fact, it's the number-one killer of postmenopausal women. One reason for female heart disease is our natural decline in estrogen after menopause, a hormone that serves as a calcium channel blocker, preventing deposits of calcium in the arteries. But the increase in heart disease is probably due to increased cholesterol production in the liver because of stress. When we're under stress, our liver manufactures more cholesterol.

Taking a Look at Stress

Living in a state of toxic emotions is draining. It leads to chronic mental stress and illness. We all know what stress feels like, but just what is it? According to pioneer biologist Hans Selye, it is "the rate of wear and tear within the body." This means that worrying about your job or a relationship produces stress, and so does traveling around the world or going on a weekend ski vacation. All stress is not bad, it's just creating wear and tear (and, along with it, a need for more nutrients to help repair both your mind and your body).

Sometimes when we're experiencing overwhelming stress we make ourselves sick so we don't have to deal with it — like getting a headache. At other times, stress causes us to use up protective vitamins and minerals that support our immune system and we "catch a cold" or get some other sickness, like heart disease or cancer. Fear and mental stress are two toxic emotional components that can lead directly to high blood pressure (hypertension) and possibly stroke.

But stress has great value for us in our lives. It can also be a pivotal point of our personal transformation. Psychotherapist Carl Jung observed that primitive people looked at illness as the strength coming from their unconscious minds that led them from one stage of life to another. Numerous people with cancer, AIDS, chronic fatigue, and other debilitating illnesses have found the quality of their lives increased greatly after facing their health issues. They adapted a different point of view and "detoxified" their emotions. They forgave people in their lives who had caused them emotional pain. They began expressing love to their friends, started doing what they wanted to do with their time, rather than what they thought they should do, and they started living life more fully. These were all benefits that came out of the stress of their illnesses.

Feeling Good With Endorphins

When you're under stress, your body uses more of certain vitamins and minerals. A lack of even some of these nutrients can alter your mood, creating irritability, mood swings, and negative thoughts. So which comes first, a diet lacking in sufficient nutrients to support your stress, or stresses in life that cause your body to be deficient in nutrients? It doesn't matter.

Endorphins are "feel good" chemicals released by the pituitary gland. Exercise helps release them. So does acupuncture. And so do certain nutrients like vitamin B_6, magnesium, and amino acids found in protein. Your thoughts do, too, through a powerful phenomenon known as the "placebo effect." Placebos are like sugar pills — worthless substances that won't change anyone's physical condition. Unless, of course, the patient believes they will. Time and again, studies have shown that when placebos were given along with the message that they would work — they did! Dr. Melvyn Werbach, author of the nutrition textbook, *Nutritional Influences on*

Illness, has stated, "We don't need better medicines, we need better placebos."

Your mind can crank out chemicals that make you feel good emotionally and even take away pain, because endorphins are chemically similar to morphine. What's the difference between them? Endorphins are hundreds of times more potent, and you have the ability to create them with your healing thoughts. Endorphins are caused by positive emotions. Toxic emotions don't stimulate their production.

Gary Schwartz, PhD, professor of psychology at the University of Arizona, has been researching emotions and health for more than 20 years. He has found that the ACE Factor (our ability to attend, connect, and express) can affect our immune systems, blood sugar, and heart in a positive way. People who repressed their emotions, Schwartz found, made too many endorphins in an effort to block out their physical and emotional pain. These excessive endorphins had a toxic effect on the body by causing high blood sugar, which promoted an emotional roller coaster, creating more anxiety and mood swings. People who had the ACE personality, by contrast, had normal blood sugar and the right amount of endorphins.

Feeling Good With Serotonin

Serotonin is a chemical manufactured in the brain that gives a feeling of well-being. One particular amino acid (part of protein) is needed to help your brain make serotonin. That amino acid is tryptophan, and tryptophan needs vitamin B_6 and magnesium to work. When you're under stress, your body uses up more B_6 and magnesium. That leaves very little of these nutrients for the brain to make tryptophan and then serotonin.

Here we have a vitamin/mineral deficiency caused by the stress from toxic emotions that creates more toxic negative feelings, which cause more stress and negativity. It's a toxic emotional roller coaster ride without an end. The only way to stop it is to recognize what you're doing and just start thinking and acting differently.

Premenstrual depression is a familiar condition to many women that has a documented link to B_6, magnesium, and tryptophan deficiencies. During our monthly cycles, those of us who are affected become more depressed and negative. We create more toxicity. The best way to stop this cycle is to balance our bodies' biochemistry.

In the past, many doctors recommended tryptophan supplementation for PMS-associated depression. Now, due to the overreaction of the

FDA to a tainted source of tryptophan that resulted in a handful of deaths (far fewer than those caused by aspirin or other over-the-counter drugs), tryptophan is unavailable except by prescription. Of course, monthly depression is not life-threatening. But it is threatening to your *quality* of life. And depression can be toxic because it often leads to lowered immunity, which can result in more serious illnesses.

To increase your body's ability to utilize the tryptophan in your foods (turkey is one of the highest foods in tryptophan, but it is found in all complete protein — both animal and vegetable), begin by raising your quantities of vitamin B_6 and magnesium. Both of these nutrients are found in whole grains and beans. And there are also some women's vitamin/mineral formulas with extra B_6 and magnesium already in them. Optivite for Women, developed by pioneer researcher and endo-crinologist, Dr. Guy E. Abraham, is one of the best (for more information, call 800-223-1601).

It is not only premenstrual depression that affects your health, but depression, in general. This depression may be caused by blood-sugar fluctuations (alcohol and high sugar intake can contribute to this), food allergies, a biochemical imbalance, nutrient deficiency, or emotional upheavals like the loss of a loved one (either death, divorce, or separation). The first step is to identify the source of your depression, then to take action to break the cycle of toxicity and neutralize any toxic emotions.

Love and Fear — Our Primary Emotions

Joan Borysenko, PhD, is co-founder of the Mind/Body Clinic in New England. She is an instructor at Harvard Medical School and a teacher of yoga and meditation. In her book, *Minding the Body, Mending the Mind*, she says that "Emotions fall into two broad categories, fear and love." Fear is the toxic emotion; love the healer.

Other toxic emotions, like guilt and shame, come out of our fears that others will learn something about us that we want to keep hidden. Anger, another toxic emotion, can come from a fear of confronting someone rationally who does not behave rationally toward us. Whether we stuff these toxic emotions deep inside ourselves or spew them out at others, they are making us sick and wasting our precious time.

Numerous metaphysicians have said that fear is the absence of love. Now more physicians and health care professionals are saying the same thing. Fear and love are not only primary emotions, they are opposite emotions. They cannot occupy the same emotional space at the same time. If you are feeling love, you have no room in that moment for fear. Sometimes all we can do is push away our fear for a few minutes. Then the fear comes back. When you accompany love with other positive emotions, like helpfulness and understanding, it stays longer.

With love comes joy, peace, and laughter. After a serious heart attack, writer Norman Cousins took charge of his life. He found, and documented his findings, that laughter has curative powers. It neutralizes toxic emotions, rendering them harmless. In *Anatomy of an Illness*, he writes: "Just as the negative emotions produce negative chemical changes in the body, so the positive emotions are connected to positive chemical changes."

Cousins and other heart patients have reversed blockages in the arteries of their heart by manufacturing more of these healing chemicals through laughter and a positive outlook. And they're not alone. Every bookstore contains dozens of books written by people with deadly illnesses who went into remission — and stayed there — using a good diet, exercise, stress reduction ... and positive thoughts. Whether or not you rent comedy videos, read funny books, or engage in friendly banter with someone you love, laughter produces healthy chemicals that neutralize the toxic ones.

Six Ways to Be More Stress-Resistant

1. Get Plenty of Sleep. Since the invention of the light bulb, people have been sleeping less and less. But this hasn't been to our benefit. In 1988, sleepiness was the cause of 41.6 percent of all reported traffic accidents — costing $37.9 billion, 769,184 disabling injuries, and 17,689 deaths. Sleep researchers have discovered that plenty of sleep helps us function better at work and in relationships and increases our ability to enjoy life. It also helps us maintain stronger immune systems. A lack of sleep is a source of stress that is detrimental at best and deadly at worst.

How much sleep do you need? Dr. Thomas Wehr, a psychiatrist and researcher at the National Institutes of Mental Health, found that with no time cues and 14 hours of darkness (as in winter), people slept 10 to 12 hours for 21 days. After snoozing off their cumulative sleep debt (about 17.5 hours), the men settled at eight hours and 15 minutes, and the women settled at an average of 9 hours and 15 minutes per night. Older persons may need less sleep.

If you have trouble getting to sleep early, try initiating a TV-free bedtime ritual to help yourself wind down. It might include a warm bath, a good book, and a calming herbal tea such as chamomile. Also, men aren't the only ones inclined to fall asleep soon after orgasm. Women are, too. Find what works best for you.

If you have trouble falling asleep and staying asleep, most experts agree it's also safe for persons age 45 and older to take low doses of melatonin, the sleep hormone, 30 minutes before you want to fall asleep. Start off with .5 mg. and increase if necessary. Try to stay under 1.5 mg. and see if taking it every other night or less is sufficient to keep you well-rested. Melatonin is preferable to other sleeping pills. It is not addictive. And, unlike other sleeping pills, it helps reestablish normal sleep cycles — what a good night's sleep is all about.

Finally, how do you get a good night's sleep when you have an infant, young child, or other family member who keeps you up at night? When my two boys were infants, I'd flee when I got too tired — spending the night alone in the guest bedroom downstairs, while my husband handled nighttime feedings upstairs! This or another creative solution is sometimes necessary to stay reasonably well-rested.

2. Eat the Best Quality Diet Possible. You should know what this means by now.... A nutrient-dense diet comprised mainly of whole grains, legumes, lots of fresh fruits and vegetables, some raw nuts and seeds for essential fatty acids, and little if any dairy foods and flesh. Comparing a meal that fits these parameters to a typical frozen, fast-food, or highly processed meal is like comparing jet fuel to low octane gasoline with water added. Our body's daily operation is fueled by the nutrients in our diets. A good, nutrient-dense diet boosts stress resistance. A poor diet is a source of stress in itself — so stressful that the Center for Science in the Public Interest estimates that poor nutrition (which includes eating habits that produce obesity) is the cause of most deaths. Be sure to drink plenty of pure water throughout the day as well — about four oz. per hour, more if you consume caffeinated beverages (which are dehydrating).

3. Take Nutritional Supplements. Start with a good, basic multivitamin/mineral. Avoid the one-a-day variety that provide only the RDA amounts. These are barely enough to prevent serious malnutrition diseases like scurvy. Instead, take the newer mega-dose multis in which the daily dose is six pills taken at three time intervals throughout the day (for maximum absorption). Remember to avoid a formula with too much calcium.

Our favorites are Maximum, which can ordered through customer service at 1-800-728-2288, and Optimox brand, which offers pre- and postmenopausal formulas and can be ordered by calling 1-800-722-9040 or writing P.O. Box 3378, Torrance, CA 90510-3378. Your multi should provide a broad base of key nutrients. From there you can add more specialized supplements, determined by you or your health care provider. Together, your multi and other supplements will provide you extra health protection and stress resistance. And always remember, they're called supplements because they're to be taken in addition to, not in place of, a good quality diet.

4. Try these homeopathic remedies for stress and anxiety:

Lycopodium: This remedy is used to soothe anxiety about a new situation, such as a new job, relocating to a new area, and even new relationships or prenuptial jitters.

Nux vomica: This is a remedy for workaholics. Often, however, their stress and anxiety is compounded by a lack of sleep, exercise, poor diet, and little or no personal life. Therefore, results are best if nux vomica is used for initial relief while positive lifestyle changes are being made.

Phosphoric acid: This remedy is for people who are normally lively, energetic, and affectionate, but have become exhausted and irritable as a result of stress.

Picric acid: This remedy is for the stress and tension that can arise from a simple case of too much work. For example, working moms who put in a full day at the office or other place of work only to leave at the end of the work day for a second work shift of shopping, cooking, cleaning, and parenting.

A few notes about using homeopathic remedies are in order. First, some prescription drugs such as birth control pills and antihistamines may interfere with the action of a homeopathic remedy. Aroma-therapy and herbs can also interfere, as can coffee, alcohol, tobacco, and strong-smelling household and personal care products such as mint toothpaste. Do not use these items a half hour before or after taking a homeopathic remedy.

Many homeopathic solutions can be found at health food stores, and some conventional pharmacies are also beginning to stock them. Follow the instructions on the label and discontinue the solution when you notice your condition is improving. If a remedy has no effect, try another. Rather than spend more time and money trying to treat yourself, however, it might be wise to visit a homeopathic doctor who can recommend a remedy based on an in-depth evaluation.

Finally, as in the case of the remedy for workaholism above, many homeopaths also encourage lifestyle changes as a complement to homeopathy. These might include more exercise, improved nutrition and posture, meditation, and professional counseling.

5. Avoid Substance Abuse. Smoking, excessive alcohol consumption, heavy coffee drinking (more than 16 oz./day), and prescription and over-the-counter medications with side effects, all place extra stress on our bodies (which, in turn, must work overtime to fight the adverse effects these substances have on our health).

6. Get Plenty of Exercise. We recently reported on the dramatic reduction in breast cancer risk that exercise produces. And the bottom-line results are even more impressive: A recent study of Swedish women ages 38 to 60 found that jobs that included moderate physical activity reduced the risk of dying by two-thirds. And moderate leisure activities reduced risk by nearly half. Exercise helps us overcome stress by keeping our bodies healthier and therefore, better able to rebound from the adverse effects of stress. Aim for a combination of aerobic and weight-resistance exercise, for at least four hours each week.

Toxic Thoughts; Toxic People; Toxic Emotions

Cancer and Toxic Emotions

Researchers are now finding that toxic emotions and personalities can encourage the development of cancer. Lawrence LeShan, author of numerous books on meditation, and one of the most prolific researchers on the cancer personality, found five factors that constituted a cancer profile.

First, the patients usually had suffered a lost relationship prior to the cancer diagnosis. Second, the patients had a "nice" personality without the ability to express hostility. Being a nice person may hold a lot of appeal for you, but the result can make you more prone to disease, especially if you fail to deal with your hostility appropriately.

Keeping your emotions bottled up is a toxic trait. Harboring anger and resentment toward your parents is toxic. Standing up for yourself and speaking out — in a calm, mature, and rational manner — is much healthier. So is forgiveness.

The third factor in LeShan's cancer profile was the patients felt unworthy and did not like themselves. Fourth, patients had tension about one or both parents. And fifth, patients experienced some kind of emotional trauma between them and a parent sometime in childhood.

Since LeShan's work, we have more studies showing that cancers can take from 10 to 30 years before they're detectable. They often grow very slowly. A leading alternative medicine oncologist (cancer specialist), who prefers to keep a low profile, has said many times, "For people who have cancer, the two aspects of treatment are to detoxify and support the immune system." And the place to begin is to eliminate or transform your toxic thoughts. So while we need to look at the early years in the life of a cancer personality, we also need to begin to make changes for any residual toxic emotions immediately. Learning to accept ourselves, focusing on your redemptive qualities, and letting go of the past, are all important parts of the process.

Accept Yourself as You Are

Toxic emotions begin with toxic thoughts that come from the dark places inside you. And toxic people who ooze negativity bring them out and reinforce them, instead of trying to help you. To heal your life, you need to focus on the positive aspects of yourself. Listen to constructive criticism, but don't let people be critical toward you.

No matter what has gone on in the past, no matter what you have done to yourself or others — or what has been done to you — you need to accept yourself as you truly are. Be honest with yourself, find the things that need to be changed, and begin working on those areas. Always remember, just as others cannot change you, you cannot change others. You can change only yourself.

If you don't think you can change and become more positive, consider this: Change is the only constant in life. If you think things will stay the same, you're fooling yourself. Whether you're thinking about your job, a relationship, or your health, they will all change some day. You may think that day is far off — and perhaps it is. But it may be as close as today, next week, or next month. Or your life may change forever with your next breath.

As difficult as this may be for you, one of the first steps to take is to forgive yourself and forgive others. The resentment and anger you have been holding inside yourself is toxic. It creates hurt, rigidity, and closes your heart. It will make you sick if it hasn't already done so. It's easier to forgive and move on with your life — even when it seems impossible to let go of the past.

Usually, people are unable to forgive when they have been hurt. Understand that no one hurt you and no one can hurt you emotionally. You allowed your feelings to get hurt. Most people do the best they can. Still, their best causes us pain when we allow the difference between their best and our expectations to hurt us. Don't allow it anymore. You've got to stop having unrealistic expectations.

Who Are You?

You are not your past. You are not your job or what you do with your life. Who you are is who you choose to be. Mother, homemaker, artist, lawyer, physician — these, at most, are only tiny aspects of who you are. They are the surface, although you may spend most of your time developing them. You are your essence; what's inside.

If you choose to focus on your positive aspects, you become a loving, supportive friend to yourself and people around you. You transform yourself into an inspiration to others — and to yourself.

Surround yourself with people who are positive, supportive, loving, and helpful. Don't be fooled by someone's potential just because you love them. All of us have potential, but that doesn't mean we'll realize it. If you are the only one in the couple working on a relationship, consider this: Relationships can be easy! They can be joyful and filled with love. But this takes the participation of each person. You can't do it by yourself, as much as you may try.

Don't over care. And don't volunteer to be a doormat, allowing people to walk all over you. There's no one but yourself for you to rescue or take care of. Even children grow and thrive best by working through problems and mistakes without excessive help from someone else. You may not want to hear this. It may not be easy. But it's the truth.

Deflecting Toxic Emotions

Many times, the key to maintaining a healthy relationship with someone who has an unavoidable toxic influence on us is to simply deflect toxic influences. The first step to deflecting is recognizing and acknowledging the unhealthy influence. Let's say an in-law or co-worker regularly belittles you. You will recognize the toxic influence because you will have negative feelings toward, or in the presence of, this person. Once you recognize this, it may be important enough for you to discuss with them what they are doing, how it makes you feel, and your desire for the cycle to end.

If they are not willing to change their behavior, you may still be able to deflect their toxic influence by changing yourself. How? Simply stop taking their actions or comments personally. This means realizing that there is nothing wrong with you. Instead, there is something wrong with them. Such a change turns the tables. It puts you in control by choosing not to react. Many times it is reactive behavior that gets us into trouble with toxic emotions. In effect, reactive behavior turns us into puppets — we are moved when someone else pulls our strings.

If we catch ourselves in the moment of decision, we can usually choose not to react: Not to take a comment or action personally. Not to let our feelings be hurt. Not to let someone take advantage of us. Not to respond angrily, but lovingly, rationally, or even with a sense of humor. In this way, we become proactive and positive. We gain the upper hand. We exercise greater control over the mental and emotional state in which we exist.

If you catch yourself frequently thinking or saying statements like "she, he, or it makes me so (fill in this blank with a toxic emotion)." You may be engaging in more reactive behavior than you realize.

Techniques for Transforming Your Toxic Emotions

Live a healthy life. Eat a good diet high in whole grains and beans for the magnesium and vitamin B_6 your body needs to make chemicals that help you feel good both physically and emotionally. Limit your intake of fats, sugar, and caffeine. They use up these and other important nutrients that contribute to your emotional well-being. Don't eat foods that make you sick. If you have food allergies or sensitivities, stop eating these substances for a few weeks. See how you can easily transform your toxic emotions into ones that heal by simply avoiding foods that are toxic to your body.

Get some exercise regularly. Whenever you feel emotionally "stuck," move your body. Put on upbeat music and dance around the house. Clean a closet that you've been meaning to get to. Go for a walk or a run, or dust off your new and unused exercise equipment and start walking, rowing, or cycling. Do 10 minutes of exercise every day, then slowly build up to half an hour or more. When you go shopping, park your car further away from the store, rather than as close as you can. Even that short walk will help.

Meditate for 10 minutes — every day you eat. That should be most days. Meditation, prayer, and relaxation exercises help center you and allow toxic emotions to melt away. You can sit quietly and simply watch your breath go in and out. Or you can say a word like "love," or "peacefulness" over and over to yourself. Or you can read one of many books on meditation and pick another technique (try Lawrence LeShan's popular and accessible *How to Meditate*). Just do it and don't expect anything.

Larry Dossey, MD, author of *Healing Words*, has done research on the effects of prayer with large groups of people. He found that when people prayed for someone, even when that person didn't know they were being prayed for, their healing accelerated. Meditation and prayer are healing because they neutralize toxic emotions and allow the body's immune system to repair itself.

Tears are also cleansing and are part of healing emotions. They actually help you get better faster. William Fry, Jr., PhD was the first biochemist to suggest that emotional distress produces toxic chemicals in the body — and tears contain other chemicals that literally wash these toxins away. He is now studying the specific chemicals in emotionally caused tears to understand this biochemical activity.

In time, we should have a better understanding of the toxic chemicals produced by stress and the neutralizing chemicals produced in tears. For now, think of your tears as cleansing, and allow yourself to cry when it's appropriate. Then adapt a positive attitude and get on with your life.

Letting Go

Transforming your health, transforming your life, is all about letting go. And let go we must. Someday you will let go of everything tangible — your possessions, your friends, your home, your pets, your life. Practice now by letting go of the negative. Use the remainder of your life feeling and expressing love. Your beliefs are powerful. If you believe you can change, you can. Begin by believing.

Forgiveness is a form of letting go. It allows you to let go of pain and negative emotions. It allows you to move on with your life. Along with forgiveness comes the ability to say, "I was wrong." We all are, at times. Admit it to yourself and others, and move on.

Be patient with yourself. Then you can be more patient with the people in your life. Recognize you're doing the best you can — and so are they — and let go of impatience.

Take Care of Yourself

Be gentle with yourself. Do nice things for yourself. Take time out to pamper yourself. Fill the tub with bubble bath and fragrance, light a candle, play your favorite music, and soak away your tensions. Take time to read something uplifting before you go to sleep. It will help you sleep better. Take yourself out to dinner or to a movie. You are not alone. You're with yourself — your best friend, your best healer.

Most of all, have fun. Every day, do something that's fun. Play with a child and become like that child for a few minutes. Remember what it felt like when you were playing happily with someone. Allow yourself to feel good for even a few minutes. Let that time expand.

Do something wonderful and unexpected for someone else. Get out of yourself. Find a group that needs your time and give them an hour a week; an hour a month. Get outside yourself and feel how good it feels to help someone else. You're helping them heal, and you're helping yourself as well. You're producing healing emotions and getting rid of some of the toxic ones that have been causing so much harm. Live each day, love each day, and enjoy every moment you can for the rest of your life.

Healing Holidays

Do you look forward to the holiday season at the end of every year? Or do they bring about a sense of dread?

I suspect more women than would like to admit it dread the holidays. We have to decorate, shop for food, cook, buy gifts, send cards and invitations, outfit the family with special clothes, try to make sure everyone has a good time, then do most of the clean up.

But even those of us who don't care for all the extra hustle and bustle are reluctant to give it up. Why? Because holidays and other occasions for rituals, offer something even more valuable. They offer the time and space to put everything else on hold, while we stop and reflect on life passages and transitions. This makes rituals powerful vehicles for healing.

In addition to giving thanks for plentiful food, the lamp that stayed lit, and the birth of Christ, the coming holidays also bestow the opportunity to rekindle and renew relationships, to show our affection and appreciation, to simply relax and laugh together, to bring the old year to a proper close, and to launch the new year with a revived sense of enthusiasm. By generating good feelings and a sense of anticipation and satisfaction, all of these activities are healing.

Anecdotal stories that attest to this healing power abound. Perhaps you know of or have heard of persons who were terminally ill and not expected to live through the holidays, yet they did, then died shortly after or even quite a while later. Death statistics support the existence of this holiday healing phenomenon. And it is available to all of us, whether we are aware of it or not. To take advantage simply requires seeking out activities that generate positive feelings. The enhanced immune system resistance you produce may help you avoid catching a cold or flu virus, help you improve an ongoing health problem, or even maintain the upper hand against a life-threatening disease.

But this isn't always so easy for those of us who are overloaded with the extra work of making holidays happen. If this sounds like you, holidays can be detrimental to your health and now is the time to plan ways to have happier, healthier, and even healing holidays. It might take a little creative thinking, but it can be done.

Here are some ideas for lightening your holiday load: buy gifts at the places you normally shop (such as the grocery store), make donations to a non-profit group in the recipients' names (great for the hard-to-buy for), give the same item to as many people as possible, have mail-order gifts shipped direct, spend half as much on gifts and use the savings toward a holiday dinner at a restaurant, help serve and then eat a holiday meal at a relief kitchen, have pot-luck holiday meals if you don't already, ask others with whom you celebrate holidays for their suggestions.

Look for simple adjustments at every turn, from decorating to clean-up, that will fit in smoothly with how you and your loved-ones already celebrate holidays. At the same time, be open to changes. Last year I told my husband it was his turn to send cards. He didn't do it and I didn't worry about it.

Last, but not least, nothing destroys the healing power of the holidays like excessive discord among family members and others. If this is a regular part of your holidays, the resulting stress and other negative feelings can actually be detrimental to health. Here again, creative solutions might be in order to help you create more positive, healing holidays. Keep in mind that the most successful rituals promote harmony by allowing everyone to contribute. For example, go around the Thanksgiving table and let everyone share what they're most thankful for this year.

Holiday-Type Healing Throughout the Year

Now I'd like to shift gears and zoom in on one of the most overlooked aspects of the coming holidays: They are a few of the many occasions for rituals that can be used to enhance our lives throughout the year. Others include our daily routine such as waking up or greeting loved-ones returning at day's end; birthday and anniversary celebrations; vacations, reunions, and other seasonal and religious events; and life-cycle rituals to share lifetime events such as birth, menarche, graduation, a new job, a new home, marriage, first-time motherhood, menopause, and death.

Of course, not everyone observes all of the above events. And all can be observed in very different ways, and can range from simple to elaborate to somewhere in-between. What's most important is the success of the experience. Was it meaningful and positive for all the participants, including yourself?

Rituals can also be included in events to give them greater depth and meaning. In the course of researching this article, I heard about a baby shower that included a motherhood ritual. In it, the mother of the expectant woman washed her feet then stood behind her. This was an enactment of the profound transition that was taking place: the arrival of a new child, the child becoming the mother, and the mother becoming a grandmother. The ritual moved them around and lined them up to illustrate this in a powerful, symbolic way that a simple baby shower never could. When Dr. Fuchs moved to her current residence, she had a house-warming party that included a blessing ritual. In it, everyone wrote a blessing — such as "may your life here be filled with love" — on a piece of paper. The papers were collected in a basket. Then the basket was passed around and everyone took out and read a blessing.

Whatever the occasion, rituals offer opportunities to enrich your life as you move through it. Even funerals can be surprisingly positive events by celebrating the goodness of the life that has passed, as well as bringing together loved-ones to support each other in their loss.

Psychotherapists are also beginning to use rituals as tools for healing. "The tragedy of our time is that our relationships are out of balance. Our lives are ruled by tasks and timetables. Much of our focus is on manufactured beliefs and external goods and goals. We're so distracted, we've lost our connection with what is essential," says Jan Boddie, a PhD and clinical psychologist at New Moon in Sebastopol, California.

According to Boddie, who creates specialized healing rituals, "Ritual brings balance back into our lives through experiences that are not dictated by logic and reason. Ritual, which is symbolic action, invites instinct and intuition, insights and imaginings to play an active role in how we live our lives. It is a way to let go of our grief and experience our joy. It puts our past into perspective and anchors us in the present. Our bodies are better able to relax, release, and renew themselves.... Rituals are available as a healing discipline for living our lives in balance and awareness."

By taking advantage of the healing powers of rituals, you too can enjoy greater wellness, starting with the coming holidays.

Editor's note: To learn more about the finer aspects of rituals, including more ideas for creating more positive ones, I recommend:

● *Rituals for Our Times*, by Evan Imber-Black, PhD, and Janine Roberts, EdD, HarperPerennial, $12.

● *Circle Left to Enter Right: A Spiritual Guide for Creating Contemporary Rites & Rituals*, by Jan Boddie, PhD, New Moon, $10, order direct by calling 707-542-4928.

Chapter 2

Female Heart Disease

What do we know about women and heart disease? An easier question to answer might be: What do we *not* know? Because the answer is: *a lot.*

We know much more about men and heart disease because most medical studies have been done with men rather than women. When it comes to some conditions — and heart disease is one of them — what works for men does not always work for women. The General Accounting Office, an investigative arm of Congress, published a booklet in 1990 that showed a bias against women in medical studies. The GAO stated that studies showing that healthy men could reduce their risk of heart attacks by taking an aspirin every other day simply don't apply to women because women were not included in the studies. Hundreds of studies on mice, rats, rabbits, and men have been conducted, but only a fraction of that amount has focused on women.

There has definitely been discrimination against women in the area of medical research until very recently. In fact, in 1993, three years after an investigation in the House of Representatives, Congress passed the National Institutes of Health (NIH) Revitalization Act. This act of Congress made it mandatory for researchers who are federally funded to include women in their clinical research trials.

In another 10 or 20 years, we should know more about women and AIDS, arthritis, irritable bowel ... and heart disease. The wheels of change move very slowly. Yet many of us don't have the time to sit around and wait for more definitive answers. We need to understand some of the reasons so many women die annually from heart disease so we don't join their numbers and become another statistic. And we need to begin today to change our lives with the information that's available now.

Fortunately, as limited as medical research is in the area of women and heart disease, there's enough out there for us to change our cardiovascular picture and improve the quality and length of our lives.

Doctors Will Eventually Learn More

The 13,000-member American Medical Women's Association (AMWA) decided in 1994 to produce a three-year program to educate doctors on women and heart disease. The program focused on a mere 100 doctors in the first year and increased the number of doctors it would reach in subsequent years. AMWA's target is our primary-care doctor who may not even be aware that there are differences between men and women in relation to cardiac disease.

Because more women in this country die from heart disease than from all cancers combined, the AMWA believes this program is imperative for our protection and health. Still, the educational process is slow. Don't expect this small group of information advocates to get to your personal doctor quickly. Become better educated yourself so you can encourage your doctor to learn more about this subject.

If doctors don't know much about women and heart disease, what do any of us know? We know that statistics from the National Center for Health, released some years ago by the American Heart Association, state that nearly 30,000 more women die each year of stroke and coronary heart disease (CHD) than men. In fact, heart disease is the number one killer of all women past menopause. Every year, about 2.5 million women of all ages are hospitalized in this country with some form of cardiovascular illness, and over 500,000 of them die of it.

We have been educated to look at our cholesterol levels to make sure they're not too high. High cholesterol is considered to be a risk for heart disease and for that reason has gotten a bad rap. *Cholesterol itself is not bad.* It is a necessary fat made up of several components, including HDL and LDL. HDL is the healthy, or "good," cholesterol that keeps cholesterol molecules from sticking to the sides of the arteries. LDL is the lousy or "bad" cholesterol that has sticky properties and can eventually slow down the flow of blood to the heart or block it entirely, causing heart attacks and death. (Here's how to remember the difference: HDL=healthy; LDL=lousy.)

Several large studies have shown that high levels of HDL in women put them at a greatly reduced level for heart disease. And low levels of the protective HDL increased their cardiovascular risk to a much greater degree than in men. In fact, these two studies indicated that low HDL is more harmful in women than high levels of sticky LDL. Low-fat diets decrease HDL in women, so it is important to include some fats, like monounsaturated olive oil, and essential fatty acids found in raw nuts and seeds (plus fatty fish if you eat flesh), and not be on a totally fat-free diet.

In summary, you want relatively higher levels of HDL; for women, over 45 is considered good and over 55 is excellent. A healthy LDL level is approximately 130 or lower. These ranges will vary somewhat among women with high cholesterol.

Women with coronary heart disease have been observed to have a worse prognosis than men with CHD. More women die after having an initial heart attack than men. Women are more likely to develop heart disease as they grow older, while in men it often starts at a younger age.

There is a reduction in our levels of many hormones, including DHEA, progesterone, and estrogen at menopause. Many in the medical community believe that a reduction in estrogen, explains in part, why so many women get heart disease, but estrogen is only one of many components. It also seems that more women fear getting breast cancer from taking estrogen replacement therapy than getting heart disease — so many women don't take estrogen.

Other women can't take estrogen. They have a family or personal history of estrogen-related cancers, like breast cancer, and would run too high a risk for getting another serious illness to feel comfortable taking hormone therapy. Other women prefer not taking it. After all, it is a medication and taking hormones requires being monitored regularly by our doctors. If menopause is not a disease, and it's not, why would all of us need to be treated? For all of us, there are many options — even with the little we know.

And we shouldn't discount the power of prevention, especially when it comes to female heart disease. Women are more likely to go untreated for heart disease, even after it develops, because doctors frequently fail to diagnose it in women. And when it is diagnosed, surgery is less likely, and effective, for women. One study from Cedars-Sinai Medical Center in Los Angeles found that the bypass-surgery death rate was 2.8 percent for men and 4.6 percent for women. Other studies confirm this discrepancy and attribute it to the fact that women have smaller arteries, which are more dangerous to operate on. Smaller-sized men have higher perioperative (during or soon after surgery) bypass death rates as well. Other studies show higher failure rates of bypass surgery in women, plus higher rates of repeat surgery.

Angioplasty surgery, bypass surgery's less expensive cousin, is also high risk, and has a similarly dismal track record when women are considered. We are 10 times more likely to die from angioplasty than men, according to a study by the National Heart, Lung, and Blood Institute. The fact that female heart disease patients are older, on average, may account for some of these deaths. Still, many are due to the fact that the surgical equipment used, such as the catheters for angioplasty, were originally developed for use on men's larger-size arteries.

Fewer bypasses and angioplasties for women may be a blessing in disguise. This sentiment is shared even by the American Heart Association, which has stated: "Women may want to think twice before asking for 'equal treatment' from their heart doctors."

It should also be noted here that many experts, including renown former cardiac surgeons Julian Whitaker and Robert Willix, MDs, question the current widespread use of heart surgery. Instead, they advocate less radical treatment first, including lifestyle modification (diet, exercise, and meditation), and in many cases, chelation therapy. This advice is especially appropriate for women in view of their poorer survival rates with conventional treatment.

What Is Heart Disease?

Coronary heart disease is a category that includes many different illnesses from atherosclerosis to stroke, cardiac arrhythmia, cerebrovascular and peripheral vascular diseases, and congestive heart failure. Since women are less likely than men to be diagnosed — for example chest pains in women are commonly written off as indigestion — women should be especially self-vigilant of any symptoms they experience.

Angina Pain

When arteries are sufficiently blocked by cholesterol, and/or calcium deposits, arterial circulation can be impaired, resulting in the pain of angina. Classic angina pain is best described as a dull pain deep within or across the chest. This pain may radiate to the left arm and/or shoulder, neck, jaw, and even teeth. Right side pain has also been reported. Sometimes angina pain runs down the back, accompanied by nausea, sweating, and shortness of breath (some women have described this as a sensation of inhaling cold air). Angina pain is often described as a sensation of tightness, heaviness, or squeezing. In women, more often than men, it can also present itself as a sharp stabbing pain.

Early-stage angina is usually fleeting and accompanied by physical exertion or emotional stress, stopping when you return to a more relaxed state. Advanced or unstable angina also occurs during relaxation.

Heart Attack

Untreated angina can result in blockage and/or a blood clot severe enough to produce a heart attack. Classic heart attack symptoms include crushing chest pain, which may radiate to the arm, neck, jaw, teeth, and back. This may be accompanied by difficulty breathing, palpitations, nausea and/or vomiting, cold sweats, turning pale and/or feeling weak, lethargic and/or anxious.

If this happens to you or someone you are with, get to an emergency room *As Soon As Possible* and demand a magnesium IV. One Orange County study of 103 heart-attack patients found that of the 50 who received a magnesium IV in the emergency room, only one died. Of the 53 who didn't receive a magnesium IV, 9 died! You can even demand a magnesium IV in an ambulance on your way to the emergency room. This is one of the most valuable life-saving tips you will ever read. Share it with your family members, friends, and doctor!

Silent Heart Disease

Thirty-five percent of all heart attacks in women are called "silent." In the Framingham study, half of these heart attacks occurred with no symptoms, while the other half were mistaken for indigestion, ulcers, arthritis, anxiety, apprehension, nervousness, and other conditions. Some patients even suspect they are having heart trouble, and share this information with their doctor, only to be told that it is something else. If this happens to you, or someone you know, you can demand definitive tests to rule out heart trouble. And remember, this is no time to let a doctor intimidate or talk you out of your desire for further investigation. If testing is negative, you will have greater peace of mind. If it is positive, you will have taken the first step toward saving your own life.

Finally, silent heart disease can also come in the form of denial of symptoms — causing women to delay seeking treatment. This is akin to playing Russian roulette: doing so results in nearly 50 percent more female than male heart-attack victims dying before they leave the hospital. Long-term survival rates also decline with delays.

Women's Mixed Signals

As you can see, symptoms of heart trouble are not always clear-cut. And being female can confuse the issue even further.

Women frequently experience harmless chest pains and rhythm disturbances. This may be a case of your heart suddenly "jumping into your throat," skipping, or beating rapidly. Then just as quickly, your normal heart rhythm returns. Sharp twinges and burning or aching in the chest are also fairly common.

Sometimes sensations are the result of overexertion caused by carrying a heavy purse, baby, child, or even heavy breasts. Exercising without warming up can also produce chest pain in women.

Another painful condition, Tietze's syndrome, is an inflammation of the cartilage between the breast-bone and ribs, and can last for weeks.

Anxiety can also produce chest pain that may wax and wane for hours. If accompanied by hyperventilation, it can produce a tingling or slight numbness of the fingertips, mouth, tongue, and even legs.

Other health problems can also produce pain similar to that experienced with heart trouble. These include hiatal hernias, gallbladder disease, and other less serious conditions.

With so many different possibilities of heart trouble presenting itself in women, a safe policy is to have any unusual sensations checked by a doctor. The good news is that, unlike men, women rarely are stricken with a heart attack without warning. If we are more informed and more vigilant over what our bodies are experiencing, we have the opportunity to identify and address heart trouble earlier rather than later. This is a case of "just do it."

Ultimately, treatment delays result in bleaker prognoses. In addition, heart attacks sometimes occur silently — without symptoms significant enough for the victim to seek treatment. If you suspect you have had a silent heart attack, your doctor can run some tests and confirm whether it happened. It is important to do this so you can know your status and receive necessary treatment.

Heart Disease Risk Factors

Lower Levels of Estrogen

As we said earlier, the primary risk factor for heart disease in women seems to be related to our production of estrogen. When estrogen production drops off, heart disease increases. Estrogen seems to have protective effects on the heart. This is why more women have heart disease after menopause than before. One reason for this may be found in a study published in the *Lancet* that indicates estrogen has antioxidizing actions, which may lower the bad cholesterol (LDL) and thus reduce heart attacks.

Of course, if you want the antioxidant protection of estrogen without the risks that come with taking hormones, you can add more antioxidants

Phytoestrogens: A Safe Alternative to Estrogen

In view of the lack of clear-cut answers about estrogen's ability to reduce heart-disease risk, a safer alternative might be to increase your consumption of foods containing phytoestrogens. These are plant estrogens, found in foods, that act similarly to estrogen in your body. There are no studies on the specific effect of phytoestrogens and heart disease. But other studies suggest that phytoestrogens do have beneficial health effects — especially on women.

According to Dr. Hermal Adlercreutz, a leading phytoestrogen researcher, phytoestrogens may reduce hot flashes and other menopausal symptoms. In other words, phytoestrogens have an effect similar to hormone replacement therapy — without the risks. Soy is the only known source of genistein, a phytoestrogen that has been shown in test tube and animal experiments to block the growth of prostate and breast cancer cells, so eating soy foods regularly may protect you against breast cancer.

In addition, Japanese men who consume lots of phytoestrogen-containing foods (like soy) have the lowest rates of heart disease in the world. The heart disease rate of Japanese women, who also consume lots of phytoestrogens, is also exceptionally low — much lower than that of American women. Phytoestrogens are found in whole grains and legumes. Soy foods such as soy milk, tofu, and miso, are also rich sources of phytoestrogens.

to your diet and supplements. This could very well give you similar beneficial results without increasing your risk for cancer, causing bleeding into your 70s, and requiring daily medication and constant medical supervision.

Another reason for estrogen's possible usefulness in preventing heart disease is that it appears to not only reduce the harmful cholesterol (LDL), but increase the helpful cholesterol (HDL) as well. And remember, low HDL is more of a risk for women than high LDL. The Framingham study, for example, found that a 10 mg/dl reduction in HDL increases a woman's risk of heart disease by 50 percent, while women with elevated LDL were only slightly more likely to develop heart disease than those with normal levels. A change in diet (low fat, high fiber) and regular aerobic exercise can improve your HDL levels without the risk of cancer that's associated with estrogen supplements.

An interesting hypothesis about how estrogen works, published in the *Lancet* in 1993, suggests that it has a long-term effect of blocking calcium. Calcium causes muscles to contract, and your heart is a muscle. Too much calcium will cause excessive contracting, and yet, we are being told we need very high amounts of calcium (especially after menopause). The problem with this is that not all calcium gets absorbed. Some unabsorbed calcium from a high-calcium diet or supplements is often stored in joints (where it contributes to arthritis) or arteries (where it contributes to atherosclerosis). *WHL* has been informing women of the danger of taking more calcium than we are able to absorb for many years.

But it is not only estrogen that blocks the absorption of the excessive amounts of calcium we're constantly being told to take. Magnesium does the same thing by helping you absorb the appropriate amount of calcium — without the risks of arthritis or atherosclerosis. And magnesium causes muscles, including the heart, to relax. Would you rather have a heart that goes into spasm (heart attack) or relaxes?

How Protective Is Estrogen, Really?

It is very important for you to understand that there is a lack of research to back up the notion that estrogen supplements prevent heart disease in women. An article published in 1994 in the *Lancet* says that "not one large-scale randomized study evaluating the benefits and risks of long-term unopposed estrogen treatment or long-term combined estrogen/progestogen treatment has ever been published." This includes the protective effects of estrogen against heart disease. Spokeswoman Cynthia Pearson of the National Women's Health Network agrees. She believes an increase in the number of women taking estrogen could result in more uterine cancer (studies show that estrogen greatly increases this risk) and breast cancer. A study from the June 1995 issue of the *New England Journal of Medicine,* and based on 65,000 women, found that those age 60 to 65 who had taken estrogen five years or longer had a 71 percent rate of breast cancer.

What we do know about estrogen and reducing heart disease in women is that the studies showing hormone replacement therapy is effective are based on observational studies. That means that a large group of women is selected, and over a period of time, is observed to have less heart disease when taking estrogen than women who didn't take it. However, there are many factors that are not being considered in these types of studies — like the type of diet and the exercise programs of the women who are being watched. Women who spend the time, energy, and money to get on hormone therapy and be checked periodically by their doctors are more likely to be eating less fats and more fresh fruits and vegetables than women who are not taking any preventive measures. They are also more likely to be exercising. It may just be that women on estrogen therapy are healthier in general than the women in these inconclusive studies who were not on hormone replacement.

If you look at the eight-year long Framingham study on estrogen and heart disease, where over 1,200 postmenopausal women were observed, the results were startling. They showed that women who used estrogen actually had over a 50 percent increase in deaths from heart disease, and twice as much risk for cerebrovascular disease, than women who did not take estrogen. So right now, the picture is cloudier than you may have been lead to believe.

It is possible that we are interpreting estrogen replacement therapy correctly as one answer to reducing heart disease, or we may be missing the forest for the trees. Whatever protection estrogen offers, it can be duplicated by other substances that offer no risks to your health (or changes in lifestyle), which could have only positive effects. Only time — and good randomized placebo-controlled studies — will tell. In the meantime, you have to decide how to protect yourself against heart disease. You may want to begin by taking a look at known risks for heart disease in women.

Cholesterol ...
Not What We Thought

As shocking as it might seem, women have been brainwashed about cholesterol. Most of the studies linking heart disease to high cholesterol have been done with men only. And we know women and men have more physiological differences than appearance alone discloses. It's true that numerous studies have shown that men who die of heart disease frequently have high cholesterol. But men with high cholesterol don't always get heart disease. Cholesterol is only one of many risk factors.

So, what about women and cholesterol? We know very little, since few studies, until recently, have been conducted on women. However, a recent survey (Buchwald, et al. *Annals of Surgery*, 1996;224(4):486-500) compiled seven large studies on cholesterol and heart disease and looked at the facts and figures, separating them by gender. The findings indicated that high cholesterol was most definitely a significant risk factor for men ... but not for women.

In spite of these findings, a large number of women with high cholesterol are being given cholesterol-lowering drugs they might not need. As a result, many women suffer serious side effects from these drugs — which shouldn't have been prescribed in the first place. Doctors are just not looking at the recent body of scientific literature. They're still treating us as if we were living in men's bodies with larger breasts and hidden genitalia!

What Is Cholesterol and What Does It Do?

Cholesterol is a fat, manufactured from the raw materials found in the animal fats, sugars, and protein we eat. It has many important functions, like keeping cell membranes from breaking (too much cholesterol) or getting too fluid and falling apart (too little cholesterol). Your liver makes most of the cholesterol in your blood, cranking it out when your diet is high in saturated fats (from animals) and sugars.

Cholesterol also is an important building block of sex hormones — like estrogen, progesterone, and testosterone — as well as adrenal hormones which help regulate our fluids, help us handle stress, and suppress inflammation. Without sufficient cholesterol, a younger woman couldn't conceive or even have enough of a libido to want to.

Bile, which helps break down and use fats, is another substance made from cholesterol. And bile carries excess cholesterol out of our bodies.

Women and High Cholesterol

This doesn't give women permission to eat a lot of fats and sugars or to ignore high cholesterol completely. After all, new information is constantly being brought to our attention, and we may find in the future that high cholesterol in women brings with it a risk factor for other deteriorating health conditions. We do know that a high-fat diet is implicated in cancers of the breast and colon.

If your doctor strongly suggests you take cholesterol-lowering medication, refer him or her to the above study before taking it. All medications have side effects, and if you don't have to take one, don't. Some cholesterol-lowering drugs suppress hormone activity, including the production of sex hormones and adrenal hormones. The adrenal glands help us handle stress. And stress contributes to high cholesterol, as well. So cholesterol-lowering drugs may lower your cholesterol, but at a high cost — especially in light of these new findings about women and cholesterol!

In addition, most drugs are approved by the FDA based on very limited testing. Afterward, when a drug is being used on a broader basis by the general public, more extensive studies are conducted. Also pre- and post-approval testing frequently focuses mainly on men, with women accounting for smaller percentages of study populations. Plus, drugs are often approved and prescribed based on an effect, such as lowering cholesterol (this is called a surrogate endpoint), not the ultimate outcome, such as lowering the number of deaths among persons with high cholesterol. One doesn't necessarily lead to the other!

Before taking a cholesterol-lowering (or other) drug, ask about specific study findings for women in your age bracket with a similar health profile to confirm whether there is a good likelihood that the drug will have the effect you're looking for. If so, weigh this benefit against the known risks. To find out about risks, request a patient package insert from your doctor or pharmacist.

Sometimes cholesterol levels run high in a family and no matter how you eat they stay high. Is that reason to ignore your diet? Not at all. A healthy diet is the foundation on which all other therapies sit. Whether or not you are on any medications for any condition, your diet needs to be a solid, healthful foundation.

Can Cholesterol Be Too Low?

Studies have shown a correlation between low cholesterol and depression. At times, this depression has led to suicide. One study of 20 women indicated a strong connection between low cholesterol following the birth of a child and postpartum depression. This small sample is an indication of a possible association that needs to be studied further. A larger study — of more than 6,000 men — showed that when cholesterol levels dropped significantly, suicide rates increased.

What about suicide and women? When a study is completed with women, perhaps we'll know more. But the postpartum depression findings at least give us an indication of an association between low cholesterol and mood changes.

Depression has been linked to low cholesterol by lowering serotonin levels. Serotonin is a "feel good" chemical produced in the brain. Low cholesterol appears to decrease the number of serotonin receptors in brain cells, meaning there's no place for serotonin to attach and allow us to feel good.

Other adverse effects of low cholesterol include an increased risk of lung cancer in older women. There have been numerous studies linking low cholesterol with increased death from various cancers. A study published in *Preventive Medicine 24* was one of the few to examine low cholesterol in women. Both men and women in this study had increased deaths from lung cancer during an 18-year period. It's possible that low cholesterol was just one marker of a suppressed immune system and was not directly responsible for these deaths. Still, it indicates that cholesterol can be too low.

How low is too low? A level lower than 140 (130 for vegetarians) may indicate a suppressed immune system and should be investigated. Once a cause of immune suppression is identified and treated, cholesterol levels should rise.

Watch Your Cholesterol

It's important to periodically check your cholesterol levels. Very high and very low cholesterol appear to be predictive of various health conditions from heart disease to depression and immune suppression. But have doctors made too much fuss over cholesterol? When it comes to women, we think so. High cholesterol may not be a problem for some people, especially when those people are women. Since most studies in the past have been conducted with men, we're not surprised there's been so much noise about lowering cholesterol at any cost, using medications with side effects.

The Fibrinogen Factor

Yet another major factor for female heart disease that is often overlooked is our fibrinogen level. A number of medical studies indicate

Cholesterol and Men

Many men eat what the women in their lives put in front of them. The rest of the time they often eat whatever they feel like eating. We do know that high cholesterol in men is a risk for heart disease. And low cholesterol in both men and women is a factor in depression and a suppressed immune system. Add to that the recent findings that low cholesterol in men is linked to increased suicides.

If the man you love is not watching his cholesterol, you may want to do a bit of prying. Keep an eye on his cholesterol levels and help him lower or raise his as needed.

What to do if cholesterol is high in spite of a good diet and plenty of exercise? Around here, we have our men drink eight ounces of low-fat soy milk a day. In a study from the University of Milan by soy and cholesterol expert C. R. Sitori, men with stubborn cholesterol replaced animal protein in their diets with soy protein. After just three weeks, the patients showed an average 21 percent decrease in total cholesterol. We've been getting similar results by simply adding soy milk to men's diets. To check whether this strategy is working, test cholesterol before and after three weeks of soy milk drinking with a home test kit.

that high fibrinogen leads to heart disease. In fact, the Northwick Park heart study from Britain reported in 1994 that elevated fibrinogen levels were more strongly linked to cardiovascular deaths than elevated cholesterol levels. Other epidemiological studies have come to the same conclusion.

Fibrinogen is a protein that is part of our blood's clotting system and viscosity (its stickiness and thickness). It also stimulates the growth and movement of some of our muscle cells into the walls of the arteries, causing these arteries to become clogged. During the blood-clotting process, fibrinogen becomes a substance called fibrin. Simply put, the more fibrin or fibrinogen you have, the thicker and stickier your blood and the insides of your arteries are likely to become. And the higher your risk for heart disease.

Between 200 and 400 mg/dL of fibrinogen is considered normal. Smoking, high blood pressure, and diabetes can cause elevated fibrinogen levels. Back in 1968, however, Framingham researchers noticed that

Cholesterol Levels in the Oldest

When you reach the age of 85, you've earned the right to relax a little, as you enter a new category that few people are privileged to enjoy called the oldest of the old. This is, in fact, the medical terminology for the later years of the longest-lived among us. If you or a loved one are in this category, should you worry about having high cholesterol? Not according to a study published in the *Lancet* (October 18, 1997) that showed death from infectious disease was the most common cause of death. And lowered cholesterol is associated with cancer and immune problems, not with cardiovascular illnesses.

In fact, this study showed that high cholesterol was associated with increased survival and longevity in both men and women. What about people in their 70s and early 80s? We don't have studies yet, but we'd caution you not to take cholesterol-lowering drugs without taking this information into consideration. And begin, always, with a healthy diet, high in beans and other soluble fiber; low in sugar. You may not need to be on medications.

Weverling-Rijnsburer, Annelies W.E., et al. "Total cholesterol and risk of mortality in the oldest old," *Lancet*, October 18, 1997.

women with fibrinogen levels as low as 334 mg/dL were still more susceptible to heart failure, heart attacks, and clot-related diseases. Higher fibrinogen can also contribute to problem varicose veins, and women comprise the large majority that suffers these. Clearly, it's better to be near the midpoint or on the low end of the current normal fibrinogen range scale for females.

For some people with varicose veins, their bodies just aren't able to break down fibrin, and their arteries get lumpy with fat and fibrin. Blood moves more slowly and pools and clots more easily. But it's not just the cosmetic condition of varicose veins that concerns us, or the pain they cause. Varicose vein complications claim over 100,000 lives annually. Veins clogged with fibrin can lead to heart attacks, stroke, and deadly pulmonary embolisms.

So if you have varicose veins or simply might want to know whether you might be more susceptible to heart disease because of higher fibrinogen, have your doctor check your fibrin levels through a blood test and keep in mind the following fibrin-lowering solutions.

The Trouble With Aspirin

Most doctors recommend taking aspirin each day to thin the blood. We don't like this idea because it has side effects and because there are more natural solutions to this problem that don't have side effects.

Aspirin has been shown to reduce the blood's ability to clot. So many doctors prescribe low doses of aspirin (325 mg/day) to reduce future heart attacks in people who have already had one episode. But according to Michael T. Murray, ND, "People who have experienced a heart attack and live through it are very likely to experience another." And a number of studies looking at nearly 15,000 heart attack survivors using aspirin for up to five years back up Dr. Murray's statement. We were very surprised to discover that these studies have not shown that aspirin lowers the death rate from heart attacks.

How can this be? Looking closely at the results of the studies, we found that while no single study showed that aspirin was effective, when all of the studies were lumped together there were fewer deaths in the people who took aspirin than those who didn't. However, all the deaths were not from heart disease! Today some doctors are beginning to suggest their patients take even lower doses of aspirin (sometimes baby aspirin) as a preventive measure, but there have been no good studies to show that lower amounts are effective, either.

What is the harm in taking aspirin, just in case? It can have serious side effects, like internal bleeding and peptic ulcers. A study published in the British Medical Journal showing the effects of various doses of aspirin — from 75 mg to 300 mg/day stated, "No conventionally used prophylactic aspirin regimen seems free of the risk of peptic ulcer complications." In other words, aspirin may give you a bleeding stomach ulcer! Some people cannot tolerate aspirin because it causes stomach pain. This pain often comes from small amounts of bleeding due to the irritating effects of aspirin.

Even if you accept the idea that aspirin reduces heart attacks, or are not willing to risk giving up trying aspirin, there's more to the story: U.S. studies on aspirin and heart disease have always used buffered aspirin. A British study used plain, unbuffered aspirin and could not replicate the findings of the U.S. studies — in which magnesium was included in the buffering agent. Knowing what we know about the medical industry, we wouldn't be a bit surprised to learn down the road that it is the magnesium in buffered aspirin, and not the aspirin itself, that reduces the blood's ability to clot. So if you still choose to use aspirin as a blood thinner, at least make sure you're getting a generous daily dose of magnesium (600 to 1,000 mg/day) along with it. In addition to helping thin blood, magnesium helps control high blood pressure and irregular heartbeats (arrythmia).

Other Natural Solutions to High Fibrinogen

Garlic, fish oils, and red wine also help break down fibrin (in a process which is called fibrinolysis) and in this way thin the blood.

Garlic is so potent that this breakdown occurs within six hours of ingestion and continues for half a day. If you add quantities of garlic to your diet, or, better yet, take garlic capsules which have higher amounts of the substances that cause this fibrinolysis, you can thin your blood and protect your heart in other ways as well. You see, garlic also lowers blood pressure and prevents the harmful cholesterol (LDL) from oxidizing. When oils oxidize, they are spoiled and create substances called free radicals that are associated with various cancers. So taking garlic protects against both heart disease and cancer.

How much garlic should you take? If it's the fresh herb, one or two cloves a day should be sufficient. If it's in capsule or tablet form, look for one that has about 4,000 mcg of allicin, one of its more protective chemicals.

Omega-3 fatty acids found in cold-water fish oils, and flax seed oil keep platelets in the blood from joining together and becoming thick. Adding several helpings of fish (salmon and herring are highest in fatty acids) to your diet each week is safer than taking large quantities of fish oils. The reason for this is that when you ingest a lot of any oil you need to also add more antioxidants to keep the oils from spoiling (oxidizing) in your body.

If you would rather not eat more fish, or if you are a vegetarian who doesn't eat any flesh, you can add flax seed capsules, flax seed oil, or grind the seeds and add flax seed meal to your cereal or breakfast drink. The latter is an inexpensive way to increase your daily intake of omega-3 fatty acids. If you're looking for something quick and easy to take, flax seed oil capsules can be found in health food stores. Or you can call AMNI (Advanced Medical Nutrition, Inc.), one of a number of good mail-order supplement companies, and they'll send you some low-cost, organic flax oil capsules. Their number is 800-356-4791.

Red wine has been in the news over the past few years as a beneficial substance in reducing heart disease. Many people choose not to drink alcohol. Drinking alcoholic beverages daily puts additional stress on the liver, the organ that is responsible for excreting the ethanol found in all alcoholic beverages. Still, if you can drink alcoholic beverages in moderation and if you enjoy it occasionally, you should know that it may be the alcohol, and not the grapes, that lowers fibrinogen levels. So other alcoholic drinks could lower fibrinogen as well.

One recent Italian study showed that 3 glasses of red wine or three glasses of alcohol diluted in fruit juice, both produced lower fibrinogen levels. We do not recommend three glasses of wine a day for anyone, especially for women. In fact, we are not in favor of drinking alcohol daily. More than two glasses of alcohol a day has been implicated in other diseases like breast cancer, fetal damage, and low blood sugar. It may have some positive qualities, but a number of cautions as well. Still we want you to know what this study found and how much alcohol was used to get these results.

There is a nutritional supplement that has been used to break down fibrin in people with varicose veins. It's an enzyme from pineapples called bromelain. The amount of bromelain used in studies has been 500 to 750 mg taken three times a day between meals. If you have high levels of fibrinogen you may want to discuss using bromelain with your doctor.

A combined program may be your best approach in reducing fibrinogen. This could consist of using high quantities of garlic or garlic extract, increasing your intake of cold-water fish or adding flax seed oil to your diet each day, and having an occasional glass of red wine. Bromelain may also be a useful nutrient to take supplementally, especially if you have varicose veins. Whatever you do, know that there are more answers — and safe ones — to the various aspects of heart disease than you may realize.

Other Risk Factors for Women

Active and Passive Smoking

When we go back to the Framingham study of 1,200 women over an eight-year period, we find that women who used estrogen and smoked had more heart attacks than women who did not smoke. While there were no more deaths in the smoking group, there was more cardiovascular disease. In the Harvard nurses study, women who only smoked between one and four cigarettes a day had nearly two and a half times the heart-disease rate of non-smoking females. That's a big price to pay for a few cigarettes. In a Mayo Clinic study, smoking was found to be the single cause of two of every three cases of severe coronary heart disease among women between the ages of 40 and 59.

This makes a lot of sense. Cigarettes contain substances that contribute to atherosclerosis and can cause you to have less oxygen in your blood stream and more carbon monoxide, making conditions ideal for heart problems. It also raises LDL cholesterol, injures the lining of the arteries, and encourages the blood to clot (a primary factor in coronary heart disease) by raising levels of fibrinogen, the blood clotting factor. In addition, cigarettes contain high amounts of the toxic mineral cadmium, which causes adverse changes in the heart tissue.

Partially because of the cadmium content in smoke and partially because other substances in it are harmful, passive smoke is also a risk factor for heart attacks and strokes. Although the studies available are not gender-specific relating to women, we mention this because if you are a mother who smokes you are not only placing yourself at an increased risk for heart disease, you are risking your child's health as well. Their small, tender bodies are more susceptible to environmental and other toxins than are adults. Their livers and lungs are less able to move these poisons out of their bodies.

In addition, all non-smokers, children and adults alike, seem to be more sensitive to smoke and have more serious effects from exposure to it than smokers. More than 35,000 deaths from heart disease have been attributed to second-hand smoke. If your partner smokes, ask that there be no smoking inside your home or car or near your children — ever. If you smoke, especially if you have children, find a doctor, acupuncturist, or naturopath who can help you stop.

Different studies give conflicting information on the subject of smoking and heart disease. We need more controlled studies with a focus on women to see what effect smoking has on incidents of heart disease and death from heart-related problems. There are, of course, no benefits from smoking. Weight can be controlled in other ways, and less harmful energy surges can be obtained with a cup of green tea with resulting benefits to weight, tumor reduction, and energy.

Caffeine and Your Heart

Caffeine is a stimulant. When you drink it, it excites your central nervous system and can cause restlessness, nervousness, anxiety, and insomnia. As little as two or three cups of coffee can increase your blood pressure and pulse rate. Coffee contains a chemical called theophylline, which can cause your heart to race (tachycardia). And although, once again, most studies on heart disease and caffeine have been conducted with men, caffeine intake has been associated with increased heart disease in women.

In a study recently published in the *American Journal of Epidemiology*, 850 women between the ages of 45 and 69 who drank coffee and had non-fatal heart attacks were compared with 850 non-coffee drinking women. Those who drank five or more cups of coffee a day had more heart attacks than women who drank less coffee or none at all.

High triglycerides, fats manufactured in the liver usually from a high-sugar diet, also increase heart disease. Other substances can trigger your liver's production of triglycerides, as well. A recent study published in

Nutrition Research reports that more than 200 mg of caffeine a day also increases triglycerides in women.

How much coffee or colas does that mean? Three five-ounce cups of percolated coffee (240 mg), five cokes (228 mg), or two coffees and two cokes (251). So try to limit your coffee to one or two cups a day and make them half decaf whenever possible. And switch to caffeine-free soft drinks (or avoid them altogether).

Although many people with heart disease have high-cholesterol levels, not everyone with high cholesterol gets heart disease. Still, cholesterol may be one predictive factor. In a large study of coffee-drinkers, both men and women, each cup of caffeinated coffee caused cholesterol levels to increase by two mg/dl. That means that if your cholesterol was 200, considered by medical doctors to be on the borderline of safe vs. unsafe (we think it's a bit too high for good health), and you drink five cups of coffee, black tea, and colas a day and reduce them to one, your cholesterol could drop to 192 by making that simple change. Decaffeinated coffee does not change cholesterol levels and, so far as heart disease is concerned, is preferable and safe.

Triglycerides and Heart Disease

Women whose triglyceride levels were over 100 mg/ deciliter had twice as many heart attacks as women whose levels were under 100. The higher the triglycerides, the greater the risk for heart attacks. Why? Because when levels exceed 190, the blood gets thicker, and less oxygen and other nutrients get into the heart.

Fish, which contain a helpful fat called omega-3 fatty acids, may help reduce your triglycerides. But limiting alcohol and foods high in sugar is probably going to get you the fastest results. When we eat too much sugar, some of the excess is stored as triglycerides. Lower your sugar intake and triglycerides usually go down pretty quickly. If this approach doesn't work well enough for you, see your doctor for additional information.

"Studies lower ideal triglyceride levels," *New York Times*, Nov. 12, 1996.

Don't Be a Couch Potato!

You don't have to train for a marathon and do heavy workouts every day to guard against heart disease. You can do housework and benefit your cardiovascular system! According to the U.S. National Institutes of Health (NIH), any activity that causes you to breathe a little harder and perspire a bit will help your heart. Try doing some physical housework like sweeping the driveway or scrubbing the floors, vacuuming or carrying unused things to the garage and storing them. If you can exercise at this level for at least 10 minutes at a time, 30 minutes or more a day, every day — you're protecting your heart. This means that doing some kinds of housework will work as well as a brisk walk. On the days when you don't do housework that meets this physical criteria, find a friend and go for a walk. Or get a yoga or aerobics video tape and give yourself a small workout each day.

If you have a sedentary job like sitting most of the day at a desk, consider a 10-15 minute walk at lunch time as part of your moderate activity. Then, when you get home, you only have 15 or 20 minutes to go. You may get away by doing this small amount of exercise each day, but staying a couch potato increases your risk of heart disease.

Increased Weight

We have known for many years that extreme obesity increases the risk of heart problems, but now we're finding that just moderate increases in weight contribute to heart disease in middle-aged women. More than 100,000 women aged 30-55 were followed for 14 years. At the end of the study, it was found that 37 percent of the incidence of coronary heart disease was related to being overweight. As little as a four-pound increase in weight was associated with an increase in heart disease. Estrogen-replacement therapy, lack of exercise, a diet high in sugars and fats, and overeating, all contribute to weight gain and an increased risk for heart problems.

The Pregnancy High-Risk Factor

Pregnancies can decrease your risk of breast cancer by giving your body a rest from producing estrogen (the longer you have estrogen in your body, the greater your risk). But pregnancies can also increase your risk for heart disease — if you have enough of them. Two studies, including the Framingham Heart Study, indicated that women who had six or more pregnancies were at a slightly higher risk for coronary heart disease and cardiovascular disease. At this time, we don't know why. With so many women working and being moms, the number of women in this category is not particularly high. Still, with so few studies on women, we wanted to include this information.

Fats and Oils Can Help or Hurt You

Not all fats and oils contribute to heart disease, but some do, like the trans-fatty acids found in vegetable oils that have been hardened through a process called hydrogenation (forcing air molecules into the fat and causing it to become solid). You wouldn't think a little air thrown into a vegetable oil would make it a harmful food, but it does. What happens during the process of hydrogenation is that the naturally occurring curved molecules get straightened out. These straight molecules resemble saturated-fat molecules, which are a known risk factor for heart disease in both men and women. Saturated fats are primarily those found in animal protein — red meat, chicken, pork, lamb, etc.

When you take a look at the Nurses' Health Study, which we've referred to in the past, you see that the trans-fatty acids in margarine, Crisco, and any other solid vegetable shortenings — and foods that contain them — increase LDL cholesterol (the bad kind) and decrease HDL cholesterol (healthy cholesterol). And they seem to be strongly associated with increased heart disease. Here's what the study said: "Women who ate four or more teaspoons of margarine per day were at higher risk of CHD than women who ate margarine less than once per month ... consumption of cookies and white bread was significantly associated with higher risk of CHD." Perhaps this is because many baked goods contain tropical oils (which also contain trans-fatty acids) or margarine, and the diets of women who ate these foods may have contained a higher total amount of trans fatty acids. Tropical oils are also often used to replace lard by many fast-food restaurants that make deep fried foods.

When buying baked goods, read the labels. What you don't want to buy are those which have the word hydrogenated on the ingredient list. Many cookies and cakes are now being made with liquid vegetable oils like safflower, canola, sunflower, and corn. These do not contain trans-fatty acids and are safer to eat.

Protecting Your Heart

Following are a number of ways to prevent and reverse heart disease. Keep in mind that many prevention techniques — such as improved diet, supplementation, exercise, and lowering stress — can also help reverse heart disease.

Antioxidants in Diet and Supplementation

Before you can understand antioxidants, you need to understand what it is they destroy. That would be molecules that circulate within our body called free radicals. Free radicals damage whatever is around them — enzymes, proteins inside cells, and the fat membrane around cells that keep our DNA coding (a code that tells the cell what to do, what to become, and how to behave) intact. Free radicals are constantly bombarding our cells. In fact, it is thought that each cell in our body gets attacked by free radicals 10,000 times each second! Obviously, our body has ways of protecting us against free radicals.

One of its protective devices is the use of antioxidants. They seek out and destroy free radicals. But once an antioxidant has destroyed a free radical it becomes inactive. So we need lots more antioxidants than free radicals.

Free radicals are produced in a number of ways. All cells in our body use oxygen, and when they do, they create free radicals. These damaging molecules are also created by cells involved in the process of detoxification. When your immune system is called upon to destroy viruses, bacteria, and parasites, it makes more white blood cells, which, in turn, manufacture free radicals to kill the foreign invaders. Finally, free radicals enter our body through environmental pollutants, medications, a poor diet, and even ultraviolet light. So the idea is to cut down on your production of free radicals by improving your diet (fresh fruits and vegetables naturally contain antioxidants, for example), eating as much organic food as possible, and breathing clean air (or at least not driving when traffic is heaviest on hot, smoggy days!).

We are at a disadvantage once again in the area of antioxidants since most studies have been done on men or do not differentiate between responses in each gender. So while we have seen many scientific studies that link antioxidants to protection against heart disease, we'd like to focus on those that specifically mention their effectiveness with women. You might still want to take other antioxidants.

Women, Heart Disease, and Antioxidants

There was one interesting 14-year-long study published in the *American Journal of Epidemiology* that indicated that women did benefit from high intakes of vitamin E, vitamin C, and carotenoids (the best known one of these is beta carotene, but the family of carotenoids includes others, as well). What is of great interest to all women is that all of these antioxidants were not only beneficial in reducing the risk of death from heart disease in men and women, but women had almost twice the protection as men. Perhaps this study infers that antioxidants in diet and supplementation is especially important for women. Fruits and vegetables contain the highest amount of these nutrients and may also contain additional protective factors (such as phytochemicals) that were not studied. The whole food, we believe, is always better than any pill, although a combined approach may be worth considering.

Looking back again on the Nurses' Health Study, we find that the women who took high amounts of vitamin E (100 IU or more) and multivitamin supplements had less major coronary heart disease than women who had a low intake of this vitamin. Long-term use of vitamin E seems to have a protective effect on atherosclerosis by reducing the LDL cholesterol (the sticky kind). The multivitamins also contained other antioxidants like vitamins A and C. If you are going to add vitamin E to your diet, we suggest you use a dry form of d-alpha tocopherol. Dry or water-soluble vitamin E is better absorbed than the oil-based variety, and d-alpha is better utilized than less-expensive mixed tocopherols or the synthetic dl-alpha tocopherol.

The Magic of Magnesium

Your doctor may be telling you to take more calcium, but studies indicate that the mineral to take more of is magnesium. Without enough magnesium, the calcium you take will not be absorbed. This doesn't mean it's harmless, either. Unabsorbed calcium that is not excreted (and most isn't) gets into the joints where it becomes arthritis or in arteries where it becomes atherosclerosis. According to a review of magnesium done back in the 1970s, taking more magnesium can prevent your blood vessels from calcifying and developing into atherosclerosis.

But it's not just hardening of the arteries that magnesium (through its natural chelating action) helps prevent. A deficiency of this mineral is also associated with a higher risk for heart attacks, cardiac arrhythmias (rapid heartbeat), hypertension, and unexpected cardiac death.

According to Dr. Alan Gaby, most of the people he sees in his practice have low levels of magnesium. A government survey shows the average American diet provides about 40 percent of the magnesium we need each day — based on the low RDA levels. Approximately 75 percent of U.S. females are magnesium deficient. And most doctors still don't check magnesium levels in sick or dying patients in hospitals who are showing signs of magnesium deficiency (cardiac arrhythmia, muscle spasms, depression, and hypertension). Dr. Jean Durlach, president of the International Society for the Development of Magnesium Research, found that throughout the world, higher amounts of magnesium in drinking water correlated with lower death rates from heart disease.

It's not easy to know if you are low in magnesium. Most blood tests are inaccurate. Red-blood-cell magnesium levels are better to check than the regular serum magnesium, according to Dr. Guy Abraham, a pioneer in the area of magnesium, PMS, and osteoporosis-reversal. If you prefer, you can just begin taking extra magnesium — up to 1,000 mg/day. Side effects from taking more than you need are loose stools. You can take the amount that will cause your stools to be loose without being runny. And you may be protecting yourself against heart disease as well as osteoporosis, stress, and other conditions.

That's magnesium in general. What about magnesium, women, and heart disease? As usual, few studies are on women only, but in a study of about 100 menopausal women with mild or moderate hypertension, none of whom were taking medication, the blood pressures of those who took oral magnesium for six months dropped significantly over those who did not take magnesium. High blood pressure leads to stroke. Other studies are not gender-specific, but indicate the broad necessity of including magnesium into the dietary and supplemental programs of all people at risk for heart disease.

Mildred Seelig, MD, a professor of nutrition at the University of North Carolina, is considered by many to be the world's authority on magnesium. She strongly suggests that magnesium be given intravenously as soon as a person has a heart attack. In the ambulance, if possible. The bottom line is don't wait until you're magnesium-deficient. Begin by increasing magnesium in your diet (whole grains and beans of all kinds are high in this mineral) and make sure any vitamin supplement you take has at least as much magnesium as calcium — and more magnesium if your bowels can take a bit more.

Green Tea and Heart Disease

Apparently, all caffeine isn't terrible for you. Green tea, which contains antioxidants that have been shown to protect us against some forms of cancer, also helps decrease total cholesterol, the harmful LDL cholesterol, and triglycerides. It also appears to increase the beneficial HDL (or healthy) cholesterol. If you like it, you might want to incorporate two or three cups of green tea into your daily program. Because of all the current research on the benefits of green tea, this beverage is now available in supermarkets, health food stores, and Asian markets.

Heart-Disease-Fighting Herbs

Herbal remedies for high blood pressure, a risk factor for heart disease, include garlic, hawthorn, Coleus forskohlii, and khella.

For angina, Michael T. Murry, ND and author of *The Healing Power of Herbs* recommends hawthorn, in the doses listed below for the various forms, taken three times daily:

- hawthorn berries or flowers (dried): 3 to 5 grams or as an infusion
- hawthorn tincture (1:5): 4 to 5 milliliters (alcohol may elicit pressor response in some individuals)
- hawthorn fluid extract (1:1): 1 to 2 milliliters
- hawthorn freeze-dried berries: 1 to 1.5 grams
- hawthorn flower extract (standardized to contain 1.8 percent vitexin-4'-rhamnoside or 20 percent procyanidins): 100 to 250 mg

Hawthorn has been shown to have low toxicity. Therefore, special caution is advised here.

For angina, Dr. Murray also recommends:
- carnitine: 300 mg, three times daily
- coenzyme Q10: 150 mg, one or two times daily
- magnesium (citrate, aspartate, or Krebs cycle chelate): 250 to 400 mg, three times daily

When treating a condition as serious as angina or heart disease with alternative and/or complimentary medicine, it's always a good idea to work closely with a naturopathic doctor, or other health care professional who is knowledgeable about alternative treatments and can track your progress with the appropriate tests.

The Chelation Solution

When I think about EDTA chelation, I usually think first about the older men I've seen getting chelation IVs at my primary care doctor's office. Let me add that they appear to be a lot friskier, too, than the older men I see in the waiting rooms at my HMO, where chelation is not offered.

Chelation, however, might be an even more valuable therapy for women. It is best known for and used primarily to treat atherosclerosis, or hardening of the arteries. To date, hundreds of thousands have used chelation to treat atherosclerosis and thus avoid angioplasty and bypass surgeries. Not only is chelation much safer, it's much less expensive.

Although most conventional doctors pooh-pooh EDTA chelation therapy for treating atherosclerosis, the actual research supporting its effectiveness is very impressive. Enough so that Julian Whitaker, MD, and founder of the Whitaker Wellness Institute believes that chelation therapy can and should be used to avert the need for bypass and angioplasty surgery for all but the most severely sick heart patients. Chelation can also improve the condition of many heart patients — enough to enable them to quit or reduce their use of heart drugs.

The survival and cost numbers for chelation are equally impressive — at least if you're the patient. To date, approximately 600,000 persons have had chelation therapy. No deaths have resulted from this therapy when the treatment was properly administered and supervised. Yet two to four percent of the 400,000 persons who have bypass surgery annually die on the table. Nearly as many angioplasty patients also die on the table. What's more, chelation therapy costs around $3,000 while bypass surgery costs around $40,000. These survival and cost discrepancies are enough to quickly put the large majority of heart surgeons out of business, if more people knew about chelation. Although insurance plans usually don't cover chelation therapy, it may be well worth the out-of-pocket cost. (If you have an 80/20 health care plan, a $40,000 bypass surgery would still cost you $8,000 out-of-pocket.)

In short, when other more conservative methods such as diet and exercise fail to produce the healing results you're looking for, EDTA chelation is frequently well worth investigating — before trying more radical measures like surgery.

For a more in-depth discussion of chelation therapy, call the *WHL* subscriber service department at 1-800-728-2288 and order *The Chelation Answer*, a highly informative book by Dr. Morton Walker. To locate a doctor who is trained and certified in chelation therapy treatment, contact the American College of Advancement in Medicine (ACAM) at: ACAM, P.O. Box 3427, Laguna Hills, CA 92653.

The Protect-Your-Heart Diet

Your best diet for preventing heart disease is one low in saturated fats found in animal protein. Monounsaturated and polyunsaturated fatty acids, found in vegetable oils, reduce your risk for heart disease. Still, all your fats should be low. Keep them below 30 percent, ideally around 20 percent, even if current fad diets tell you to eat more fats. More than 30 percent will not help prevent heart disease. But don't eat a very low-fat diet or a fat-free diet, because while they will lower you harmful LDLs, they'll also lower your helpful HDLs. And low HDL levels put women at a higher risk for heart disease. In addition:

- High fiber is a necessity, and you can get enough if you eat plenty of whole grains, beans, and vegetables. Constipation is frequently a sign you are not. Aim to eat enough fiber to have one bowel movement daily. (This will also significantly lower your risk of colon cancer.)
- Vegetable protein is better than animal protein. Tofu, lentils, and beans of all kinds turn into a complete protein when you eat them the same day as grains. You need not eat both at the same meal.

- The best animal protein for heart protection is cold water fish that have high amounts of omega-3 fatty acids, which help your fat metabolism. However, cold water fish, like salmon, which are farmed and not fed their usual diet of sea vegetation, are not high in these protective fatty acids. Make sure the fish you eat come from the ocean. When in doubt, ask.
- Keep your refined-sugar consumption low. In some people, it promotes atherosclerosis. In others, it raises cholesterol while lowering HDL. If you limit refined sugar to 10 percent of your caloric intake, you can still enjoy an occasional dessert, cookie, or muffin and have a healthy heart.
- Include raw nuts or seeds in your diet as well. One study of Seventh Day Adventists found that those who ate a handful of nuts a few times a week had significantly less heart disease. Nuts contain omega-6 fatty acids, and walnuts are one of the richest sources. Omega-6 and omega-3 are called essential fatty acids. Your body must have them for optimum performance. Yet it can't manufacture them — they must come from an outside source.
- Keep caffeine low and drink green tea instead of coffee when you can.
- If you can handle just a little alcohol and want to include it in your diet, limit yourself to one glass of red wine a day. If you have any liver disease, past or present, don't drink daily. Just 1 ½ drinks a day can raise a woman's risk for breast cancer by 60 percent. Carefully weigh the data and make your choice a wise one. You can reduce stress by meditating and with exercise, and get antioxidants into your body in other ways. Daily alcohol may prove in time to not be as safe as it appears to be today. Caution is advised here.

Protective Supplements

Numerous vitamins, minerals, and fatty acids appear to be helpful in preventing heart disease, so take a good multivitamin/mineral with equal amounts of calcium to magnesium, or a greater amount of magnesium. Folic acid is now in the news in relation to heart disease, but deficiencies of vitamin B_6 and B_{12}, chromium, copper, selenium, and others are also linked to heart disease. Don't wait for new studies to be published. A good multi is good, inexpensive insurance.

Do not be misled by the one-a-day type vitamins that provide 100 percent of various Recommended Daily Allowances. This is barely enough to prevent serious nutritional deficiency diseases such as scurvy. Your best bet is the newer mega multivitamin/mineral formulas that have a daily dose of six capsules, taken at three intervals throughout the day for best absorption. One brand we like, Optimox, has pre- and postmenopausal formulas and can be ordered by calling 1-800-722-9040. Another is Maximum by Healthy Resolve, which can be ordered by calling 1-800-728-2288.

Add magnesium to bowel tolerance. After you have modified your diet to include more whole grains and beans, after you have taken a good multivitamin/mineral for a month or so, increase your magnesium to an amount that gives you comfortable bowel movements. As you protect yourself from heart disease with magnesium you will be eliminating constipation and the resulting illnesses it often brings.

De-Stress

In the '60s and '70s, researchers expected heart disease rates to climb among women as they began climbing corporate ladders. That didn't happen. The explanation for this surprise is that the increased personal satisfaction and higher levels of self-esteem that come with professional success appear to mitigate female stress.

Feelings of frustration and powerlessness among pink-collar workers, on the other hand, has been identified as a cause of higher heart-disease rates. In fact, female pink-collar workers suffer three times the heart disease rate of female white-collar workers. A study of the Cynomolgus Macaque monkey provided a biological explanation for this phenomenon. Researchers found that lower social status suppressed estrogen among this species, robbing them of the hormonal protection against heart disease that was enjoyed by the higher-status dominant female monkeys. Just last year the *Journal of the American Medical Association* published the results of a Duke University five-year study that concluded mental stress is more dangerous to the heart than physical stress.

If you find yourself frequently feeling frustrated, anxious, tense, edgy, restless, overwhelmed, or powerless, these feelings of stress may be increasing your heart disease risk. You may be able to lower heart-disease risk, however, with stress reduction techniques. The ultimate stress-reduction technique may be meditation. In 1978, researcher and physiologist R. Keith Wallace of the University of California at Los Angeles discovered that a group of meditation practitioners experienced 80 percent less heart disease (and over 50 percent less cancer) than those in a control group.

The simplest way to meditate is to find a quiet place to sit comfortably, close your eyes, and direct your attention to your breathing. Repeat one word, such as "calm" slowly and continuously. As thoughts come into your mind, let them go. Do this 15 minutes or longer. The goal is to be still, physically and mentally, until you feel extremely relaxed and peaceful. After stopping, try to keep the relaxed feeling with you. Some people find it helpful initially to receive more formal meditation instruction. Numerous meditation groups across the country offer this. Or pick up a copy of *How To Meditate* by Lawrence Leshan. All forms of meditation work, even when you aren't sure initially whether it's working.

Five More Ways to Overcome Mental Stress

The following list of ways to reduce mental stress is not comprehensive. You may have some lesser-known favorites of your own, such as listening to music, relaxation tapes, or just getting away by yourself for a while. For best results, use the combination of techniques that works best for you:

Get Thee to a Cultural Activity

For years, we've been encouraging readers to be sure to include plenty of fun activities in their lives. By reducing deadly stress, more fun — in the form of movies, concerts, plays, artistic events and even sporting events — appears to actually increase longevity. That's what researchers in Umea, Sweden recently discovered when they surveyed more than 12,000 people about their lifestyles in 1982 and 1991. They found that those who regularly attended such activities were half as likely to be among the subjects who died during the study period. Lead researcher Lars Olov Bygren speculated that these types of activities can have a greater influence on longevity than education, income, physical activity, and even smoking, because they elicit strong positive emotions that provide a powerful boost to the immune system.

Forbes FYI, Summer 1997

Laughter. Have you ever laughed so hard you nearly fell out of your chair? And what about the ultra-relaxed feeling you had afterward? Whether we realize it or not, laughter is a powerful stress-relief tool. This probably explains in large part why prime-time TV is dominated by sit-coms — they help us unwind and de-stress. Other tools for regular laughter include funny movies, books, and taking a humorous approach whenever possible. Medical research has confirmed the healing power of laughter and includes many reports of persons actually healing themselves with intensive laughter therapy.

Fun and Games. A Swedish study found that persons who regularly attended cultural activities — movies, concerts, plays, artistic events, and even sporting events — were half as likely to die as persons in a control group who didn't. The lead researcher of this 12,000-person study even speculated that such activities have a stronger influence on longevity than income, physical activity, and even smoking by eliciting strong positive and healing emotions that, like simple laughter, boost the immune system's ability to fight stress.

Togetherness. Sexual arousal and orgasm, and just being with others also boost stress resistance. Numerous studies show that persons with the strongest ties to family, friends, church, and other community groups enjoy significantly greater longevity. Strained, unpleasant, and abusive relations with others, however, create stress.

A Positive, Proactive Approach. If you're prone to negativity, a little mindfulness can go a long way in helping you overcome it, and the dysfunctionality and illness it breeds. The reward? Your stress resistance, effectiveness as an individual, and enjoyment of life will soar. Remember the famous saying of Jeanne Calment, the upbeat French woman who lived to age 122. She said, "if you can't do anything about it, don't worry about it." If necessary, get professional help to overcome excessive negativity or fatalism.

Change Your Life

Protecting yourself against illness always changes your life. If you haven't already, be sure to include regular exercise — aerobic, five times a week when possible — and stress-reduction techniques into your life. If you don't have time for exercise or 10 minutes of relaxation exercises or meditation a day, how will you find time to recover from heart disease? Do you have time to spend sitting in doctors' offices waiting for appointments, tests, and prescriptions for medication?

Begin slowly. Start today by exercising for 10 minutes. Tomorrow, meditate or play a tape with a guided meditation or relaxation technique on it. Do this for 10 minutes. Each day, do one or the other for 10 minutes. At the end of a week or two, increase to 15 minutes. When you are up to 20 minutes a day, do 10 minutes of exercise and 10 of meditation. Eventually, gèt your exercise up to 20-30 minutes five times a week. Walks with friends count. So does housework and gardening. Get active. Make your heart work a little harder at times. And open it up more with meditation, relaxation exercises, and prayer.

Protecting Yourself Against Heart Disease

To Drink, or Not to Drink? That Is the Question.

People who want to drink argue that the French, who drink wine daily, have a low incidence of heart disease. This is true. They also have a high mortality from alcohol-related liver disease. The amount of alcohol consumed seems to be the most predictive factor for prevention of heart disease vs. other harmful effects. Japanese men, however, are proof that red wine consumption is not a must for heart disease prevention. They have a lower incidence of heart disease than French men, yet drink little, if any wine. (They do drink lots of green tea, and eat a lot of fish and tofu, as recommended earlier.)

If you drink wine, look at other toxic substances you're ingesting in addition to alcohol. It takes the liver about three days to remove the ethanol from a glass of wine. A primary function of your liver is to remove harmful substances. If alcohol is one of many, drinking daily may cause you more problems than it solves. If your diet is clean (without a lot of additives, preservatives, pesticides, etc.) one or two glasses of wine a day could help you guard against heart disease.

What kind of wine is best? Again, we're not completely certain, but preliminary data suggests that red wine is more protective than white wine. Red wine seems to contain more flavonoids, naturally occurring antioxidants that protect against LDL cholesterol. Some studies have indicated that red wine contains antioxidants, while white wine contains pro-oxidants. But a very recent study indicates that if white wine comes in contact with grape skins while it's being made, it contains more antioxidants. To be safe, stick with one glass of red wine a day.

Or take vitamin C! One gram (1,000 mg) of vitamin C has a 22 percent antioxidant status at the end of one hour and 29 percent at the end of two hours. Red wine contains 18 percent and 11 percent, respectively; while white wine has only four percent and 11 percent of an antioxidant action.

In the area of alcohol and its protective effects on heart disease, we must remember that many people cannot drink just one or two glasses of alcohol. People with a genetic predisposition to alcoholism, or people who cannot control their intake for emotional or other reasons, should not even consider drinking a glass of wine as a preventive measure.

Not surprisingly, there is little data on women, alcohol, and heart disease. Most studies have been conducted on men. It is thought that the protective effect of alcohol appears to be that it raises levels of the protective HDL cholesterol (and women tend to have higher levels of HDL than men). In addition, women's livers are more sensitive to the effects of alcohol than are men's.

One study of over 120,000 nurses, conducted over a 10 year period of time, gives us at least a beginning look at this subject. It showed that women over the age of 50 who have one glass of wine or beer a day have fewer heart attacks and less heart disease than non-drinkers. They did, however, seem to have a higher risk for brain hemorrhages, which might be associated with both drinking alcohol and smoking. We just don't know at this point.

Still, the idea of having one glass of wine a day is appealing to some women. It may be causing beneficial results for two reasons: the antioxidants in the wine and the relaxation that having a drink at the end of a stressful day may produce. In both cases, options other than alcohol exists for women who do not drink alcohol.

Homocysteine and Your Heart: The Missing Link

At one time, not so long ago, we heard about the connection between high cholesterol levels and heart disease. Then cholesterol was broken down for us into HDL and LDL. One is healthy (HDL), one is not (LDL).

The ratio of the healthy, slick cholesterol to the unhealthy, sticky stuff was, we were told, a predictor of heart disease.

Next came the role of hormone replacement therapy (HRT), which kept calcium deposits on arterial walls at bay. Nutritional studies later showed, however, that this calcium build-up was due to unabsorbed calcium, and that magnesium, the mineral that helps with calcium absorption was an effective blocker of these deposits and also helped keep the heart muscle relaxed.

Then we heard about fibrinogen, a protein that is part of our blood's clotting system and viscosity (its stickiness and thickness). It stimulates the growth and movement of some of our muscle cells into the walls of the arteries, causing these arteries to become clogged. During blood-clotting, fibrinogen turns into fibrin. The more fibrin or fibrinogen you have, the thicker and stickier the insides of your arteries are likely to become. And the higher your risk for heart disease.

It seemed that we had to watch our cholesterol and boost the HDL with a low-fat diet and regular exercise, and either take HRT after menopause or increase our magnesium intake in diet and supplements. Then add a few nutrients like omega-3 fatty acids and a glass or two of red wine to lower fibrinogen levels. Now we hear there's more: homocysteine levels need to be factored into the equation. With all the aspects that need to be addressed to keep our heart healthy, no wonder there's so much heart disease!

As much as you may not want to hear one more thing to take into consideration concerning your heart, we've chosen the month in which we celebrate Valentine's Day to give you some of the latest information on homocysteine, because heart disease is still the biggest killer of postmenopausal women. And until the numbers drop, we must look at all aspects of preventing this deadly disease. Besides, we have more information, so let's use it to our advantage and put all the parts of the puzzle together.

Homocysteine: What Is It?

Homocysteine is one of the sulfur-containing amino acids, a chemical component of protein. It is closely related, chemically, to methionine, another sulfur amino acid known for its antioxidant properties. With the help of other nutrients, homocysteine is made from the breakdown of methionine, which is found in meats, legumes, soy, fish and eggs, as well as garlic, onions, corn, rice, and other grains. With the help of such nutrients as betaine, vitamins B_6 and B_{12}, and folic acid, homocysteine is then converted into other chemicals and then either turned back into methionine or excreted.

High amounts of homocysteine damage cell membranes, make collagen unstable, and lead to the formation of atherosclerotic plaques. End result: heart disease. Methionine helps prevent cholesterol deposits in the arteries.

One of the earliest researchers in the link between high homocysteine levels and heart disease is Kilmer S. McCully, MD, author of *The Homocysteine Revolution* (Keats Publishing, 1997). His book offers an extensive explanation of this formerly obscure amino acid and its effects on heart disease, aging, and hormone levels in both men and women. If you're looking for a more thorough explanation, you'll want to read this book.

How Do We Get Too Much Homocysteine?

Dr. McCully explains that aging is a factor in high homocysteine levels. For one, as we age our diets contain less of the vitamins B_6, B_{12}, and folic acid needed to convert harmful homocysteine into helpful methionine. Studies have shown that elderly people in the Framingham (Mass.) Heart Study had lowered consumption and blood levels of these nutrients. I'm not surprised. Try going to New England and finding lots of vegetables in restaurants. They're not there. Green leafy vegetables are the primary source of folic acid (the name comes from "folate," or leaves). What would a study of elderly people in Southern California show? Or a study of vegetarians who eat plenty of fresh produce?

Folic acid has been found in some studies to be the nutrient deficiency most associated with high homocysteine levels. In a European study, normally healthy people with elevated homocysteine who took one mg/day of folic acid responded with lowered homocysteine during the first five days of treatment.

Vitamin B_{12} is often low in older people, because it needs a substance called "intrinsic factor," which comes from gastric juices, to be absorbed. Intrinsic factor is made in the large intestines. Intestinal bacteria also affect the amount of intrinsic factor. If you have digestive problems or not enough friendly bacteria like acidophilus and bifido, you may not be producing enough intrinsic factor to have sufficient vitamin B_{12}.

Other Risk Factors

While men usually have higher levels of homocysteine than women, as we age, our homocysteine levels rise. This means that postmenopausal women usually have more homocysteine than premenopausal women.

Genetic factors can cause high homocysteine in people of any age. Barring this inborn genetic error, smoking cigarettes combined with drinking eight cups of coffee or more a day, raises your levels. So will just drinking this amount of coffee without smoking. What about tea? Remember, folate is an important nutrient in lowering homocysteine, and folate comes from leaves. So does tea. Authors of a Norwegian study found that all caffeinated coffee contributed to elevated homocysteine, while caffeinated tea did not.

Helpful Foods

As complex as all this may seem, it's really not. We've been telling you for years to drink a couple of cups of green tea daily, increase your intake of soy (high in methionine), and to eat plenty of fresh green leafy vegetables. We've been telling you that smoking is more harmful than just affecting your lungs, and that too much coffee is not good for you. We've also stressed the importance of having enough friendly bacteria in your intestines. This is what it takes to lower homocysteine levels.

How to Test for Homocysteine

Many laboratories are now performing blood tests that show whether or not your homocysteine level is high. This test must be done after you have fasted for about 12 hours (nothing but water from 9:00 p.m. until you have your blood drawn in the morning). If you have a clear-cut high homocysteine level, this test will be accurate. If you don't, and many people do not, a more reliable test is called a methionine-loading test. You take 100 mg/kg of methionine and have your blood drawn six hours later to test for homocysteine levels. Speak with your doctor about either of these tests.

More on Homocysteine

In the past five years, more than 1,000 articles on homocysteine have been published in scientific journals. Elevated homocysteine has been implicated in neural tube defects, rheumatoid arthritis, diabetes, and is suspected to be connected to osteoporosis. Later, we'll explore these connections and give you some specific foods to add to your diet that are especially high in folic acid — thought to be the key nutrient needed to regulate homocysteine.

Why Women Need Low Homocysteine Levels

You've now seen that when the amino acid homocysteine is high, cell damage occurs and plaque builds up in the arteries of the heart, leading to atherosclerosis. But there are more reasons for wanting your homocysteine levels to be low, especially since you're a woman. High levels have been implicated in neural tube defects, osteoporosis, diabetes, and rheumatoid arthritis — conditions which, when added together, affect just about all women.

Homocysteine and pregnancy: Folic acid supplementation is now being touted as the nutrient that will prevent both neural tube defects and miscarriages. Research currently in progress in the Netherlands suggests that a defect in the metabolism of methionine and homocysteine may be both the cause of these problems and the reason folic acid corrects them.

Homocysteine and bone loss: The connection between high homocysteine and osteoporosis is less well-defined. A number of authors of scientific studies have suggested that because children with genetically high homocysteine commonly have osteoporosis, the same pathway that causes this condition in children may well contribute to bone loss in adults. At present it is only a theory, but one based on sound scientific principles. Until there are further studies we won't know for certain. But this connection may explain the reason for more osteoporosis in women whose homocysteine levels rise after menopause. Until we have more information, the wise approach would be to keep your homocysteine levels low, especially after menopause.

Homocysteine and diabetes: In the case of diabetes, homocysteine metabolism seems to be impaired in people with non-insulin-dependent diabetes mellitus (NIDDM) — as opposed to those with type I diabetes.

Safer Angioplasties

Two large studies have found that, as in many other things, there's no substitute for experience when considering a doctor for angioplasty. The studies, which appeared in the June issue of the American Heart Association's journal *Circulation*, compared angioplasty outcomes with the number of these procedures doctors performed each year. Both studies found that in general, the more angioplasties a doctor performs each year, the lower the rate of complications.

The first study, from the Cleveland Clinic, found that major complications were suffered by 9.3 percent of the patients of doctors who performed 69 or fewer angioplasties a year, compared to only 2.9 percent among patients whose doctors performed more than 270 angioplasties a year.

The second study, from Duke University Medical Center, found that doctors whose patients did less than 25 angioplasties a year had higher rates of emergency bypass surgery and death than patients whose doctors performed over 50 angioplasties a year.

In 1992, the American Heart Association and the American College of Cardiology said doctors should perform a minimum of 75 angioplasties a year to maintain competency. These studies now provide hard data to back up this position. Angioplasty is a high-risk procedure and over 400,000 were performed in the U.S. in 1995. Still, cardiologists need no special training or certification to perform an angioplasty. This makes it a big money-maker for cardiologists.

If you or someone you know will be hiring a doctor for an angioplasty, it would be best to investigate the track records of as many doctors in the area as possible. Ask about the total number of procedures performed and compare this to the total number of emergency bypasses and deaths. If you can't get this information, the safest choice is to select the doctor who performs the most angioplasty procedures each year — whether it's your regular doctor or not.

The Duke study found that more than half the doctors performing angioplasty in 1992 were unlikely to have met professional competency standards.

This can lead to diabetic retinopathy, since elevated homocysteine is also a risk factor for this eye condition. Remember, high homocysteine causes cell damage, and injured cells within small vessels like the eyes appear to lead to retinopathy, as well as heart disease.

Homocysteine and arthritis: Rheumatoid arthritis patients also tend to have high homocysteine levels. When a number of them were given an arthritis medication that assists the conversion of homocysteine to methionine, their homocysteine levels dropped and their pain was reduced. Again, it's too early to do more than postulate, but for those of us who don't have the time to wait for research on these diseases, it is clear that there are numerous benefits in lowering homocysteine levels, especially as we grow older.

Nutrients You Need to Lower Homocysteine

Folic acid may be the most important nutrient to keep your homocysteine levels lower. Folic acid is most abundant in legumes (beans) and green leafy vegetables, and few people eat them daily. A salad plus a serving of broccoli, spinach, or chard is an easy way to get plenty of greens. The way you cook vegetables can also either reduce or retain folic acid. When you stir fry, you seal in a number of nutrients and retain more folic acid. Aim for a total folic acid intake of 400 to 800 mcg/day. For information on the amount of folic acid and other nutrients in various foods, look up the foods you eat in the *Nutrition Almanac* (John D. Kirschman, McGraw-Hill), an excellent reference book found in most bookstores and many health food stores.

While your diet could contain sufficient folic acid, some drugs block its absorption. These drugs include oral contraceptives, alcohol, nicotine, anticonvulsants, antibacterials, and some chemotherapy agents. If you are on medications, check with your doctor, pharmacist, or the *Physician's Desk Reference* to see if the medication you are taking or have taken blocks folic acid metabolism.

Alcoholics tend to have twice as much homocysteine as nondrinkers. And what you drink seems to influence your levels, as well. People who drink wine and hard liquor tend to have higher homocysteine than people who drink beer. However, all alcoholics have low folate levels, which could be the reason their homocysteine is high. If you drink regularly, keep your vegetable intake high and supplement your diet with a multivitamin.

Vitamin B_6 also helps lower homocysteine, according to the Framingham Heart Study, the lengthiest evaluation of heart problems and nutrients ever conducted. In this study, low folic acid and vitamin B_6 correlated with high homocysteine in people who had heart attacks. Vitamin B_6 is found in meats and whole grains, but the amount in food may not be enough to lower your homocysteine. Consider taking a multivitamin with 25-50 mg of B_6.

Vitamin B_{12} is also needed to keep homocysteine low, and this vitamin is lacking in a vegetarian diet. However, many vegetarians have sufficient B_{12} due to a healthy digestive system. The amount of B_{12} found in most multivitamins is sufficient to meet your daily needs of 5-8 mcg a day. In fact, one cup of black tea contains 9 mcg.

The primary problem with vitamin B_{12} is that it is absorbed in the large intestines. If you have digestive problems, including a lot of gas, you may not be absorbing this important nutrient, since a chemical called "intrinsic factor," manufactured in the large intestines, is needed for vitamin B_{12} absorption. This means you need to pay attention to your digestion as part of a homocysteine-lowering program. To correct digestive problems, begin by chewing your food well. Next, consider taking enzymes and/or hydrochloric acid. Check with your health care practitioner about these supplements before taking them.

Check It Out!

You can have your homocysteine levels tested through a simple laboratory blood test. Talk to your doctor about this, and take the necessary dietary precautions for reducing homocysteine if yours is high. These dietary changes will contribute more to your health than simply lowering homocysteine. Bottom line: if your homocysteine level is high, you're not eating properly, or your lifestyle needs to be adjusted a bit.

Are You at Risk for Heart Disease?

How susceptible to heart disease are you? Knowing can save your life.

To help you assess your personal vulnerability, researchers at the Arizona Heart Institute have compiled the following test. It was designed specifically for women based on our unique disease development patterns and physiology. The test covers all those risk factors that have been proven time and again to influence women's risk in a predictable way.

Take the test, total your score, and find out your risk level at the end of the test.

Heart Test for Women

Age

50 and over	5
35 to 50	2
34 and under	0

Family History

If you have parents, brothers, or sisters who have had a heart attack, stroke or heart bypass surgery at:

Age 55 or before	5
Age 56 or after	3
None or don't know	0

Personal History

Have you had:

A heart attack	20
Angina, heart bypass surgery, angioplasty, stroke, or blood vessel surgery	10
None of the above	0

Smoking

Current smoker: how many cigarettes per day?

5 or more	20
4 or fewer	10

If you are a smoker currently taking oral contraceptives and are:

Under 35 years old	2
35 years old and over	5

If you are a previous smoker who quit less than two years ago: how many cigarettes did you smoke?

5 or more	10
4 or fewer	5

Blood Pressure

If you have had your blood pressure taken in the last year, was it:
Elevated or high (either or both readings
above 160/95 mmHg) 6
Borderline (between 140/90 and 160/95 mmHg),
Normal (below 140/90 mmHg),
or don't know 0

Hormone Status

If you have undergone natural menopause, your age at its start:
41 or older 1
40 or younger 2

If you have had a total hysterectomy, your age when it was done:
41 or older 1
40 or younger 3
If you take an oral estrogen supplement .... -2
If you are still menstruating .... -1

Exercise

Do you engage in any aerobic activity, such as brisk walking, jogging, bicycling, or swimming for more than 20 minutes:
Less than once a week 6
One or two times a week 3
Three or more times a week 0

Blood Fats

If you have had your cholesterol and blood fat levels checked in the last year, score your risk here:
Over 240 mg/dL 6
200 to 240 mg/dL 3
Cholesterol under 200 mg/dL 0

If your HDLs are lower than 45 1

Or if you do not know your cholesterol and blood fat levels, use this section to score your risk: Which of the following best describes your eating pattern:

High fat: red meat, fast foods, and/or fried foods daily; more than seven eggs per week; regular consumption of butter, whole milk, and cheese 6

Moderate fat: red meat, fast foods, and/or fried foods four to six times per week; four to seven eggs weekly; regular use of margarine, vegetable oils, and/or low-fat dairy products 3

Low fat: poultry, fish, and little or no red meat, fast foods, fried foods, or saturated fats; fewer than three eggs per week; minimal margarine and vegetable oils; primarily non-fat dairy products . . 0

Diabetes

If you have diabetes (blood sugar level above 140 mg/dL), your age when you found out:

40 or before 6
41 or older 4
Do not have diabetes 0

Body Mass

Calculate your body mass index with the following formula:
Weight (lbs.): __x 0.45= __(W)
Height (inches):__x 0.025= __(H)
W/(HxH)=your Body Mass Index (BMI)
If your BMI is 27 or greater 2
If your BMI is below 27 0

Now measure your waist and hips and divide your waist measurement by your hip girth to calculate your hip to waist ratio:
(waist) _____/(hips)_____=_____
If your waist to hip ratio is 0.8 or greater 1
If your ratio is 0.79 or less 0

Stress

Are you easily angered and frustrated:
Most of the time 6
Some of the time 3
Rarely 0

What Your Score Means

15 points or below: Low Risk

Congratulations! Maintain your heart healthy status by watching your weight, blood pressure, and blood fat (cholesterol and HDL) levels; get regular check-ups and don't smoke. Retake this test every year to monitor your heart-health risk profile.

16 to 32 points: Medium Risk

Our experience indicates that your medium risk level warrants attention. Personal factors or lifestyle habits may be increasing your vulnerability to heart disease. We strongly recommend you schedule an appointment with your doctor for an evaluation, and take this test with you to get advice on how you can improve your heart-health status.

33 points or above: High Risk

Your potential for experiencing a heart attack or stroke is significant. You must take action NOW. If you are not already being treated for heart disease, we urgently advise that you see your doctor immediately and take this test with you. You must seek ways to reduce your risk!

Chapter 3

Osteoporosis and the Calcium Controversy

Is calcium the culprit behind the increasing rates of osteoporosis, premenstrual syndrome, arthritis, and heart disease among American women?

Some 25 million Americans, 80 percent of them older women, suffer from osteoporosis, or "brittle bone" disease. Unfortunately, most women find out they have osteoporosis when it's too late — usually after a fracture of the wrist, hip or spine, loss of height, or curvature of the spine has occurred.

Like high blood pressure, osteoporosis is a silent, underlying condition, usually symptomless, with potentially devastating consequences. All of us lose some bone as we age, but people with osteoporosis lose an excessive amount. Their bones become fragile and their skeleton is weakened to the point where even a minor fall can result in a fracture.

Osteoporosis leads to some 1.5 million spine, hip, and wrist fractures in the U.S. each year, of which about 40 percent are spinal, 25 percent are hip, and 15 percent are wrist. Spinal fractures will affect one out of every three women in their lifetime, while wrist and hip fractures will happen to one out of six.

Osteoporosis is like high blood pressure in another way, too. In many cases it can be prevented and treated with a combination of lifestyle, diet, and therapeutic approaches.

Osteoporosis-related fractures can affect any bone in the body. But it is particularly critical to do everything possible to prevent hip fractures, because they can lead to loss of function and independence. A woman's frequency of hip fracture — three times that of a man's — is more serious than most of us realize. One hip fracture alone can total more than $30,000 in direct medical costs. Half of those affected lose the ability to walk independently, and up to a third become totally dependent. Studies have shown that within one year, up to 20 percent of hip fracture patients die from conditions related to the fracture or to fracture-related surgery.

Do We Have Enough Information?

Your risk of developing osteoporosis-related hip fracture is equal to your combined risk of developing breast, uterine, and ovarian cancer. Nevertheless, a survey of women between 45 and 75 showed that most are not aware of the widespread nature of the disease. Nearly three-fourths of the women thought they were knowledgeable about osteoporosis, but eight out of ten didn't connect the disease with hip fracture. Yet, ask an older woman what she most fears, and chances are fracture will be high on the list.

Doctors themselves are often not knowledgeable about the disease. One study, for example, found that only four percent of a group of people entering long-term care were diagnosed with osteoporosis, although nearly all of them had it.

Calcium and Kidney Stones

Small amounts of calcium are normally stored in the kidneys, but large amounts, in the form of calcium oxalate crystals, can result in problematic kidney stones. Now a 12-year study of over 90,000 women shows that dietary calcium decreased the risk of stones, while calcium supplementation may have increased them.

The theory for this phenomenon is that dietary calcium reduces the absorption of calcium oxalate in the intestines, so it can't get trapped in the kidneys.

Once again, Mother Nature triumphs. By getting your nutrients from foods you get balanced nutrients. Harmful substances may be contained in a food, but blocked from being absorbed. Can you get enough calcium from food alone? Yes, if you count broccoli (1 cup = 178 mg), tofu (1/2 cup =258 mg), and white beans (1 cup =121 mg). Even a cup of butternut squash has 84 mg of calcium. Whole grains and beans also contain both calcium and magnesium, the mineral that helps get calcium into your bones, where you want them.

"News in brief," *Lancet*, April 5, 1977, p. 1002.

In addition, most doctors insist that high doses of calcium, hormone therapy, and the newer bisphosphonate drugs are the only effective ways to prevent osteoporosis. They are ignoring many of the more current studies which indicate there are much more effective (and safer) options.

Bone: It's Not What You Think

Most people think of bone as a hard, permanent substance — the skeletal "infrastructure" of our bodies. But bone is living tissue that constantly undergoes remodeling — an alternating process of the removal, or resorption of old bone, and formation, the laying down of new bone. In healthy tissue, bone-removing cells carve out cavities in the bone's surface, while cells that form bone fill in these cavities. Thanks to this remodeling process, about a fifth of your skeleton is replaced each year.

During your first 30 years, more bone is formed than is lost. Sometime in your early 30s, peak bone density is reached and the balance begins to shift to the loss column.

Bone loss is a natural part of the aging process. By age 70 or 80, women will have lost about a third to a half of their bone mass. (In men, bone mass also declines as a natural part of aging — about 20 to 30 percent by comparison — but the decline is slower and begins from a point of higher density.)

In osteoporosis, however, the loss is much greater. Too little bone is formed or too much is removed — or both. As a result, bones become fragile and break easily, leaving people vulnerable to pain and injury.

The Overlooked Mineral: Magnesium

Since the 1950s, American women have been told by the medical profession that increasing the amount of calcium in our diets can greatly reduce the risk of developing osteoporosis. Advertisers and the media have emphasized the importance of this one mineral over all others — suggesting that calcium is enough to prevent bone loss. And as a result, sales of calcium supplements have skyrocketed and the consumption of dairy products has soared as well.

Still, a number of health problems that are the result of calcium-related imbalances, including premenstrual syndrome, arthritis, heart disease, and osteoporosis, continue to escalate.

Why?

We all need calcium for a variety of bodily functions including good colon health and building strong bones. But all recent studies do not agree that a high calcium intake has a positive effect on bone health. And it's no wonder. The more calcium one ingests at any given time, the smaller the percentage of calcium that is actually absorbed. And there is research that has shown that when we adapt to a low calcium diet, we actually excrete less of it in our urine and increase our absorption.

What's more, in 1988 the National Women's Health Network announced that women who lived in countries where calcium intake was low had less osteoporosis than women in this country who are on a high calcium diet.

And indeed, a great number of studies support the idea that lowered calcium intake may benefit American women as well. A Dutch study published in 1960 was one of the first to caution that excessive calcium could result in soft tissue calcification, or arthritis, and one possible beneficial nutrient to help counteract this effect would be magnesium. Recently, a study published in the *Journal of Applied Nutrition* showed an increase in bone density in postmenopausal women who took more magnesium and less calcium than has been generally recommended.

Magnesium's Role in Preventing PMS, Arthritis, Osteoporosis, and Even Heart Disease

One greatly overlooked factor in calcium absorption is the importance of having enough magnesium.

When women take large amounts of calcium, either in supplements or by eating diets high in dairy products and low in whole grains and beans, calcium is elevated in the blood and stimulates the secretion of a hormone called calcitonin. At the same time, it suppresses the secretion of the parathyroid hormone (PTH). These hormones regulate the levels of calcium in the bones and soft tissues and are related directly to osteoporosis and osteoarthritis. PTH draws calcium out of the bones and deposits it in the soft tissues, while calcitonin increases calcium in the bones.

But the optimum execution of these two delicate functions is dependent upon having sufficient magnesium. Because magnesium suppresses PTH and stimulates calcitonin, it helps move calcium into our bones. This chemical action helps prevent osteoarthritis and osteoporosis.

A magnesium deficiency, however, will prevent this chemical action. And more calcium is not the solution, because while magnesium helps the body absorb and utilize calcium, excessive calcium prevents the absorption of magnesium. Taking more calcium without adequate magnesium — and what is adequate for one woman may be insufficient for another — may either create calcium malabsorption or a magnesium deficiency.

Only additional magnesium can break this cycle, as was demonstrated by a study reported in *International Clinical Nutrition Review*. Volunteers on a low magnesium diet were given both calcium and vitamin D supplements. All subjects were magnesium-deficient, and all but one became deficient in calcium, as well, in spite of the fact that calcium had also been added to their diet. When they were given intravenous calcium infusions, the level of calcium in their blood rose for the duration of the intravenous feedings. When intravenous calcium was stopped, blood levels of calcium dropped again. However, when they were given magnesium, their magnesium levels rose rapidly and stabilized, and their calcium levels also rose within a few days even though they had not been given any additional calcium.

In addition to helping move calcium into the bones to reduce the risk for osteoporosis, magnesium is helpful in battling premenstrual syndrome. That's because magnesium helps the body utilize B vitamins, as well as inactivate excessive estrogens. And it is these conditions, low quantities of B vitamins and high estrogen to progesterone ratios, that have been found to contribute to premenstrual moodiness and irritability.

In most studies of women and heart disease, the magnesium factor is also being overlooked. In fact, magnesium may even be more important than calcium in reducing our incidence of heart disease. Consider this: Calcium causes muscles to contract. Magnesium, on the other hand, causes muscles to relax — and your heart is a muscle.

A recent randomized, controlled trial using magnesium in about 4,000 patients with acute myocardial infarction (heart attacks) showed that there were fewer deaths in people who were given magnesium than in those who did not take this mineral. The study recommends giving magnesium to all patients during acute heart attacks, and suggests this long-overlooked mineral may be beneficial when it is added to traditional medical treatments.

Postmenopausal women, those at highest risk of heart disease, would be wise to consider a diet higher in magnesium (whole grains and beans) and lower in calcium (dairy products). Nutritional supplements can be found that contain equal amounts of calcium and magnesium. Some, formulated specifically for postmenopausal women, already contain more magnesium than calcium.

Finally, high calcium diets may actually increase the risk of stroke, another leading cause of death in women as well as men. A UCLA study recently reported in the *Journal of Clinical Investigation* suggests that artery wall cells are able to form bone tissue and high calcium diets may contribute to such growth. In turn, this bone growth may contribute to the development of hardening of the arteries and blockages, which can cause strokes.

How Did This Trend in Magnesium Deficiency Begin?

Women's obsession with weight control may be at least partially responsible for much of our current magnesium deficiency. We have been assured that high quantities of non-fat dairy products, like milk and yogurt, were both safe and beneficial. But when you increase dairy products, even those without fat, you are upsetting your body's balance of calcium and magnesium.

The high protein content of dairy, especially when combined with other animal products, can pull calcium from the bones where it's needed. One study, reported in the *American Journal of Clinical Nutrition* of 1,600 women found that those who followed a vegetarian diet for at least 20 years had only an 18 percent loss of bone mineral by age 80, while meat eaters had a 35 percent bone mineral loss!

Also, dairy products contain nine times as much calcium as magnesium. If you have been eating a lot of dairy products, along with few or no grains and beans (which are rich in magnesium), you have probably upset your calcium/magnesium ratio even further.

In addition, most nutritional supplements contain twice as much calcium as magnesium. But again, because we've eaten so much dairy and so few grains and beans, our bodies have come to need as much magnesium as calcium, or even more. To bring yourself back into a chemical balance you would have to eat three cups of brown rice every day to compensate for one small serving of dairy. Because white rice has most of its magnesium removed, along with fiber and many other nutrients, you would need ten cups to balance one portion of calcium-rich foods.

Restoring Your Calcium and Magnesium Balance

What can you do to help eliminate PMS symptoms, protect yourself against osteoporosis, heart disease, stroke, and reduce your risk of arthritis?

Begin with a magnesium-rich diet. Many of the foods we eat have been refined, and magnesium is one nutrient removed in the refining process and not added in "enriched" products. Increase your consumption of whole grains like brown rice, millet, buckwheat (kasha), whole wheat, triticale, quinoa, and rye, as well as legumes, including lentils, split peas, and all varieties of beans. A whole grain cereal or bread in the morning, a cup of bean soup at lunch, a snack of whole grain crackers or popcorn, and a serving of brown rice, millet, or other grain with dinner should go a long way to help increase your magnesium intake.

More Soy Benefits

A six-month study conducted at the University of Illinois found that women who ate large quantities of soy protein had increased bone density in the spine as well as in other bones. Other studies have shown that soy can help lower cholesterol and protect against coronary heart disease, stroke, and menopausal hot flashes. Numerous international studies claim soy may also help prevent various forms of cancer. The reason seems to be the high concentrations of isoflavones, chemicals found only in soybeans.

We have found that the natural estrogenic effect of soy can reduce menopausal symptoms including vaginal dryness. Since soy products are easy to obtain, from soy protein powder to Boca Burgers (the best veggie burgers we've tasted!) to tempeh and edamame (frozen green soy beans found in Asian markets), we suggest that unless you have a sensitivity to soy, you include it in your diet — often.

Erdman, Dr. John W, Jr. "Short-term effects of soybean isoflavones on bones in postmenopausal women," Division of Nutr Science, Univ of Ill; "Disease prevention with soy," HSR *Supplement Industry Insider*, November 6-9, 1997, Scottsdale, AZ.

Eat plenty of fresh vegetables, too. Fresh produce and whole grains will, in addition to calcium and magnesium, provide your body with many other essential minerals. And it's especially important for you to not overlook one vitamin or mineral for another, since all work together to supply you with the nutrients you need.

Reduce your consumption of refined sugar and alcohol as well, to prevent excessive magnesium from being excreted in the urine. You may think your chocolate cravings are due to a sweet tooth, but they may be an indication that you have a calcium/magnesium imbalance. Cocoa powder contains more magnesium than any other food, so you may be a chocoholic if your body needs more magnesium, less calcium, or both.

But don't rush out and stock up on candy bars and other chocolate-rich foods. If you do, you're creating even more of an imbalance. You already know that chocolate contains an excessive amount of sugar. Not only does sugar cause magnesium excretion, but it also causes calcium to be leached out of your bones. In this way, diets that are excessive in sugar contribute to premenstrual bloating and weight gain. When you increase your magnesium and decrease calcium, eventually the chocolate cravings will leave and chocolate will be more a flavor you enjoy than a craving that drives you.

Another extremely important step is to evaluate the amount of dairy in your diet. If it has been high — more than a serving or so a day at most — reduce it at the same time as you increase magnesium-rich foods. Oriental and Indian diets contain little or no dairy, and arthritis and osteoporosis are not major health problems in these cultures. By featuring greater amounts of green vegetables, grains, tofu (soy bean curd), and seafood, these diets contain twice as much magnesium as the average American diet.

In addition, keep your animal protein (fish, chicken, meats) low, since a diet high in phosphorous, a mineral found in animal protein, can cause lowered calcium levels. Vegetable protein (grains with any beans) in any amount is safer, since a diet high in soy protein maintains calcium levels.

And if you've been taking vitamin/mineral supplements which are higher in calcium than magnesium, you may want to reverse the proportions to take more magnesium than calcium.

Can Soft Drinks Promote Osteoporosis?

Yes — this is one of the unhealthful effects of soft drinks. Some of them, mostly colas, contain phosphorus (in the form of phosphoric acid) which is added to keep the bubbles from going flat. But unfortunately, too much phosphorus in the diet can cause calcium to be leached from bones — hastening the development of osteoporosis.

In one survey, soft drinks containing the highest amounts of phosphorus included Tab, Coke, Diet Coke, and caffeine-free Coke. Phosphorus-free soft drinks included Pepsi Free, Diet Pepsi Free, 7-Up, and Mountain Dew. Others are low in phosphorus.

It's a good idea to limit any soft drinks that contain phosphorus to one a day. An excellent alternative is carbonated mineral water. The only phosphorus it contains is found naturally in water — and therefore, an amount more appropriate for human consumption.

How Much Magnesium?

How much magnesium does your body need? According to Dr. Mildred Seelig, executive president of the American College of Nutrition, we need about 200 milligrams more than we get in an average diet. She suggests that geriatric patients on a good diet take between 700 and 800 milligrams of magnesium supplements each day. This is considerably more than the Recommended Daily Allowances (RDA) of 350 milligrams per day for women of all ages.

Can you take too much magnesium? It's unlikely, according to Melvyn R. Werbach, MD, author of *Healing Through Nutrition* (HarperCollins, May 1993) and *Nutritional Influences on Illness*, a health practitioner's reference book. His research into medical studies has not found any cases of magnesium toxicity from taking it in the form of oral supplementation.

Guy E. Abraham, MD, a research gynecologist and endocrinologist in Torrance, California, has given postmenopausal women from 200 to 1000 mg of magnesium a day to strengthen their bones. He based the amount he gave each woman on bowel tolerance — enough magnesium to cause soft stools, but not diarrhea. These women showed an average bone density increase of 11 percent in one year, by adjusting their diets to increase magnesium (600-1000 mg/day) and lower calcium (500 mg/day).

Another study touting the benefits of magnesium for postmeno-pausal women, this one from Israel, also suggests that it is magnesium, not calcium, that protects our bones from the thinning characteristic of osteoporosis as we age.

In the Israeli study, 31 postmenopausal women were given from 250 to 750 mg of magnesium each day for two years. In almost 75 percent of the women, their bone density actually increased — in some, as much as eight percent. Women who refused additional magnesium had a loss of bone density from one to three percent — an expected decrease according to most medical doctors.

Most studies on the effect of increasing the amount of calcium in the diet show that calcium merely slows the rate of bone loss by an average of around 50 percent, but does not prevent or reverse osteoporosis.

For many women, getting sufficient magnesium is the missing link to reducing the risks of osteoporosis, heart disease, and arthritis, as well as eliminating PMS symptoms.

Reduce Your Risk for Broken Bones

There's one simple way you can lower your risk for osteoporosis: reduce the number of soft drinks you consume. A recent study reconfirmed what we've heard before: The phosphoric acid in soft drinks draws calcium out of bones and makes them more brittle and easier to break.

Interestingly, this study showed that the increase in bone fractures was limited to the girls in the study, not the boys. Because women are at an increased risk for osteoporosis later in life, it's important to avoid or stop any dependency on soft drinks as early in life as possible. Diet or decaffeinated soft drinks are not any safer. The phosphorus is the culprit.

Is one soft drink every once in a while a problem? Probably not. Most studies showing the harmful effects are concerned with large quantities ingested daily over a period of time. But if you're a cola addict and drink two or more a day, it could be wise to break this addiction.

Since high sugar diets also leach calcium from the bones, be sure you don't simply switch from sugar-sweetened colas to sugar-sweetened non-cola drinks!

Journal of Adolescent Health, 1994; 15:210-215.

The Estrogen Puzzle

The rapid bone loss many women experience as they go through menopause is due to the drop in estrogen, a hormone that regulates menstrual periods and plays a role in our bones' ability to absorb calcium from the bloodstream. Women who choose estrogen replacement therapy often do so for symptomatic relief of such menopause-related symptoms as hot flashes, vaginal dryness, and depression.

Studies have shown that estrogen intervention, particularly in the years immediately following menopause when the rate of bone loss can be as high as five percent a year, can decrease the risk of hip fracture by 25 to 50 percent and vertebral (spinal) crush fractures by perhaps as much as 50 to 75 percent. Estrogen, which blocks the process of bone resorption, has been shown to increase bone density three to five percent in the first year. In the long run, however, studies show that estrogen merely slows the rate of bone loss by an average of around 50 percent.

Although some studies strongly suggest that estrogen also provides protection from cardiovascular disease, there are as yet no definitive answers. Heart disease in postmenopausal women may come, in part, from increased calcium intake. Preliminary results from a study currently in progress show blood clots and heart disease actually developed in women taking estrogen, but not their placebo counterparts. It's very possible that doctors and drug companies jumped too early, concluding that since estrogen tends to lower cholesterol, it also lowers heart disease risk. Not necessarily!

There is also evidence that estrogen replacement therapy increases the risk of breast and endometrial cancer as well as stroke and gall-bladder disease. Many women, such as those who have had breast cancer, or whose mothers had breast cancer, should not take estrogen. Others choose not to for a variety of reasons.

Side effects, which may be difficult to tolerate, can include migraine headaches, breast soreness and swelling, bloating, mood changes, and cramping. Women on estrogen therapy report that ERT increases weight and contributes to the body's thickening, but medical doctors tend to deny this phenomenon.

In women who do take estrogen and have not undergone a hysterectomy, the increased risk of endometrial cancer may be offset by taking progesterone. The estrogen-progesterone combination, referred to as hormone replacement therapy (HRT), usually results in menstrual bleeding, which some women regard as a disadvantage.

Many women are reluctant to undertake hormone therapy, including progesterone, because the research on long-term effects is so limited. Their health care providers cannot give them clear and definitive answers, positive or negative.

We do know long-term estrogen use significantly increases breast cancer risk. A Harvard study reported in the Journal of the American Medical Association found a 71 percent increase in breast cancer risk among women aged 60-65 who had taken estrogen for five years or more! (There is also a disturbing lack of long-term safety studies for progesterone.) Many physicians advise that women limit therapy to 7 to 10 years. Others recommend it for longer, depending on a woman's individual situation. It is important for women to understand that once therapy stops, the increased rate of bone loss that marks the early postmenopausal years resumes. There is no carry-over in the protective effect.

Although studies show that women who take estrogen for at least seven years between menopause and age 75 reduce their risk of fracture by half during that time, recent studies show little difference after age 75, the period when women are most at risk. When women over the age of 75 who had taken estrogen for ten years following menopause were compared with women who had not taken estrogen, there was only a two percent

---

Calcium, Aluminum, and Kidney Failure

While calcium citrate is an easy-to-absorb form of calcium, we have said many times before that increasing your calcium without sufficient magnesium could lead to problems like PMS, muscle spasms, and even bone loss.

Now a South African study brings up another concern. As little as four grams of calcium citrate increases the absorption of aluminum, a mineral that has lead to kidney failure and is suspected to be linked to Alzheimer's disease. Calcium citrate can be found in some antacids, effervescent calcium, and buffered vitamin C supplements.

Are you safe if you take calcium citrate and are not taking any of these products which may contain aluminum? Yes. It's an excellent form of an essential mineral. Just be sure you're not cooking in aluminum pots and pans or using a deodorant with aluminum.

Nephron, 1994; 68:197-201.

difference in bone density. This suggests two types of bone loss — estrogen-dependent in earlier years and age-dependent later on.

Better Than Estrogen

A new type of plant estrogen, called isoflavonoids, has been so successful in trial studies in Europe that a drug containing this substance, Ipriflavone, is now an accepted treatment for osteoporosis in Italy, Hungary, and Japan. Since the drug is a derivative of a naturally occurring substance, women in this country should know that natural isoflavonoids can be found at their local markets. Soy products are high in this natural estrogen, making soy beans, tofu, and miso soup (the soup found in Japanese restaurants) desirable foods for women concerned about bone loss.

It's interesting to note that the lower incidence of osteoporosis in Japanese women has been attributed in part to their high consumption of soy products. If you aren't familiar with soy foods, we recommend Earl Mindell's *Soy Miracle* ($12, Fireside Books) for ideas on easy ways to incorporate them into your daily eating, and a wide variety of recipes.

The New Osteoporosis Drugs: Bisphosphonates

This new family of drugs acts to decrease bone loss by preventing bone resorption. These drugs, called bisphosphonates, are mineral compounds whose structures have been altered to act selectively on bone. Two popular bisphosphonate drugs go by the trade names Etidronate and Fosamax.

In a double blind placebo controlled study of Etidronate therapy in 135 postmenopausal women without osteoporosis, at the end of 7 to 10 years, women taking the drug showed a 3.42 percent increase in lumbar spine bone mineral density, compared to a .38 percent decrease among the placebo group.

What about Fosamax? Five controlled clinical studies, involving more than 1,600 postmenopausal women with osteoporosis, showed that patients treated with Fosamax experienced 29 percent fewer fractures of the hip and other bones (excluding the spine), compared to patients who took a placebo. Fosamax was also shown to reduce the incidence of new vertebral fractures by 48 percent.

In two, three-year trials with 994 postmenopausal women with osteoporosis Fosamax built bone. Women taking Fosamax had an increase in bone mineral density of 8.2 percent at the spine and 7.2 percent at the hip, compared with patients treated with a placebo, in whom bone mineral density decreased by between .065 and 1.16 percent.

Like many popular prescription drugs, the long-term safety of bisphosphonates has yet to be established.

Current advice from the manufacturer, Merck, is that patients with low levels of calcium in their blood, severe kidney disease, or who are pregnant or nursing should not take Fosamax. The manufacturer also urges that caution be used when Fosamax is given to patients with active upper gastrointestinal problems. Apparently Fosamax can irritate such problems. The most commonly reported drug-related side effects in patients taking this drug are musculoskeletal and abdominal pain, and other digestive disturbances such as nausea, heartburn, and irritation or pain of the esophagus.

The severity of the digestive disturbances should not be underestimated. Fosamax users frequently complain of horrible burning that wasn't helped by either Tums or Maalox. The manufacturer is very aware of this and has made the unprecedented move of distributing special drug warning stickers for pharmacists to adhere to prescription bottles. The stickers warn patients to take Fosamax 30 minutes before breakfast with water (coffee, orange juice, and other acidic beverages will contribute to digestive problems) and not to lie down for at least 30 minutes after taking the drug (this also can aggravate digestive problems).

In the absence of long-term safety testing, these dramatic digestive problems may very well be the body rebelling against even greater unknown threats. Nausea, for example, can be a warning sign for potential liver damage. Beware!

Users should also be aware of how these drugs work — by inhibiting bone resorption. This process, in which calcium moves into and out of the bones to other parts of the body, helps maintain healthy levels of calcium elsewhere throughout the body for important functions, including nerve cell communication, contraction of muscle cells, blood-clotting efficiency, enzyme function, and production of certain proteins. If calcium is not allowed to move around freely in it's normal manner, will any of these functions be adversely affected? Currently lacking long-term studies may provide an answer. The fact that patients with low levels of calcium in their blood are presently advised not to take Fosamax might be an early clue to a yes answer.

In view of these concerns, taking bisphosphonates to prevent osteoporosis may be a much riskier proposition than doctors and drug companies are letting on. It might be wisest to reserve use of these drugs for cases of advanced osteoporosis, when other safer therapies aren't enough, or in temporary conjunction with other therapies when circumstances require fastest results.

Attention to Prevention

More and more of us are finding out how much we benefit from exercise. Young women reap the greatest benefit, since they can build bone mass up until their 30s. After that, exercise is critical to maintaining bone mass or slowing the rate of loss.

Exercise that forces the body to work against gravity (weight-bearing exercise) like jogging, walking, aerobics, dancing, and team sports, strengthens the skeletal system. Non-weight-bearing activities like cycling and swimming do not strengthen bone, but are important for cardiovascular health.

You don't have to train like an athlete — in fact, it's better if you don't. A good guideline is 30 to 60 minutes of exercise three or four times

It's Never Too Late!

A six-month study of two dozen women over the age of 75 (the average age was 79), reports that exercising an hour a day twice a week can improve balance, other muscle coordination, and muscle strength. The exercise included warm-up, light aerobics, and calisthenics.

Loss of balance as we age is one of the most predictive risks for falls and broken bones. While more frequent exercise could improve your heart, preventing falls and broken hips ranks high on our "to do" list. Consider starting before you're 75! Join a gym if you're not disciplined, or buy a video tape or two for bi-weekly workouts.

Okumiya, Kiyohito, MD, et al, "Effects of exercise on neurobehavioral function in community-dwelling older people more than 75 years of age," *Journal of the Amer Geriatric Soc*, 1996;44(5):569-572.

a week. Impossible? Even three 10-minute walks over the course of a day help.

As we age, we lose muscle mass as well as bone. Weight training can improve muscle strength and tone, which contributes to bone health, as well. There have been studies in the past that suggested heavier women have greater bone density than thinner women. A more recent study, however, now suggests it's not a person's weight, but the amount of muscle, that is the determining factor.

A group of nearly 250 healthy premenopausal women had their bone density examined. Those who had the highest amount of both fat and muscle had the most dense bones. Those with flabby muscles had low bone density — whether they were heavy or thin.

While it's possible to say that bones that are dense before menopause will continue to remain strong and healthy after menopause, this study strongly suggests that weight alone will not protect you against osteoporosis. All women, whether heavy or light, should increase their muscle mass through regular weight resistance exercise.

You're never too old to benefit from exercise, either. One study that appeared in the *New England Journal of Medicine* compared mobility and strength of 100 nursing home residents between the ages of 72 and 98. Half the seniors participated in a 10-week weight resistance training program. At the end of this short time, their muscle strength had increased by an average of 113 percent, compared to the non-exercisers. Significant improvement in mobility was also seen which made these seniors less prone to bone-breaking falls — a very significant achievement in view of the fact that 80 is the average age of persons suffering hip fractures.

Exercise is essential to good bone health, but it is far more effective when coupled with absorbed calcium. For women entering menopause, however, it is important to note that reduced estrogen, not calcium, is the primary cause of bone loss in the first five years beyond menopause. Women who do not get enough calcium (less than 400 mg./day), however, may lose even more bone mass.

When coupled with vitamin D and magnesium, calcium has shown tangible benefits. One study showed a reduction in hip fractures in a nursing home population whose average age was 85.

Another study published in the *Journal of Applied Nutrition* showed a reversal of osteoporosis in postmenopausal women who adjusted their diets to increase magnesium (600-1000 mg/day) and lower calcium (500 mg/day). These women showed an average bone density increase of 11 percent in one year.

Although this and other similar information has appeared in medical publications, most doctors still ignore it and attempt to frighten their patients into taking 1500 milligrams of calcium a day. The majority of nutritional supplements contain twice as much calcium as magnesium, perpetuating the myth that calcium prevents osteoporosis. Numerous studies, however, show that most of this calcium does not get into the bones.

Boron and vitamin D are also necessary for calcium absorption. Many older people need vitamin D since it is harder for them to absorb calcium. Many house-bound older adults get less sunlight — the major source of this essential vitamin — and consume fewer vitamin D-rich foods, such as fatty fish, liver, and egg yolk.

Recommended daily amounts of vitamin D are 200 to 400 IUs (international units) but no more than 800. A good quality multivitamin/mineral may have both, and offers good insurance toward having adequate quantities of many other important nutrients your body needs to maintain optimal bone health.

In the future, health care providers may have a test to determine who is genetically at risk for developing osteoporosis. Recently, Australian researchers discovered that women with two copies of the variant of the gene for the body's vitamin D receptors reached a "fracture threshold" eight years earlier than women with two copies of the normal gene.

Are You at Risk?

Why do some of us develop osteoporosis? We need much more research to understand the causes, but some factors have been identified.

● Genetics plays one of the strongest roles. The signs to watch for in older relatives include loss of height with aging, curvature of the spine, fractures, or chronic back pain.

● Loss of estrogen. Women are most vulnerable to osteoporosis when they go through menopause, whether it occurs naturally or is surgically induced. During these years, the body is changing the way it makes estrogens and as the amount of estrogen produced declines, bone loss increases significantly. This is particularly true in the first five to seven years after menopause when we can lose from two to five percent of bone mass each year. After that the annual rate of loss slows to about one percent.

● Cessation of menstrual periods. Hormone imbalance, often characterized by lack of menstrual periods, may also contribute to bone loss. High-performance athletes are at risk. One study found that 40 percent of competitive women skaters do not have a menstrual period. Many young women who diet excessively or suffer from eating disorders like anorexia are at similar risk.

● Smoking and alcohol. Researchers have found strong links between smoking and reductions in bone mass, resulting in a deficit of 5 to 10 percent in some cases. Because it decreases levels of calcium and vitamin D in the body, moderate to heavy alcohol use can also reduce bone mass.

● Diet. Women may also be more vulnerable to osteoporosis in midlife if their calcium absorption has been low since childhood. The recommended amounts for children and young adults range from 800 to 1500 mg/day. Vulnerability increases even more in later years as our bodies become less able to absorb this essential mineral.

Steroids and Osteoporosis

The American College of Rheumatology, admits that one out of every four patients who uses steroids to counteract the inflammation of arthritis and rheumatism eventually gets a fracture from thinning bones. In fact, bone wasting is most rapid during the first six months of steroid therapy. How much steroid contributes to osteoporosis? Just 7.5 mg of prednisone a day is enough to cause thinning, brittle bones, and eventual fractures.

Doctors are being told to use topical or inhaled steroids, rather than those that are ingested, whenever these forms are appropriate. We'd like to add that there are anti-inflammatory agents that do not have side effects of bone loss, like vitamin C and glucosamine sulfate. Explore with your alternative health care practitioner other, safer, anti-inflammatory medications.

Some topical creams containing capsaicin, a chemical found in cayenne pepper, reduce the pain and inflammation from arthritis and rheumatism. They're either going to work for you — or not. But they won't cause bone loss.

McCarthy, Michael. "Guidelines issued for steroid-induced osteoporosis," *Lancet*, Vol. 348, November 2, 1996.

Although as we age we have more difficulty absorbing calcium, doctors and the media still insist we increase our intake, both in our diet and supplements. This increase in unabsorbed calcium often leads to heart disease (the biggest killer of women past menopause) and arthritis.

Diets high in sugar, protein, phosphorous (found in colas), and caffeine cause calcium to be excreted from the bones, contributing to osteoporosis. Some nutrients help the body absorb calcium into the bones, helping to prevent osteoporosis.

Magnesium contributes to calcium absorption. It is found in abundance in whole grain foods such as brown rice, oatmeal, corn tortillas, and whole grain breads, as well as legumes such as split peas, lentils, soy products, and beans.

Lack of vitamin D, which also helps the body absorb calcium, is a critical factor, particularly for older people who may not get enough sunlight, a primary source of the vitamin, and do not take vitamin supplements which include this vitamin.

In general, the better *all* nutrients in your diet are balanced, the more your bones will benefit.

● Immobility. Use it or lose it. People who are bedridden or in a cast for any length of time show evidence of bone loss from lack of use. An example of this is the astronauts who spend time in a weightless

Calcium, Bone Loss, and Caffeine

It takes more than calcium and other minerals to prevent or reduce osteoporosis (bone loss) in women who are past menopause. You need to also take a look at how much caffeine you're drinking. A study in the *American Journal of Clinical Nutrition* showed that women who drank two to three cups of brewed coffee or more (450 mg of caffeine) could have increased bone loss from their spines, especially if their calcium intake was less than 800 mg a day.

It would be interesting to determine in a medical study whether or not women who take additional calcium are absorbing it, since calcium absorption is inhibited as we age and our stomachs produce less acid. Antacids contribute to calcium malabsorption. Perhaps it is not the amount of calcium but our body's' ability to absorb it that is the major factor. Still, it is important that women understand that more than one cup of brewed coffee may contribute to bone loss. Instant coffee and tea (especially green tea) have less caffeine per cup.

environment and get osteoporosis from their time in space. Women who exercise too little lose bone strength as well, placing them at greater risk for osteoporosis-related fractures.

● Ethnicity and body type. Caucasian and Asian women are more likely to develop osteoporosis than members of other ethnic groups. Although studies show that fewer African-American and Hispanic women experience the disease, they are still at risk and should take the same preventive measures. Thin, petite women are also more vulnerable. Although heavier women produce more estrogen and are thus better protected against osteoporosis than thin women, they also need to take their risk for the disorder seriously.

● Medications. Some medications given for other disorders may cause osteoporosis. The most common are glucocorticoids (steroid medicines), generally prescribed for diseases such as arthritis, asthma and ulcerative colitis. As research progresses, we are learning that other medications, such as high doses of thyroid hormone, may also increase bone loss. Ask your health care provider if any of your medications fall in this category and what, if anything, can be done about it.

Why Calcium Makes
Bones More Brittle

Would you like your bones to be as brittle as chalk or as strong as ivory? You may have a choice in this. In fact, without realizing it, you may be opting for exactly what you don't want — brittle bones. This section addresses bone flexibility versus brittle bones, and answers a number of other questions relating to osteoporosis prevention and reversal.

The husband of one of our readers used to drink two gallons of milk every week, thinking that it would keep his bones strong. Then he developed definite signs of osteoporosis. He stopped drinking milk and is now taking magnesium to help the calcium in his diet get into his bones better.

She wanted to know why magnesium sometimes causes loose stools? Which is the best form of magnesium to take? And whether or not it should be taken with calcium or alone? She also asked what causes magnesium to make bones more flexible and less prone to fracture?

An Expert Says ...

The media is bombarding you with appeals to consume massive quantities of calcium. We tell you to ignore this hype and concentrate on a high magnesium intake, and that this will actually enable you to absorb more calcium into your bones. Who should you believe?

To help better convince you of our position, we called on one of the country's leading experts on the subject, Dr. Guy Abraham. Dr. Abraham is a research gynecologist and endocrinologist in Southern California where he heads Optimox, Inc., a small supplement company that designs some of the most often copied nutrients on the market: Optivite PMT, a formula that has been shown to eliminate PMS; and Gynovite, a multivitamin/mineral that has been shown to reverse osteoporosis in a small but significant study.

Yes, he does have a vested interest in selling his products, but not in whether or not women (or men) use more magnesium and less calcium in general. He just advocates magnesium over calcium because he and others have found through scientific studies that it makes the most sense. He's an expert in the field who is always happy to give us general information we can pass on that's based on sound scientific studies.

First, why might magnesium cause loose stools? Because it's not well absorbed. Unabsorbed magnesium that enters your large bowel causes diarrhea. So you want to be able to utilize this mineral before it gets to your gut. This means you need enough hydrochloric acid (HCl) in your stomach to begin breaking it down. Antacids neutralize stomach acids. Taking antacids along with magnesium is counterproductive and can contribute to loose stools. Just as taking an antacid prevents calcium (which is in some antacid tablets) from being absorbed, it prevents magnesium absorption as well. Chew your food well to stimulate your body's natural production of HCl, and remember that as you age, your body produces less of this digestive juice, so don't overeat.

Next, find a well-absorbed form of magnesium. Dr. Abraham's Mag 200 contains 200 mg of magnesium oxide and has been designed specifically to be well tolerated because it is so well absorbed. If you get loose stools from taking even 100-200 mg of magnesium, try switching to any brand of magnesium oxide. If another brand causes loose stools you might want to try Dr. Abraham's. (Optimox, Inc., 800-722-9040). According to Dr. Abraham, a well-absorbed form of magnesium should be tolerated at levels of around 600 to 800 mg/day.

When you want to increase the bone-strengthening effect of magnesium, take it alone, not with calcium. You may have a supplement that contains both minerals, but which has insufficient magnesium to meet your requirements (several studies have shown that 500 mg of calcium and 600-1000 mg of magnesium can reverse osteoporosis). In this case, take additional magnesium alone.

Making Bones Strong: Chalk vs. Ivory

Let's address the subject of bone flexibility, since this may be the determining factor in whether or not your bones break when you fall as you get older. The more flexible your bones, the less likely you are to break them. Bone density is only one part of osteoporosis — the part we can now easily measure. Bone flexibility may be even more important, though. And we have no sophisticated tests to let us know whether or not our bones are brittle. This is why doctors only talk about how dense your bones are.

Calcium contains properties that makes them brittle, while magnesium binds to protein in your bones and keeps them supple. Take a look at two substances in nature with relationship to these properties of suppleness and brittleness: chalk and ivory. Chalk is pure calcium carbonate, the stuff they put in mineral supplements to help you meet your daily requirements. Take a new piece of chalk and drop it. Watch it break. Then compare it with a piece of ivory the same size taken from an elephant's tusk. The ivory is a combination of calcium and magnesium. Now, which do you need, more calcium or more magnesium?

Dr. Abraham believes we can get sufficient calcium from our foods without taking additional amounts in supplement form. His supplements, which have been shown to improve bones, are lower than most in calcium. We suggest you may need more magnesium to make your bones more like ivory and less like chalk. And that you find a product that will allow you to increase your magnesium to 600-800 mg/day while limiting calcium supplements to around 500 mg. You'll get even more calcium as well as magnesium in whole foods like whole grains (millet is especially high), beans, nuts and seeds, dark green leafy vegetables, as well as tofu and soy products. The minerals you take are not just in pills. They're in your food, as well.

So when your doctor suggests you take more calcium or consider taking hormones or other prescription drugs to increase your bone density, ask him or her what they suggest to make your bones more flexible. If they don't have an answer, tell them about magnesium.

Beware of Bone-Density Testing!

Doctors' offices across the country are being filled by a new breed of diagnostic machines. These new machines measure your bone density and they sound like a good idea — especially if you're interested in preventing osteoporosis.

But watch out! If you're old enough, you're virtually guaranteed that one of these machines will convince your doctor that you have, or are at dangerous risk of developing osteoporosis. Then, before a meaningful discussion can take place, your doctor will likely write you out a prescription for one or more osteoporosis drugs — such as Fosamax or Premarin. But is this the best course of action?

It used to be that osteoporosis was diagnosed when an older person with brittle bones actually suffered a fracture.

In recent years, however, the definition of osteoporosis has changed. In 1991, a panel of medical experts, in a report that appeared in the *American Journal of Medicine*, redefined osteoporosis as: "A disease characterized by low bone mass and microarchitectural deterioration of bone tissue, which lead to increased bone fragility and a consequent increase in fracture risk." In plain English, this new definition of

---

Be Wary of Tums!

An article in the *American Journal of Epidemiology* (vol 145, 1997) published the results of a two-year study of over 9,000 women aged 65 or older. They found "no important associations between dietary calcium intake and the risk of any of the fractures studied." In fact, taking calcium supplements proved to increase the risk of hip fracture. What about Tums? Again, an increase in bone breakage. The authors conclude that they can find no benefit of calcium on the risk of fractures. If your doctor insists you take calcium, or Tums, refer him or her to this study. And make your own decision.

Cummings, R.G., et al. "Calcium intake and fracture risk: results from the study of osteoporotic fractures," *Am J Epidemiol* 1997;145:926-934.

osteoporosis simply means you have an increased risk of fracture, not that you had a fracture or will definitely get a fracture.

But doctors are now diagnosing osteoporosis by completely disregarding your bone's flexibility, fragility, and micro-architecture (in the above definition), and instead are heavily relying on bone density, which can be easily measured using various machines. Some of these machines are more accurate than others, though there are accuracy problems with all of them.

In addition, many are inadequate for precisely monitoring your progress, including the results of any therapy you are using to prevent osteoporosis. Yet doctors persist in using these machines for this purpose as well. Urine tests, which measure the rate of bone break-down as reflected in various markers, are also problematic. They can produce day-to-day variations of up to 40-50 percent. Unfortunately, there are no tests to measure bone flexibility vs. fragility.

In addition, bone density is not always the same throughout your body. A high or low density reading in one area, say the heel or lower spine, doesn't necessarily mean you have similar density elsewhere in more critical locations such as your wrist, hip, or upper spine, where fractures are most likely to occur.

Finally, to complicate matters even more, deposits of unabsorbed calcium — perhaps from arthritis — can result in overreads, in which machines report higher density than actually exists.

The bottom line on test results is this: Don't make assumptions. Instead, get straightforward answers from your doctor about the accuracy and real meaning of any bone-density and bone-loss testing.

Impossible Standards Are Also Deceptive

One reader recently wrote, "I am trying to decide which estrogen to take. My bone density is at 85 percent and I'm 55 years old."

It's easy to understand how, upon first hearing that your bone density is 85 percent or even 60 percent or another percent less than 100, you might be concerned. But when we take a closer look at exactly what these numbers mean, it's easy to see that (even if test results were completely accurate) their value and importance is still limited.

That's because all test results are compared to the peak bone density of a typical pre-menopausal female, not other women in your own age group, including the ones who are actually getting fractures. This is akin to telling postmenopausal women that they are estrogen-deficient and therefore diseased simply because their estrogen levels are not comparable to those of premenopausal women. This is ridiculous. Estrogen levels do decrease after menopause. Bones do lose some of their density. But this doesn't mean they are going to break.

Rather than taking age-related differences into account, however, doctors compare your bone density to pre-menopausal peak levels to determine your T score, in which the T stands for fracture threshold. Now here's the catch. According to the National Osteoporosis Foundation bone-mass chart, by age 80 nearly every woman will have bone density below the fracture threshold. Once your bone density falls below this fateful line, you are deemed to be at increased risk of fracture, and therefore are diagnosed as having osteoporosis.

Doctor Susan Love, a leading authority on female health care, summarizes the predicament this way: "The level of bone density that [now] defines osteoporosis has been set rather high, with the result that most older women will fall into the "disease" category — which is very nice for the people in the business of treating disease."

Osteoporosis Is Now Big Business!

In spite of the fact that only 39 percent of older women will ever suffer a fracture....

Or the fact that the large majority of these fractures will be minor and have no permanent long-term consequences*....

---

* Most people who suffer osteoporosis-related fractures recover and return to their normal lives. Actual fracture risk among Caucasian women (there is a general lack of data for women of color who tend to have even lower fracture rates) is estimated as follows:

Wrist fracture. Estimated lifetime risk is 16 percent; the average age at time of fracture is 67; an estimated 1.9 percent of wrist fracture sufferers becoming dependent as a result of the fracture.

Vertebral fracture. Estimated lifetime risk is 15 percent; the large majority of these fractures are painless and often undiagnosed; dowager's hump may occur with multiple fractures; an estimated 1.5 percent of vertebral fracture sufferers become dependent.

Hip fracture. Estimated lifetime risk of fracturing one or both hips is 17 percent; average age at time of fracture is 80; an estimated 10.2 percent of those who suffer hip fractures will become dependent on a long-term basis.

Or the fact that a combination of frailty, weakness, and other considerations such as slippery or poorly lit walking surfaces, poor balance, and a lack of mental alertness (often a side effect of prescription drugs), also frequently contribute to the occurrence of disabling or life-threatening fractures....

Most researchers now advocate that women whose bone density is nearing or already below the fracture threshold need treatment — which usually includes prescription drugs.

Is it possible that health conscious women are being marketed a disease that requires them to load up on lots of expensive doctor's appointments, diagnostic testing, and prescription drug treatments?

Merck, the maker of the popular osteoporosis treatment drug Fosamax, wrote in its 1995 Annual Report that "We have been aggressively working to educate consumers about the disease and the importance of early diagnosis and appropriate treatment with organizations such as the National Osteoporosis Foundation, the Older Women's League, and members of the European parliament. We have established the Bone Measurement Institute, a non-profit organization, to increase the accessibility and affordability of bone measurement technologies. Merck has also provided funding for the first world summit of osteoporosis societies."

This excerpt basically says that Merck is helping to fund the distribution of bone-density testing machines around the country. So wherever you are, it will be easier for you to get to one of these machines, get diagnosed with osteoporosis, and maybe even start taking Merck's drug Fosamax. (Remember that annual reports are about profits, not public service.)

What's more, during the next two years, you might not have to go out of your way at all to get your bone density measured. As I was writing the above paragraph, I received a phone call and long fax from a public relations firm being paid to tell me about a newly formed group called The Osteoporosis Business Coalition, and the new osteoporosis public awareness campaign this coalition is launching. The campaign will offer free bone-density testing at work sites, as well as other locations including the National Association of Realtors State Conventions and Dress Barn clothing outlets.

More prominent members of this coalition include Wyeth-Ayerst Laboratories, the maker of today's best-selling estrogen supplement (Premarin), which happens to slow bone loss; and Proctor & Gamble

Pharmaceuticals which is getting ready to launch a new osteoporosis treatment drug called Actonel. (I'll report the scoop on Actonel after it gets final FDA approval.) In other words, here are more businesses promoting bone-density testing that stand to profit when women are found to have low bone density. And the National Osteoporosis Foundation is in cahoots with this coalition, as well.

In the midst of current and coming propaganda that plays on our fears of becoming disfigured and disabled with osteoporosis, it will become increasingly easy to get the idea that if your bone density is low, you're destined to become a hunched-over little old lady who eventually falls, breaks a hip, and spends the remainder of her days in a convalescent home. Although this serious and life-threatening, worst-case scenario does indeed happen, it's not as likely to happen to you as vested interests would like you to believe.

For a more realistic perspective, take a closer look at the older women around you in your community and your family. What do you see? Few, if any, women stooped over with dowager's humps, and probably a good number of healthy, active older women. What's more, there's a lot more you can do — besides taking potentially harmful drugs — to help ensure you have healthy bones in your senior years, even if you're already in them.

Here's a parting thought on the importance of bone density that you might share with your doctor: Asian women are living proof that bone density is of highly limited value in determining fracture risk. Their bone density averages are so low that simply being Asian is frequently listed as a risk factor for osteoporosis. Yet Asian women have far fewer hip fractures than Caucasian women. Asian women also consume little, if any, dairy foods.

Parts excerpted from "A Status Report on Osteoporosis: The Challenge to Midlife and Older Women," *Older Women's League*, June 1994.

Chapter 4

Making the New Hormones Work for You

Currently, the National Institutes of Health (NIH) spends approximately $9.8 billion on research, yet virtually none of this is spent on researching one of the most intriguing topics in health today: natural hormones.

When we think about age-related hormone declines, we usually think about falling estrogen levels, and perhaps progesterone declines as well. In reality, however, our bodies are teaming with hundreds of hormones — all of which decline as we age.

Increasingly, attention is turning from estrogen and progesterone to other key hormones: DHEA, melatonin, testosterone, pregnenolone, and human growth hormone. And a small but growing number of researchers and doctors are now advocating full-spectrum hormone supplementation as a means to delay aging and ultimately increase longevity, as well as prevent disease and treat advanced disease.

Some of these hormones, including DHEA, melatonin, progesterone, and pregnenolone are now available to consumers over-the-counter. But one important fact we need to keep in mind when considering any type of hormone supplementation is that, whether a prescription is needed or not, all hormones are powerful drugs.

Another key concern to keep in mind as you consider using hormones is that, in general, there are many unanswered questions regarding whether these supplements are safe for long-term, human use. Only time and additional human studies will provide specific answers.

Still, used cautiously, and under the supervision of a knowledgeable doctor, these hormone supplements may be highly beneficial. But used carelessly, they may wreak havoc with our health. To avoid the latter, follow these general guidelines:

1. If you are premenopausal, still have your ovaries and uterus, and have good hormonal balance, be especially cautious about taking hormone

supplements. Since hormones work interdependently and are carefully balanced against each other, taking a hormone supplement when no imbalance exists can result in hormone imbalance, and actually create health problems. Using melatonin (the sleep hormone) occasionally, such as to overcome jet lag, may be harmless.

2. Use hormones only under a knowledgeable doctor's supervision.

3. To locate a knowledgeable doctor near you, call the American Holistic Health Association at 714-779-6152, or one of the compounding pharmacies listed in the Resource Guide at the end of this report.

4. Pursue non-drug, and non-hormonal therapies as a first line of action.

5. If these do not produce satisfactory results, work with your doctor to have your hormone levels tested. In addition to estrogen and progesterone levels, testing should also check the levels of testosterone, thyroid, pregnenolone, and DHEA. Any hormone supplementation should then be based on the results of these tests. For increased longevity, the goal is to replenish key hormone levels back to more youthful levels.

6. If you start taking hormones, monitor yourself closely for any adverse reactions and report these to your doctor right away. Also, continue to have your hormone levels checked regularly — every six months or so. This is the most prudent way to track your progress. It will also help protect you against one of our foremost concerns regarding women taking hormone supplements: Even if you don't take estrogen supplements, other hormone supplements can increase your estrogen levels. And increased estrogen levels have been linked to an increased incidence of breast cancer. Therefore, always include estrogen in your hormone level tests.

7. Take the lowest dosages possible to achieve desired results. In the case of hormones, more is not always better. In fact, overly high dosages can be highly detrimental to your health.

To what extent you wish to use hormones, if at all, is a decision that should be made with great care and attention. Although much is known about hormones. Much is also left to be learned. One way to minimize unnecessary adverse risks, however, is to maintain superior health without hormones as long as possible. Then if and when you do decide to begin taking any hormones, keep dosages as low as possible to achieve the desired benefits.

That said, here is an introduction to the key full-spectrum hormones available for prevention, advanced healing, and increased longevity.

DHEA

The hormone DHEA (dehydroepiandrosterone) leads off our list because it is considered by many to be the "mother of all hormones." It's produced by the brain, the adrenal glands, the skin, and is the most abundant steroid hormone in the body. Its behavior is very unique and until the last decade or so, DHEA was probably the most misunderstood key hormone.

This chart graphs typical DHEA levels throughout the human life span. Note the dramatic surge between the onset of puberty and the early 20s. For women, levels then decline steadily through the fifth decade, our 40s. It's interesting to observe that around age 40, our DHEA levels are comparable to the level right before puberty. Between age 50 and 70, our DHEA level typically drops, then rises slightly. Then in our 70s, the decline continues and finally around age 80 levels out at a level 1/6 the peak for women, and 1/8 the peak level for men.

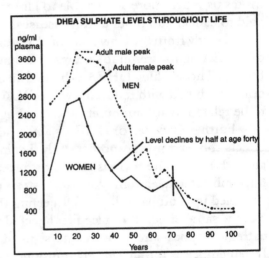

Studies to date have found that DHEA lowers cholesterol and prevents blood clots, improves memory, strengthens the immune system, prevents bone loss, fights fatigue and depression, enhances feelings of well-being, increases strength, reduces body fat, increases libido, and alleviates menopause symptoms. DHEA may also protect against diabetes and autoimmune disease. And important research is currently underway into DHEA's ability to prevent cancer.

Perhaps DHEA is best-known, however, for its overall energizing effects. In a six-month study conducted at the University of San Diego, participants taking DHEA reported a "remarkable* increase in perceived physical and psychological well-being." (*In medical jargon, remarkable means significant.) They also reported sleeping better, feeling more relaxed, being less affected by stress, and experiencing relief from joint pain (among arthritis sufferers).

In a series of experiments with mice, by Dr. Raymond A. Daynes at the University of Utah School of Medicine, DHEA proved to have remarkable revitalizing effects on the immune system, providing old mice with immunity comparable to that seen only in young mice. Among other things, these studies suggested that it's DHEA's ability to block the body's production of stress hormones that produced this revitalized immune response.

While further in-depth study is needed, DHEA's apparent ability to reduce stress and, in turn, boost immune system function should not be missed or underestimated. Study after study has shown that high stress makes us much more susceptible to illnesses, ranging from the common cold to cancer and other deadly diseases.

A study from the University of Tennessee that investigated the effects of DHEA on the immune systems of women made this important cancer finding: Those taking DHEA exhibited an increase in cancer-fighting NK cells, combined with reduced levels of IL 6 cytokines (which are believed to be related to autoimmunity and other age-related diseases).

Further evidence of DHEA's ability to mitigate stress and its deadly effects comes from yet another study that investigated the effects of stress and DHEA on the thymus glands of mice. The thymus glands of those mice subjected to extreme, long-term stress eventually ceased functioning, shriveled up, and basically died. Injecting the mice with stress hormones had the same effect. But mice first injected with DHEA, then exposed to extreme physical stress showed no signs of damage to the thymus gland. It, remember, is the all-important producer of T-cells, which help protect us from infection and disease.

Alan Gaby, MD, president of the American Holistic Medical Association and medical editor of the *Townsend Letter for Doctors and Patients*, often recommends five or 10 mg of DHEA daily to some patients. According to Gaby, "Sometimes hot flashes get better; sometimes mood changes improve; sometimes vaginal dryness improves; sometimes the combination of [natural] progesterone cream plus DHEA works better than either one alone. In another study that appeared in late 1993 in the *American Journal of OB/GYN*, healthy women took DHEA at the time of menopause and their immune function improved. Usually, this declines at menopause.

Dr. Gaby also uses DHEA with his patients as a remedy for certain age-related conditions; "People who come in who are in their 70s or 80s or even with premature aging in their 60s, with loss of muscle mass, loss of memory, diminished appetite, depression, weakness, fatigue — their DHEA levels are usually low or below normal, sometimes even well below normal and you just give them a little bit and they gradually come back to life. You see a dramatic change. After a year, you look at them and they're just a completely different person," says Gaby.

Both blood and saliva tests can be used to check DHEA levels. Dr. William Regelson, a researcher and co-author of *The Super-Hormone Promise*, recommends taking DHEA supplements in the morning, in keeping with the body's natural DHEA production pattern. A month or so after beginning DHEA, your doctor should recheck your DHEA level to make sure your dosage is correct. Then this level should be monitored every six months. This periodic level checking is advisable with any hormone you are taking.

In addition, your doctor should also monitor any other medical concerns that may be affected by hormone supplements. For example, DHEA supplementation can reduce the need for insulin among diabetics.

A Question About DHEA

Q: When I was 40 years old I had a hysterectomy and started having hot flashes. I've found that 5 mg of DHEA a day prevents them. Why isn't DHEA recommended for postmenopausal symptoms? — *K.D.V., Bartlesville, OK*

A: Taking 5 mg of DHEA is probably very safe. Most people, unfortunately, believe that more is better and take from 25 mg to 50 mg of this hormone every day. We think this isn't wise. Ray Sahelian, MD, author of *DHEA: A Practical Guide*, agrees.

Dr. Sahelian has become aware of people who used 25-50 mg of DHEA a day who developed cardiac arrhythmias. One person had been previously very healthy. After taking 50 mg of DHEA a day, he had to be hospitalized for tachycardia. Another person, a woman, had heart palpitations the first day she took 50 mg. Low doses of DHEA taken under medical supervision seems to be the safest way of improving your health without harming it.

Black cohosh, an herb found in Remifemin (a natural formula found in health food stores) or HMC hesperidin (a bioflavonoid), also help eliminate hot flashes without any negative side effects.

Pregnenolone: Food for Thought

A second hormone that has recently appeared for purchase over-the-counter is pregnenolone. It is a key brain hormone, credited with memory enhancement and concentration improvement, as well as being a fighter of mental fatigue and reliever of arthritis. In the opinion of many experts, pregnenolone is the most potent memory enhancer available.

The body uses cholesterol to make pregnenolone (as well as other steroid hormones including DHEA, testosterone, and estrogen). It is possible that high cholesterol in some older persons is the result of the body not converting this cholesterol into steroid hormones, as it did during younger years.

In addition, pregnenolone is the first hormone the body makes from cholesterol in what is known as the "steroid pathway." Excess pregnenolone is converted into DHEA, from which estrogen and testosterone are then made.

Human studies have confirmed pregnenolone's ability to improve mental functioning. Additional research also suggests that this is the result of increasing testosterone levels in men (who show improved ability to perform visual spatial tasks), and estrogen levels in women (who show improvement in verbal recall), rather than a simple across-the-board increase in pregnenolone. Instead, pregnenolone is broken down and used differently by men and women.

Another promising use of pregnenolone is to treat depression. A study from the National Institutes of Mental Health found that people with clinical depression have subnormal levels of pregnenolone. Hormone expert Dr. Regelson, is highly optimistic about pregnenolone's potential to treat age-related depression and advocates its use to treat mild cases, before higher-risk drugs such as Prozac are considered.

Finally, half a century ago, pregnenolone was successfully used to treat rheumatoid arthritis, with patients reporting feeling less pain, fatigue, and more strength. Since it is a naturally occurring substance, however, pregnenolone cannot be patented and therefore held little profit potential as a treatment. When synthetic cortisone was discovered in the late 1940s, it became the drug industry's preferred answer to arthritis suffering. It was patentable, offered much greater profit potential, and the devastating side effects (including immune system suppression and excess bone loss) wouldn't be discovered until many years later, after cortisone use was well-established in the medical community as a first-line treatment for arthritis.

Theoretically, it is reasonable to think that pregnenolone may be the only supplement anyone would need. This is not the case, however, because enzymes and other substances are needed to convert pregnenolone into other hormones. In short, there are many fine points to take into consideration. In some cases, pregnenolone and DHEA supplementation alone can achieve desired results. Different bodies respond differently. It is always prudent, in any event, to have your doctor check pregnenolone and other hormone levels before, as well as after, you start taking any supplements. This will alert you to any adjustments that may be in order, as the course of your therapy progresses. According to Dr. Regelson, the usual dose for pregnenolone is 50 mg daily taken in the morning. Modest improvements in mental function are often evident within hours of taking pregnenolone. For arthritis pain, improvement is usually seen within a few weeks.

The Strong and Sexy Hormone, Testosterone

Although testosterone is considered a male hormone, women's bodies produce and use testosterone, too. Women who have had their ovaries removed are often testosterone deficient. And a deficiency can occur even when the ovaries are still intact. In the event of a true deficiency (documented through testing), natural (not methyl) testosterone supplements to correct the deficiency can help protect against heart disease and other problems associated with a lack of testosterone. The risk is believed to be minimal. Testosterone creams and gels are also available and some women and their doctors prefer these. For best results, also get total and HDL cholesterol levels checked regularly, since too much testosterone can adversely affect these levels.

In addition to boosting your libido, testosterone can also be used to treat depression, increase energy, and strengthen muscle and bone tissue, and even relieve menopause symptoms. While higher testosterone levels are traditionally associated with greater aggressiveness, this isn't necessarily bad: Women with higher testosterone levels tend to be higher achievers.

An interesting study by Dr. Barbara Sherwin of McGill University in Montreal found that premenopausal women who had undergone hysterectomies, fared better receiving a combination estrogen and testosterone supplements, than those supplemented only with estrogen. Other studies have found that the estrogen/testosterone combination is more effective than estrogen alone against osteoporosis.

Another Important Energizer: Thyroid

Too cold in the winter and too hot in the summer. Fatigue, in spite of plenty of sleep. Low energy, slow metabolism, constipation, and difficulty losing weight. Fertility, miscarriage, menstrual and menopause problems. Forgetfulness and depression. Hair loss and brittle nails. Susceptibility to colds and frequent infections. High cholesterol. And little interest in sex.

These are some of the many signs of hypothyroidism, or failure to produce enough thyroid hormone. Actual symptoms may vary. But because the symptoms are commonly experienced with other conditions, many doctors miss diagnosing hypothyroidism. It is frequently passed on genetically, so if your mother had thyroid problems there's a good chance you will, too. Ultimately, it can leave you feeling and looking like you're continually stuck in low gear, barely able to muster the energy to get through an easy day.

As we age, increasingly less thyroid hormone is produced. And by age 60, 17 percent of women and nine percent of men have signs of low thyroid function. Many more simply have vague symptoms that doctors generally attribute to normal aging. And many cases of hypothyroidism go untreated because conventional blood tests used for diagnosis are inadequate. Antibodies and other factors can result in an error rate of as high as 40 percent. Therefore, even if blood tests have shown that your thyroid function is normal for your age, if you have symptoms, you may still benefit from further investigating the matter.

Building on the fact that low thyroid function and low body temperature go hand-in-hand, Broda Barnes, MD, developed the Basal Temperature Test for measuring thyroid function. It is performed by shaking down a thermometer and leaving it on your nightstand before going to bed. The next morning, immediately upon waking (and even before going to the bathroom), put the thermometer securely in your armpit for 10 minutes. It is critical not to engage in any other activity or movement that will raise your body temperature and result in an elevated reading. This test should be repeated for 7 to 10 consecutive mornings, when you're not menstruating and don't have a cold or infection. Then figure your average. The normal range for the underarm temperature is 98.2 to 97.8. A reading of 97.4 or lower, according to this test, is a sign of thyroid dysfunction. Persons with borderline readings may also benefit from treatment. The bottom line is how you feel before and after adequate treatment.

Researchers from Johns Hopkins University, writing in the *Journal of the American Medical Association* (July 24, 1996) recommend routine thyroid testing starting at age 35. Over the years, even minor changes can alert you well in advance to serious potential trouble. From a preventive care point of view, this enables you to take corrective action sooner rather than later when treatment may be more difficult. Here's why thyroid function is so important.

Thyroid deficiency signals immune deficiency. In his book *Solved: The Riddle of Illness*, Stephen E. Langer, MD writes, "Subnormal body temperature and too little thyroid hormone can reduce the strength and resistance of every cell, including the billions involved in the immune system. One of the most common results of hypothyroidism which I see daily in my office is recurrent colds, throat and nose infections, and other respiratory ailments."

In older persons, of course, a simple chest cold can easily develop into fatal pneumonia. So, as we grow older and thyroid activity declines, we need to be extra vigilant about supporting optimal thyroid function to help maintain strong overall immune resistance. This is because the thyroid gland stimulates lymphocytes, the cells that attack viruses, bacteria, fungal, and other foreign invaders that threaten us.

An Energy Catalyst

One of the most common complaints of sufferers of low thyroid activity is fatigue. This is because T3 and T4 are vital to our body's ability to produce energy. Each cell in the body contains mitochondria. They function as the body's furnaces by burning oxygen to produce a type of fuel or energy called adenosine triphosphate (or ATP). And it is T3 and T4 that fire up the mitochondria to burn oxygen.

When less thyroid hormone is available, our bodies burn up less oxygen. Leftover oxygen can then form free radicals, which can ultimately contribute to the development of cancer, heart disease, diabetes, Parkinson's, cataracts, arthritis, and other serious disorders. High doses of antioxidant vitamins such as A, C, and E, help "mop up" these free radicals, and thus minimize their damage. But optimal thyroid function helps minimize the creation of free radicals in the first place.

Just as our bodies need energy for optimal performance, so do our brains. This is why hypothyroidism can also result in mental sluggishness. Doctors frequently dismiss the resulting lack of alertness and even confusion as a normal part of aging. Often, however, it is related to thyroid function. Some experts even believe that depression in seniors and the elderly is often the result of an under-active thyroid. Certainly the difficulty and challenge of functioning with insufficient energy, day in and day out and in spite of our best efforts, is discouraging at best and can easily lead to the general lack of interest that frequently characterizes depression.

But there is a biochemical connection as well. The thyroid hormone T3 also interacts with neurotransmitters in the brain to affect mood and emotion. According to Gillian Ford, author of *Listening to Your Hormones*, thyroid hormone supplements may be the most appropriate first line of treatment for women with hormone-related depression. She also reports that a number of physicians she knows use low-dose thyroid to treat PMS.

Rev Up Your Thyroid ... And Your Life

The first step toward revving up your thyroid is an optimal diet. Such a diet will include adequate amounts of vitamins A, C, E, B vitamins, the trace elements zinc and copper, and essential fatty acids like flax seed oil or borage oil (1 to 2 teaspoons, or 2 capsules, 2 times a day may be sufficient). These are so critical to thyroid function that many doctors prescribe them, along with natural or desiccated thyroid, for their hypothyroid patients. If your thyroid function is borderline low, say 97.5 or 97.6, dietary improvements and nutritional supplements may quickly bump thyroid function back up into the normal range.

A supportive diet includes emphasis on foods that are high in iodine such as fish, kelp, vegetables and root vegetables (such as potatoes), and foods that are high in B vitamins (including whole grains, raw nuts and seeds, dark green and yellow vegetables).

Some foods slow thyroid function and should be reduced, including cabbage, brussels sprouts, mustard greens, broccoli, cauliflower, turnips, kale, spinach, peaches, and pears. Sulfa drugs and antihistamines should also be avoided. In other parts of the world, hypothyroidism is commonly the result of iodine deficiency. This is rare in the U.S. since iodine is added to most table salt. Still, if you have a very low salt diet, increasing salt intake might provided you with needed iodine.

Other Self-Help: Moderate aerobic exercise, as well as qigong and yoga, will also stimulate metabolism, body temperature and in turn, thyroid function. Some cases, especially milder ones, can be remedied with herbal bitters. Look for Swedish bitters to take before each meal, or standardized capsules or extracts of gentian and/or mugwort and take according to label instructions. Hot and cold water therapy is another option. Rotate ice and hot water packs directly over the thyroid gland, and if you can take it, consider a hot-cold shower rotation with water directed at the thyroid (the change in shower water temperature can stimulate overall body circulation and metabolism as well.) Fasting may stimulate thyroid function. The homeopathic remedy calcarea carbonica (calcium carbonate) at the 1M strength can boost thyroid function. Finally, many alternative practitioners recommend tyrosine amino acid supplements and animal glandulars, such as thymus, which contains low doses of thyroid hormone. Most herbal and other remedies mentioned here can be purchased over-the-counter at well-stocked natural pharmacies and foods stores. If this list sounds overwhelming, try the options that you feel most comfortable with.

Professional Care Can Be Very Worthwhile

For more stubborn cases that don't respond to self-care, or if you'd rather skip developing your own self-care regimen, professional care may be more appropriate. With the increasing popularity of alternative practitioners, there's a wide range of treatment courses to pursue. For hypothyroidism, consider traditional Chinese medicine (including acupuncture), an osteopath, naturopath, or homeopath. These doctors can give you extra help in treating parasite-related thyroid dysfunctions. Doctors specializing in environmental medicine report success in treating allergy-related underactive thyroid. To find a doctor of any of these disciplines in your area, call the American Holistic Health Association at 714-779-6152.

Doctors usually treat hypothyroidism with thyroid hormone supplements. Several types are available, and finding the one that works best for you should be your top priority. Doctors with more wholistic treatment approaches usually prefer natural or desiccated thyroid, made from animal sources. These contain the full range of thyroid hormones that humans produce, including calcitonin.

Synthetic thyroid medications include Synthroid, which contains only T4, and Cytomel, which contains only T3. Some doctors prefer these preparations because dosage strength is more reliable. Also, Synthroid very closely resembles human T4, but takes around five to six weeks to reach peak effectiveness. Therefore, finding the right dosage can take a while. The results of taking animal thyroid, on the other hand, can be felt almost immediately. A final consideration is that, for our bodies to make use of Synthroid or T4, our bodies must break it down into T3. If the necessary enzyme, 5-deiodinase, is lacking, Synthroid will be ineffective and Cytomel or T3 may be the better choice.

Regardless of which type of thyroid medication taken, your doctor will want to carefully monitor you to make sure your dosage is right. This is very important. Too much thyroid can cause a condition known as "thyroid storm." In the most severe cases, the resulting rapid heart rate can bring on a heart attack. Other symptoms of adverse reactions to thyroid medication include changes in appetite, diarrhea, fever, headache, irritability, nausea, nervousness, sleeplessness, sweating, and weight loss. These and any other symptoms should be reported to your doctor immediately. Long-term use of too much thyroid can result in osteoporosis by increasing osteoclast activity.

Hypothyroidism also frequently co-exists with other hormonal problems such as estrogen, progesterone, and adrenal insufficiency, according to Pat Puglio of the Broda Barnes Foundation. Therefore, if thyroid treatment doesn't produce satisfactory results, don't give up. Instead, look at other hormone levels.

If a self-care or doctor-supervised course of treatment for hypothyroidism is working for you, you will know it because the results can be truly dramatic. Within weeks, most people with an underactive thyroid will experience a renewed sense of energy and vitality, along with an overall improvement in their general health and sense of well-being.

The Fountain of Youth May Flow
With Human Growth Hormone

When other hormone supplement regimens aren't enough, many enthusiasts claim it's time to try human growth hormone. It is by far the most controversial, perhaps the least understood, and definitely the most expensive — somewhere in the market of $9,000 to $12,000 a year — although this could soon change. It does boast capabilities that other key hormones don't, including the ability to revive a dying heart and stave off kidney failure.* It also holds promise for persons experiencing wasting syndrome, which is often seen in elderly convalescent home populations and persons with AIDS. While much remains to be understood about growth hormone, scientists do know that growth hormone stimulates production of another hormone called insulin-like growth factor (IGF-1). This is what makes growth hormone a particularly promising therapy for life-threatening, late-stage diabetes.

Currently, substances called Growth Hormone Releasing Agents are in development and may soon be available to offer the benefits of growth hormone without the side effects. Drug-maker Merck is developing an agent for treating immune problems and the diseases that accompany them, such as cancer. Release of growth hormone can also be stimulated with vigorous exercise, and estrogen supplements for women and testosterone supplements for men.

As the name implies, human growth hormone is what makes children grow. It is produced by the pituitary gland throughout our lives, but like other hormones, the level declines with age. In adults, growth hormone has a rejuvenating effect. A 1990 study reported in the *New England Journal of Medicine* that men taking growth hormone just 6 months experienced the equivalent of reversing 10 to 20 years of aging, with significant increases in muscle and bone mass accompanied with a 15 percent reduction in body fat.

According to Dr. Edward Chein of the Palm Springs Life Extension Institute in California, "Only growth hormone can actually reverse

---

* Research on growth hormone therapy to treat kidney failure is being conducted by Dr. Aengtake Bengtsson, at the Research Center for Endocrinology and Metabolism at Sahlgranska University Hospital in Sweden. To date, he says the therapy has produced excellent results.

biological aging. Lung capacity improves, body fat decreases, muscle mass increases, cardiac function improves, kidney function improves, bone density increases, fingernails and toenails grow faster, the skin is more resilient, the immune system improves — antibody production goes up, natural killer cell activity is restored."

Another MD, Dr. Sam Baxas, founder of the Swiss Rejuvenation Centre in Basel, Switzerland, and who also has extensive experience treating patients with growth hormone, says this: "Growth hormone brings you back to a youthful state in which the organs are returned to ... the size they were at age 25 or 30. Nothing else can do this."

As glowing as these reports may sound, there are also reports of severe side effects — so much so that studies have fairly high dropout rates because many cannot tolerate growth hormone. Known adverse effects include carpal tunnel syndrome, diabetes, and severe fluid retention. Many doctors continue to defend growth hormone, though, explaining that these adverse effects are the result of improper dosage. There is probably some validity to this since studies usually give the same dose to everyone across the board. In hormone therapy, however, individualized dosage, based on test results, is of utmost importance. This is definitely an area where one size does not fit all.

Resetting Your Biological Clock With Melatonin

While melatonin appears to be best known as a sleep aid, top researchers claim it does much more. Dr. William Regelson writes in *The Melatonin Miracle* that there is only one hormone "that can actually reverse aging by resetting the body's aging clock ... melatonin."

A few years ago, melatonin's potential as an age reverser caught public attention by storm with the release of the above book in which co-author Dr. Walter Pierpaoli's mice studies were reported. These studies showed that when pineal glands (which secretes melatonin) of young and old mice were surgically switched, the young mice quickly grew old, while the old mice were restored to youthfulness.

The pineal gland, you may recall, regulates many important body systems, including the endocrine (hormone) system, which controls maturation. This includes the high rate of growth during childhood, the onset of puberty, menarche, menopause, and beyond.

To prove that extra melatonin was responsible for the above old mice growing youthful, Dr. Pierpaoli conducted another series of experiments in which the nightly drinking water of 19-month-old mice (the human equivalent of 65 years) was spiked with melatonin. Within five months, the control group of mice that wasn't receiving melatonin showed the expected signs of advanced age including bald spots on their coats, cataracts, and weak, toneless muscles. The melatonin mice, however, looked and behaved like teenagers in perfect health, and lived an average of 30 percent longer — to the human equivalent of 105 years.

Further study revealed that the melatonin mice had stronger immune systems, with more disease fighting cells. They also had more youthful levels of thyroid hormone. Thymus glands that had shriveled with age, grew back, complete with a greater number of high-functioning T cells; stronger antibody responses; higher disease resistance; and greater resistance to the debilitating effects of stress including mitigation of the stress hormone cortisteroids. One group of mice, which was genetically prone to developing cancer, remained cancer-free. Finally, the latter years of the melatonin mice were not unproductive. They were healthy and vigorous years.

Studies into melatonin's cancer-fighting ability have also produced promising results. It has been shown to interfere with breast cancer development in both test tube cultures and animals. And at the San Gerardo Hospital in Monza, Italy, Dr. Paoli Lissoni has been combining high-dose melatonin therapy and conventional chemotherapy together. In colon cancer patients, he has increased short-term survival threefold. Melatonin also appears to significantly reduce the side effects of chemotherapy.

Initial investigations into melatonin's ability to fight heart disease are also encouraging. These include the benefits of lowering cholesterol, high blood pressure, and the incidence of clot formation.

Finally, for sleep problems, melatonin may be the best solution available today for jet lag, insomnia, and unrestful sleep. The usual dose is 0.5 to 5.0 mg. taken 30 minutes before bedtime. In general, take the lowest dose possible to achieve the desired results. And the younger you are, the less you should require. Unlike many sleeping pills, melatonin doesn't produce grogginess the next day, is not habit forming, and actually restores normal sleep cycles.

Taking Melatonin: For age reversal, Dr. Regelson recommends the following doses of melatonin taken at bedtime: age 40 to 45, 0.5 to 1.0

mg.; age 45 to 55, 1 to 2 mg.; age 55 to 65, 2 to 2.5 mg.; age 65 to 75, 2.5 to 3 mg.; age 75 and over, 3.5 to 5 mg. These dosages are based on human equivalents used in mice studies. Time-release formulas are preferable since they more closely mimic the body's natural melatonin release that occurs throughout the night.

What Every Woman Must Know About Estrogen Replacement Therapy

"Menopause is not a disease," says medical anthropologist Margaret Lock in a 1991 article in the *Lancet*, the esteemed weekly British medical journal, "but a life-cycle transition to which powerful symbolic meanings, individual and social, are attached."

That's not what most medical doctors believe, however. And their beliefs are making thousands of sane menopausal women crazy with confusion.

Chances are your doctor looks at menopause as an estrogen deficiency disease. This disease concept originated in 1966 in a book, *Feminine Forever*, written by Robert A. Wilson, MD His theory — and that's all it was — is now accepted as fact by many medical doctors. This is understandable, although unfortunate for women, because doctors are trained to treat diseases with drugs and hormones, not to look at natural life transitions and offer drug-free solutions to uncomfortable menopausal symptoms.

Since the majority of women live long enough to go through menopause, doctors have a ready market of hundreds of thousands of women every year who are potential patients. Pharmaceutical companies have lined up with hormones, antidepressants, and other medications to help solve your menopausal "problems," like hot flashes, osteoporosis, and heart attacks.

What if you didn't need these drugs and hormones? The majority of women, after all, report little if any menopausal discomfort. And what if most of the discomfort could be addressed through dietary and lifestyle changes? Well, you can be sure the drug companies wouldn't want you to find out. But, fortunately, you can.

This is a big relief for the many women who cannot or decide not to use estrogen replacement therapy (ERT). All medications have side effects, and some women are simply not candidates for this approach. We're not saying that ERT is bad for everyone. But we disagree with the medical model that says drug intervention is necessary to prevent unwanted health and beauty changes. And we are not satisfied that it's as safe as some people say.

Menopause and Society

Germaine Greer's book, *The Change*, mentions a study on the effect of estrogen replacement on a woman's personality. According to the study, estrogen keeps us less outwardly aggressive, but more inwardly hostile. This may be good for motherhood, but it stifles our outward creativity and our ability to be more assertive. Estrogen replacement therapy may be greatly responsible for the high-level female bonding among older women we're seeing in our society today, says Cheri Quincy, D.O. (Doctor of Osteopathy).

But those women who don't take ERT may be much more likely to use their *increased individual power* to get out in the world and accomplish things they had put off while raising families.

Dr. Quincy also notes that "Economic power in old age is one of the most important predictors of both longevity and health. The retirement plan, the golden parachute, the vested annuity; these are rewards for those who work outside the home." With the hormone shifts of menopause comes the opportunity for a woman to enter parts of society she may have avoided by necessity when higher estrogen levels and the circumstances they created gently nudged her into nesting with family and close friends.

Dr. Susan Love promotes the idea of menopause mirroring puberty: Like puberty, menopause is a transition into a new hormonal state.

Anthropologist Margaret Mead coined the term "post-menopausal zest" to describe the leading characteristic that provides us direction and meaning as we make the symbolic transition from mating-and-mothering mode to matriarch.

Forever Young

To avoid this transition and help keep us "feminine (as defined by our reproductive years) forever," there is a wide selection of estrogen replacement therapy (ERT) products available to us. They are taken to supplement and thus counteract the body's natural decline of estrogen and progesterone production that takes place at menopause. Let's take a good look at these estrogen supplements.

Traditional ERT (Estrogens and progestogens — synthetic progesterone): Most hormones currently on the market are synthetic. In the case of Premarin, the most widely studied and prescribed estrogen supplement for women, it is made of horse estrogen, not human estrogen. One of the most important things every woman needs to know about these hormones is that they are not exactly identical to any form of estrogen or progesterone normally found in the human female body.

This also means that the term estrogen replacement therapy, (when applied to these hormones), is a misnomer. When these hormones are taken, your hormones are not being replaced. Instead, a more accurate way to describe ERT would be to call it similar estrogen supplementation. In essence, the synthetic hormones used in ERT mimic your hormones. But they don't always do a satisfactory job. And they certainly aren't the real thing.

If synthetic hormones were identical to naturally occurring hormones (those found in your body), their marketing potential would be too poor to interest drug manufacturers. Since the synthetic hormones are all slightly different than the real thing, however, they are patented. This gives the manufacturer exclusive rights to sell a particular synthetic hormone — at very impressive prices.

This makes synthetic estrogen pills a near-perfect product for pharmaceutical companies: You don't have to be sick to take them. Instead, every woman is a potential customer from the time her menopause begins. And you can take these pills for as long as you like! The longer you take them, the more money the manufacturer makes. And if you stop taking them, you have menopause symptoms. In short, millions

---

☞ TIP ☜

If you decide to take estrogen supplements, di-estrogen (estriol and estradiol) or estriol alone might be the safest way to go. Limited studies suggest that estrone (found in tri-estrogen) increases breast cancer risk. On the other hand, other limited studies suggest that estriol may be anticarcinogenic. In one study of women with breast cancer, 37 percent saw their cancers reverse or stop growing when they took estriol supplements.

of healthy women taking synthetic hormones every day adds up to one of the highest profit potentials of any drug ever approved for the U.S. market.

Drug companies are keenly aware of this and their marketing efforts reflect this fact. Consider *Seasons* magazine, which is published by Wyeth-Ayerst — America's largest estrogen supplement manufacturer. This magazine is not available by subscription. Instead, it is available only to women who have prescriptions to Premarin (Wyeth-Ayerst's estrogen supplements). All it takes is one quick examination of this magazine, however, and it's easy to see that this magazine is an expensive propaganda tool — designed to brainwash women into taking Premarin indefinitely.

Seasons magazine even misleads women about what exactly Premarin is made of. It states that Premarin is made of "natural substances." This is technically true. Premarin is horse estrogen from real horses. But, *Seasons* magazine and other promotional literature conveniently omit the fact that the main natural substances are extracted from the urine of pregnant mares. In fact, the name Premarin is derived from the phrase "PREgnant MARe urINe" and was probably approved for use by top marketing executives because it sounded pleasant. They knew that if they gave it a more truthful name, such as horse-pee-in-a-pill, they would quickly lose the interest of millions of potential lifetime customers.

If this weren't bad enough, there's more. To collect the urine, horses are impregnated, fitted with a rubber device, and made to stand for most of their pregnancies, so the urine can be collected. Places where this happens are called pee farms. As you can imagine, animal rights activists are very upset about the goings-on at these places.

Around here, though, we are more concerned about what these hormones do to women's bodies. Numerous studies have linked them to breast cancer. One large study that appeared in the *New England Journal of Medicine* (mid-June 1995) found that women aged 60 to 64 who had taken estrogen five years or more had a 71 percent higher breast cancer risk than those who didn't take estrogen. Taking progestin boosted risk even higher.

Other health problems for which studies suggest traditional ERT increases risk include asthma, lupus, endometrial cancer, ovarian cancer, brain cancer, depression, rheumatoid arthritis, and heart disease. Some of these will be discussed more, later in this book.

Names of Synthetic Female Hormones

Synthetic Estrogens Pills: Estrace, estratab, Ogen, Estinly, Estrovis
Synthetic Estrogen Creams: Premain, Estrace, Ogen, Ortho Dienestrol
Synthetic Progestogens (man-made versions of progesterone): Provera, Curretab, Cyrin, Amen, Aygestin, Norlutate, Norlutin, Megace, Oveerette, Micronor, Nor-Q.D.

Note: New hormone products continue to be approved for marketing. To be absolutely sure about what an unlisted hormone is made of, ask your doctor or pharmacist.

Compounded Estrogens

Compound estrogens are forms of estrogen that are chemically identical to the real thing found in the body. They include:

tri-estrogen — contains three forms of estrogen: estrone, estriol, and estradiol.

di-estrogen — contains two forms of estrogen that have not been linked to breast cancer — estriol and estradiol.

Like synthetic estrogens and progestogens, compounded estrogens are available by prescription only. Are they safe? It's impossible to say because of a lack of research.

Natural Progesterone

The type of progesterone that's traditionally been used most often by doctors in the past is called progestogen. It is synthetic (or man-made) progesterone. Provera is a brand of progestogen. Progestogens act just like progesterone with one exception: They are absorbed well orally, while progesterone itself is not absorbed well in the intestines. Progestogens have numerous side effects, including abnormal bleeding, weight gain, nausea, insomnia and depression, and increased breast cancer risk to mention a few.

Natural progesterone, made from plant sources, including wild yam (different from our cultivated varieties), appears to be well absorbed orally and through the skin. However, several doctors we have spoken to do not believe wild yam extracts are effective in raising progesterone levels or in eliminating menopausal symptoms. We think natural progesterone has fewer side effects than synthetic progestogens, but we don't know. There aren't any long-term, double-blind studies — even with the synthetic hormone.

The best study on natural progesterone was done by Dr. John R. Lee, a physician in Northern California who became interested in its possibilities in the early 1980's. His are the only long-term studies, and they are observational, not scientifically designed double-blind studies. Dr. Lee observed a reduction in osteoporosis with only occasional side effects (slight vaginal bleeding and one case of uterine cancer) in a few women.

Out of at least 20 natural progesterone creams, only eight contain more than 400 mg of progesterone. Some are fortified with USP grade natural progesterone, which is not extracted from wild yam as many think, but instead is taken primarily from soybeans. We are disturbed and concerned that these companies have not funded independent studies to prove the long-term safety and efficacy of natural progesterone (from wild yam as well as other sources). Instead, they're sitting back and watching women jump on the natural progesterone bandwagon without sufficient scientific data to justify the trend.

Natural Progesterone — Safe or Not?

We wish we had the answer about the safety of natural progesterone, but no one does, not even expert advocates like Dr. John Lee. Why? Because there have been no studies showing short or long-term negative effects, even though synthetic progesterone is known to be potentially cancer-causing — linked to breast cancer. An absence of studies on natural progesterone may not be enough to make you re-evaluate using the more natural product, but a recent article in the *Archives of Pathological Laboratory Medicine* (vol 120, 1996) raises some important questions.

Some forms of breast cancer are estrogen receptor-positive, some are progesterone receptor-positive. This means these are receptor cells in breast tissue that can cause tumors to grow. They are receptive to either estrogen or progesterone.

This published study showed that among 300 women with breast cancer, women who were estrogen receptor-negative, but progesterone receptor-positive, they were more likely to have other incidents of breast cancer or cancer-related deaths. This means that progesterone, not estrogen, was the contributing culprit.

The authors of this study were very concerned that so many health care providers are suggesting that women use natural progesterone without studies showing its safety. Indeed, natural progesterone might be safe. It also may not be. When the maker of Progest, one of the more popular natural progesterone creams, recently called here to promote their products, we requested it provide us safety data about Progest. We're still waiting. And if it comes through, we'll be pleasantly surprised.

In the meantime, remember that progesterone (natural or synthetic) is a hormone. All hormone therapies should be carefully monitored by a doctor who uses them cautiously in the lowest possible doses. We have heard numerous reports from doctors and patients attributing weight gain, depression, and other problems to the use of natural progesterone.

However, we *believe* natural progesterone may be an effective product in some cases. We don't think it causes serious side effects, but no one

Potency of Commercial Progesterone Creams

More than 400 mg. Progesterone/oz. cream: Pro-Gest (Prof. & Tech. Services, Inc.), Bio Balance (Elan Vitale), Progonol and Ostraderm (both from Bezwecken), Pro-Alo (Healthwatchers Systems), Phytogest (Karuna Corporation), NatraGest (Broadmoore Labs, Inc.), Happy PMS (HM Enterprises), Equilibrium (Equilibrium Lab), Pro-G (TriMedica), ProBalance (Springboard)

Between 2 and 15 mg progesterone/oz. cream: Gin Yam (Bezwecken), Pro-Dermex (Gero Vita Int'l.), Endocreme (Wuliton Labs), Life Changes (MW Labs), Progestone-Plus (Prof. Health Products), Novagest (Strata Dermatologics)

Less than 2 mg progesterone or no progesterone/oz. cream: Yamcon (Phillips Nutritionals), Born Again (Phytopharmica), PMS Formula (PMS Relief, Inc.), Menopause Form (PMS Releif, Inc.), Femarone (Wise Essen. Inc.), Nutri-Gest (NutrSupplies, Inc.), Progerone (Natures Nutr., Inc.), Wild Yam Cream (Alvin Last, Inc.), Progesterone-HP (Dixie Health, Inc.), Woman Wise (Jason Natural Cosmetics)

* prepared by Aeron LifeCycles, November 1995

really knows. Just because a product is natural doesn't necessarily mean it's safe. Some physicians claim natural progesterone does not raise blood hormone levels, but still relieves menopausal symptoms. Others have seen side effects or no effectiveness with their patients.

If you do decide to try any form of ERT, with or without progesterone, we suggest you do the following: Have a base-line bone density test to know what's going on inside your bones. While bone density isn't everything (bone fragility may count for a lot more), it's all we can measure. Next, have your hormone levels tested either by blood or saliva tests. Many complementary physicians prefer saliva tests as being more accurate. One lab that does saliva tests is Aeron Life Cycles at 800-631-7900. Consult your health care practitioner and discuss the amount and type of natural progesterone or other hormones for you to try. Keep a record of any health changes, positive or negative. Be monitored periodically to assess its effectiveness. Remember that any hormone you take, either natural or synthetic, constitutes hormone replacement therapy. Use it cautiously and judiciously.

Myths About Postmenopausal Health

If you listen to the media and look at advertisements for calcium supplements, you may believe that you're destined to be a bent-over old woman with a wrinkled face and fragile bones unless you take a lot of calcium and hormones. This is not necessarily true. There are, in fact, a number of myths surrounding how you will look and feel after menopause with or without ERT. The first myth is one on which other myths are built. It contends that menopause is an estrogen-deficiency disease.

Anthropologist Margaret Lock disagrees. She points out that people have lived into old age for thousands of years. The idea that modern women are living longer lives and for that reason alone require estrogen replacement is simply invalid. She also says, "Most women do not seek help at menopause, and this part of the life cycle is not subject to medical attention to the same extent as childbirth."

Susan E. Brown of the National Women's Health Network supports Margaret Lock's position. She states that "blaming osteoporosis on an estrogen deficiency is just a little less absurd than blaming heart attacks on a deficiency of bypass surgery. Surgery might solve the problem for a while, but it is not a deficiency of the operation that caused the problem."

Calcium and Bones Loss

Another prevalent myth is that postmenopausal women need high amounts of calcium to prevent bone loss — about 1,500 mg/day. Yet a 1985 study by Gordan and Genant, which has been duplicated many times, showed that 1,500 mg of daily oral calcium supplement has no preventive effect on bone loss. We can think of several reasons why a lot of calcium doesn't prevent osteoporosis. One is that calcium is poorly absorbed unless you have sufficient acid in your stomach, and post-menopausal women often have lowered concentrations of hydrochloric acid.

Many people think that because vitamin C is made from an acid (ascorbic), it should help calcium be absorbed. But an alarming study published just last year in the *Journal of Epidemiology* showed that women who took large amounts of both calcium and vitamin C — what looks like a winning bone-strengthening combination — had a higher incidence of hip fracture than women who took only one of these supplements.

We've said it before and we'll say it until every woman who's interested hears it: just because you take calcium or eat calcium-rich foods doesn't mean this mineral gets into your bones. This is a myth perpetrated by vested interest groups who sell calcium supplements and dairy products.

Research gynecologist and endocrinologist Guy E. Abraham, MD conducted a prospective study with Dr. Harinder Grewal that was published in the *Journal of Reproductive Medicine* in 1990. This small, double-blind study showed that postmenopausal women who took more magnesium than calcium had an average increase in bone density of 11 percent after just one year. These women took only 500 mg of calcium and from 600 to 1,000 mg of magnesium. A higher magnesium intake seems to be correlated with increased bone density.

This isn't news. It was discussed in 1988 in an article in *Bone Mineral* written by Rosalind Angus. She found that there was no significant correlation between calcium intake and bone mass. Instead, iron, zinc, and magnesium intake were indicators of stronger bones. Add boron to that list, based on studies by Forrest H. Nielsen, and you'll better understand why vegetarians have a lower risk for osteoporosis than meat eaters. Boron, like magnesium, is high in plant material and low in animal products.

ERT and Heart Disease

Another myth surrounding menopause is that estrogen replacement is necessary to prevent heart disease. It's true that heart disease is the number one killer of postmenopausal women. But it's also true that unabsorbed calcium — from high-calcium diets and supplements — can collect in the arteries and become atherosclerosis (build-up in, and blockage of, the arteries). It's also true that numerous dietary and exercise factors contribute to a higher or lower risk for heart disease. If you don't want to take ERT, you need to exercise regularly and eat well.

Most physicians believe that ERT reduces a woman's heart disease risk. Yet, to date, studies that support this idea have neglected to take into account the fact that women who take estrogen also tend to eat healthier foods, get more exercise, and, in general, usually take better care of themselves than other women.

Preliminary results for the first three years of a more equitable study were published in the *Journal of the American Medical Association*. This study is comparing 875 healthy postmenopausal women who are taking either a placebo or one of four estrogen regimens.

The preliminary results are impressive:
1. The women receiving ERT had more favorable cholesterol ratios.
2. Five new cases of heart disease developed among the ERT groups, yet none developed among women in the placebo group.
3. Ten women in the ERT groups developed blood clots, yet none in the placebo group developed blood clots.

Overall, in spite of "better" cholesterol ratios, the ERT group didn't fare any better than their placebo-taking counterparts when it came to heart disease. Instead, the ERT group experienced worse side effects, with a combined total of 15 new cases of blood clots and heart disease — while not a single woman in the placebo group developed either problem.

ERT is neither good nor bad. It's one option. But you shouldn't be frightened into taking it. It should be your choice after looking at both sides. And this includes looking at its benefits.

The Benefits of ERT

Estrogen and progesterone replacement offers relief from temporary menopause symptoms, such as hot flashes and severe mood swings.

Proponents also claim that, in the long run, it helps protect women against osteoporosis, heart disease, and strokes. Estrogen appears to lower the bad cholesterol (LDL) through its antioxidizing actions. Other antioxidants, however, are found naturally in foods. Vitamins A, C, and E, for instance, are found in abundance in fresh fruits, vegetables, and vegetable oils. This gives you a choice of where you get your protective antioxidants.

One more reason doctors suggest women take hormones is to protect brain function. But you may be being brainwashed about taking estrogen replacement therapy (ERT) to lower your risk for memory loss and Alzheimer's. Yes, studies are showing that ERT may protect your brain. But are these good studies? We think not. For one, vested interests can heavily influence results of scientific studies by omitting or adding data that throws off the results.

For example, one large study conducted by Annlia Paganini-Hill at Leisure World in Southern California linked ERT to a lower risk for dementia. The study was funded in part by Wyeth-Ayerst, the pharmaceutical company that makes Premarin. And Premarin is the most widely used form of estrogen at Leisure World, as well as in the United States. Also, the new nine-year Women's Health Initiative study on hormone therapy now in progress is being funded 100 percent by Wyeth-Ayerst. Don't be surprised if the results say ERT prevents dementia.

An article in the National Women's Health Network newsletter, *The Network News*, points out that "the failure to control for socio-economic status (SES) in the conduct of this research is its greatest shortcoming." It has been found that the less money a person has, the higher the incidences of Alzheimer's. We think this is because women with less money are less likely to use hormones due to their expense. So women who were most likely to get any form of dementia are least likely to use hormones. Women on a limited income are also more likely, we believe, to ignore information

---

☞ TIP ☜

"What I'm noticing in my practice is that the women with the most bone loss and those who have already had hip fractures at a fairly young age are women who had undergone total hysterectomies and have been taking Premarin alone for the past 10 to 15 years. These women have never used synthetic or natural progesterone." Alan Gaby, MD.

on the aluminum content of underarm deodorants and the absorption of aluminum from cooking utensils. And, if we were to search further, we would no doubt uncover other associations between possible dementia and low income.

But perhaps most important is for us to realize that Alzheimer's is not a woman's disease. There is no evidence to show that more women get Alzheimer's than men. And there is no conclusive evidence that ERT prevents this disorder. At present, there have not been any long-term studies that show ERT prevents dementia. And the nine-year study currently in progress is funded by a pharmaceutical firm.

The risks associated with ERT often greatly outweigh its benefits for many women. And few benefits exist with short-term use. If you take ERT for menopause symptoms, these will reappear as soon as hormones are stopped. And conventional treatment for osteoporosis and heart disease prevention requires decades of usage. If you plan to use ERT, plan to use it for many years.

ERT Side Effects

As long as you use ERT your estrogen levels will remain high, placing you at an increased risk for breast cancer. Studies on the relationship between ERT and breast cancer show this may be as much as a 30 percent overall increase in risk. The longer you have high estrogen levels, the greater your risk for breast cancer. We don't believe hormone therapy would be made available to men if it increased their risk for prostate cancer by 30 percent. Why is it safe for us?

Nearly 70,000 nurses over a period of 14 years showed an increased risk for lupus, an inflammatory disorder of the connective tissues that occurs mostly in young women. It can attack any organ of the body from the liver to the heart. People with lupus appear to have estrogen metabolism abnormalities. In this nurses' study, the increased risk for lupus coincided with an increased use of estrogen, primarily Premarin. Your risk for lupus may increase proportionally with the length of time you use hormones.

If you take hormones, you may continue to menstruate into your 70s and 80s. And you may increase your risk of blood clots and gallstones. Since blood clots can lead to strokes or heart attacks, you may not be helping your heart with ERT.

Painful uterine fibroid tumors and endometriosis will shrink when your estrogen levels decrease naturally at menopause. But they will continue to grow if you are on ERT. In some cases, this means they will need to be surgically removed.

Breast tenderness, depression, liver problems, blood sugar imbalances, nausea, headaches, fluid retention, and weight gain are all side effects of taking estrogen. In a study of over 36,000 postmenopausal women during a 10-year period, women who used estrogen had a higher incidence of asthma than those who never used it. In fact, side effects are so severe that the ERT compliance rate is quite poor: Approximately 50 percent of those who take it, end up discontinuing it because of unwanted side effects.

ERT is most often given to prevent osteoporosis (brittle, thinning bones that lead to fractured wrists, hips, and legs). Let's look at how bones are made and look at other protective options.

Calcium and Your Bones

You've probably heard that bones are living tissue that are constantly changing. Bones are built by cells called osteoblasts which make new bone tissues, while other cells called osteoclasts break down old bone tissue. This breaking down process is called bone resorption.

Your bones are made out of mineralized collagen fibers, and numerous nutrients are needed for both the collagen formation and its mineralization, which strengthens the collagen. The mineral used in the greatest quantity in building bone is calcium. But calcium can't be absorbed without sufficient hydrochloric acid in your stomach (antacids neutralize this acid, rendering calcium useless), vitamin D, and magnesium (a mineral that helps carry calcium into the bone).

In order to get into your bones, calcium needs vitamins, minerals, and certain hormones. In women, these hormones are estrogen and progesterone. The final factor in building bones is bone-stressing exercise like walking, running, biking, tennis, etc. Swimming is not bone-stressing and, while a good exercise, is not as protective against osteoporosis.

Building Strong Bones Before Your 30s

The best time to build bone density is when you're young. After your mid-20s, it's more difficult to get calcium into your bones. Children and teens build strong bones better than people in their 50s and 60s. But they may also cause excessive calcium to be leached out of their bones if their diets are not good.

Diets high in table salt, sugar, and colas cause calcium excretion in the urine of pre-teen girls. Salt is found in lots of foods popular with children and teens: French fries, popcorn, chips, cheese, and burgers. Low-sodium chips with low-sodium salsa or bean dip, and just going easier with the salt shaker, can go a long way to preserve and build bones in girls and young women.

Are You at High Risk for Osteoporosis?

Michael T. Murray, ND (Naturopathic Doctor), has developed a questionnaire to determine your risk for osteoporosis. If you score higher than 50 points, your risk is high, especially if you have never had any children (this gives the body a break from estrogen production) or had an early or surgical menopause.

We'd like to add to Dr. Murray's questionnaire. First, all soft drinks do not contribute to bone loss, just those with phosphoric acid. In plain English, this means all colas. Non-colas are fine. Phosphorus, which leaches calcium from the bones, is also contained in processed meats. If you rely on lunch meats like salami and bologna, you're upping your phosphorus levels.

The same goes for sugar, if you consume large quantities. This doesn't mean your daily blueberry muffin is contributing to bone loss, but lots of candy, soft drinks, cookies, ice cream, and frozen yogurt every day will.

While a sedentary lifestyle means you're not stressing your bones and keeping them strong, excessive exercise, like training for a marathon or two hours of heavy workouts a day can use up calcium needed by your bones. If you do regular, long, intensive exercising, you need to take a little extra calcium to make up for this.

In addition to steroids and anticonvulsants, antacids contribute to osteoporosis. Both calcium and magnesium (the mineral that helps calcium get into your bones) require acid in order to be absorbed. Antacids neutralize the hydrochloric acid in your stomach, rendering these minerals useless. At this point, calcium can collect in your arteries and become atherosclerosis, or get into your joints and become arthritis. And if you think you're preventing osteoporosis by taking antacids with calcium, think again.

Chronic kidney disease, endocrine problems, and an overactive thyroid can all contribute to a higher risk for osteoporosis. But don't jump to conclusions if you have one or more of these conditions. Check with your physician to see if he or she believes it is severe enough to be considered.

Do not underestimate the effect smoking has on osteoporosis. Women who smoke a pack a day stand to lose two percent of their bone density every 10 years over non-smokers. This means that if you begin smoking in your 20s, by the time you reach menopause (around 50), you've already lost six percent of your bone density compared to someone who hasn't smoked at all with similar risk factors.

Osteoporosis Questionnaire

Choose the item in each category that best describes you, and fill in the point value for that item in the space to the right. You may choose more than one item in categories marked with an asterisk.

	points	score
frame size		
small-boned or petite	10	____
medium frame, very lean	5	____
medium frame, average or heavy build	0	____
large frame, very lean	5	____
ethnic background		
Caucasian	10	____
Asian	10	____
other	0	____

activity level
How often do you walk briskly, jog, engage in aerobics, or perform hard physical labor, of a duration of at least 30 minutes?

seldom	30	____
1 to 2 times weekly	20	____
3 to 4 times weekly	5	____
5 or more times per week	0	____

smoking (cigarettes per day)

smoke 10 or more	20	____
smoke fewer than 10	10	____
quit smoking	5	____
never smoked	0	____

personal health factors*

family history of osteoporosis	20	____
long-term corticosteroid use	20	____
long-term anticonvulsant use	20	____
drink more than 3 glasses of alcohol per week	20	____
drink more than 1 cup of coffee per day	10	____
seldom get outside in the sun	10	____
had ovaries removed	10	____
premature menopause	10	____
had no children	10	____

dietary factors*

consume more than 4 ounces of meat on a daily basis	20	____
drink soft drinks regularly	20	____
consume 3 to 5 servings of vegetables per day	-10	____
consume at least one cup of green leafy vegetables each day	-10	____
take a calcium supplement	-10	____
consume a vegetarian diet	-10	____

total score ____

Lowering Your Risk for Osteoporosis

You've lowered your risk if you happen to be either muscular or overweight. The latter generally means your body is storing extra estrogen, and estrogen stimulates the absorption of calcium in your intestines. Unfortunately, obesity lowers your life expectancy.

If you take estrogen for more than a year after menopause you also have a lower lifetime risk for bone breakage. The problem here is that the added protection that ERT provides wanes away around age 75. Yet the average age for suffering a hip fracture is age 80. In other words, ERT doesn't provide osteoporosis protection when your bones need it the most.

Fortunately, there are better ways to protect your bones.

Estrogen Alternatives for Osteoporosis Prevention

Begin at the beginning: Have good digestion. You need acid to help break down and absorb calcium. Your stomach, when digestion is normal, produces enough hydrochloric acid (HCl) to help utilize calcium. With poor digestion, or if you're taking acid-neutralizing antacids, you may have low production of HCl, or the HCl may be neutralized, and the result is poor calcium absorption. Signs of poor digestion include anemia, lack of appetite for protein, feelings of constant hunger, tiredness, and gas or bloating after eating. To improve digestion eat slowly while sitting down, chew foods well, and drink fewer liquids with meals. Then, if you still think your digestion may need improvement, try taking the digestive enzyme Beano (sold in most food stores) before meals — or talk to your health practitioner about taking HCl supplements.

Increase your magnesium: Several studies, including one from Israel, show that higher magnesium levels increase bone density. Magnesium is high in whole grains and legumes (all beans). Increase your dietary sources of magnesium and consider taking 250 to 1,000 mg of magnesium a day. The side effect from taking too much magnesium is loose stools. Postmenopausal women who are constipated may find they are improving their health in more ways than bone density by increasing their magnesium intake. Dr. Guy E. Abraham, who has published numerous articles on PMS and osteoporosis, believes postmenopausal women should take magnesium to bowel tolerance. That is, however much you need to not be constipated and without creating stools that are uncomfortably loose.

Specific fats protect your bones: Essential fatty acids, like omega-3 fats found in fish oils, protect against osteoporosis. You can take fish oil capsules (one or two, twice daily) or add fatty fish like salmon to your weekly diet. If you are a vegetarian or not a fish lover, essential fatty acids are also found in high amounts in flax seeds (grind 1-3 tablespoons in a coffee grinder and add to your cereal or breakfast drink) and walnuts.

It's soy good for you! The plant estrogen called isoflavonoid found naturally in soybeans is very similar to synthetic phytoestrogens and tamoxifen, chemicals that have been shown to reduce bone loss. Lowered osteoporosis in Japanese women has been attributed to their high consumption of soy products like green soybeans, dried soybeans, miso soup, and tofu. In Europe, a drug containing isoflavonoids is accepted treatment for osteoporosis. In this country, many natural progesterone creams contain progesterone extracted from soybeans.

Increase your consumption of soy products. Try a soy-based protein powder if you make a breakfast drink. Or you can take low-fat tofu (Mori-Nu brand comes in little waxed paper boxes that don't have to be refrigerated until after you open them. And they have some that are one percent Lite rather than 50 percent fat like most tofu). Blend it in your blender and add it to your soups, stews, sauces, and salad dressings. Soy has very little taste. It takes on the flavors that surround it.

Hot Flashes and Your Hypothalamus

If you have uncomfortable periods of menopausal hot flashes, chances are it's because your hypothalamus is having a difficult time adjusting to your new levels of hormones. The hypothalamus is part of your brain and sits above the pituitary gland. It regulates body temperature, sleep patterns, your stress reactions, metabolism, moods, and libido — and it releases pituitary hormones, as well. To work properly, your hypothalamus needs substances called endorphins.

Athletes think of endorphins as "feel good" chemicals, because when you exercise your body produces more of these chemicals that bring a feeling of well-being. They act as natural antidepressants (when you're feeling low, get out and exercise!) and relieve pain. They also allow the hypothalamus to work properly.

Exercise, diet, and certain supplements can help balance the hypothalamus. Or you can use ERT. What if you do nothing? Will mother nature balance your hypothalamus? Of course it will. But why be hot and sweaty longer than necessary? Here are some safe and effective ways to speed regulation of your hypothalamus.

Natural Solutions for Hot Flashes

Fats and sugars increase body heat. So keep your dietary fats low and reduce your sugar intake. Decrease heat-provoking spices like cayenne and other hot peppers. At least temporarily lower the spiciness of the foods you eat one or two notches.

Eat foods high in phytoestrogens (plant estrogens). They help balance your hormones. Fennel root and fennel seed are high in phytoestrogens. So are celery and parsley. Try adding these to a vegetable juice or just increase their use in salads and soups. Soy products eaten on a daily basis have been shown to lower hot flashes in Japanese women. (In fact, menopause is such a non-event in the lives of Japanese women that the word "menopause" doesn't exist in the Japanese language.) Tofu wieners (Smart Dogs are one tasty variety) and soy-based veggie burgers (we love fat-free Boca Burgers — juicy and flavorful and in most frozen food sections of supermarkets) may decrease your hot flashes while their animal-based varieties increase the heat.

Vitamin E and evening primrose oil have both been used to reduce hot flashes. Eight capsules daily of evening primrose oil (take four in the morning, four at night) or 800 IU of a dry or water-soluble vitamin E for best absorption. Reduce your vitamin E to 400 IU after your hot flashes have subsided.

One of our favorite solutions to hot flashes is a flavinoid found in citrus fruits called hesperidin. Hesperidin appears to act directly on the hypothalamus, turning off the "hot" switch in your brain. We have seen a great deal of success with women taking 500 mg of HMC hesperidin (hesperidin methyl chalcone — another flavinoid from citrus) twice a day. Michael T. Murray, ND suggests hesperidin be added to 1,200 mg of vitamin C a day. While vitamin C with bioflavinoids does usually contain hesperidin, the amounts are too small to be effective in this form. Check

---

☞ TIP ☜

Robert Atkins, MD and author of the popular diet books, suggests that women who do use natural progesterone cream apply it to their faces — where it may help reverse some of the effects of aging.

your health food stores for this safe answer to hot flashes. If you have difficulty finding HMC hesperidin, you can also order it by mail from Dr. Fuchs at 707-824-1123. (She keeps a limited supply available for patients and will screen you for free to make sure it's a good choice for you.)

Herbs have also been used to reduce menopausal symptoms including hot flashes: Dong quai (Angelica sinensis), licorice root (Glycyrrhiza glabra), chaste berry (vitex agnus-castus), and black cohosh (Cimicifuga racemosa). In the Orient, where herbs have been used extensively, herbal combinations have been found to be more effective than taking any one of them individually. These four herbs appear to have mild estrogenic effects on the hormone system. Remifemin, an herbal remedy for hot flashes and other menopausal symptoms, contains a standardized amount of black cohosh and has scientific studies to back up its effectiveness. All of these can be found in health food stores.

Vaginal Dryness

As we age, our tissues begin to thin. This includes the vaginal lining, which is called atrophic vaginitis, and is another reason many women take estrogen replacement. However, soybeans will give you the same results. Michael T. Murray, ND, says that one cup of soybeans contains about 300 mg of isoflavone. This is equal to about 0.45 mg of conjugated estrogens or one tablet of Premarin. The difference is that soybeans will not increase your risk for cancer like Premarin. If you're troubled by vaginal dryness during intercourse, a personal lubricant will usually help.

Postmenopausal Heart Disease

It's true that the number one killer of postmenopausal women is heart disease and that estrogen seems to have a protective effect on cholesterol levels. Studies have shown that it increases the good cholesterol (HDL) and lowers the bad cholesterol (LDL). After menopause, with lower estrogen, HDL levels drop and LDL levels rise. If you're not prepared to exercise and eat well, you may want to look at ERT. But there are other problems connected with postmenopausal heart disease that we believe have not been sufficiently addressed, and we think there are other options to ERT.

Along with higher levels of calcium intake, there has been an increase in heart disease among postmenopausal women. As you've seen, much calcium is not absorbed. If you put it in your mouth and it doesn't get into your bones, where does it go? Dr. Guy E. Abraham suggests, "It gets into the joints and causes arthritis or into the arteries and becomes athero-sclerosis." That calcium buildup in your arteries appears to be increasing your risk for heart disease.

Calcium also causes muscles to contract, while magnesium relaxes them. Your heart is a muscle. You want it to be as relaxed as possible. Therefore, it makes sense to increase your dietary magnesium and keep calcium levels reasonable — not too high. Dr. Abraham's study showing a reversal of osteoporosis indicated that 500 mg of calcium with 600-1,000 mg of magnesium was sufficient. And all the women in his study ate food that also contained more magnesium than calcium. Since whole grains and beans also have calcium, much of which is well-absorbed, a healthy diet will give you additional minerals your body can use, not store.

Natural Prevention for Heart Disease

Particular fats, like margarine, increase your risk for heart disease if you eat more than four teaspoons of it a day. That's not a lot. The trans-fatty acids found in margarine increase the bad cholesterol over the good. So do many of the oils used commercially — especially in baked goods and to deep fry foods. Even butter was better than margarine for reducing heart disease risks. Your best solution is to eliminate all the hydrogenated and trans-fats in your diet, such as margarine and shortening. In their place, use fresh oils such as extra virgin olive oil and flaxseed oil. These should be kept refrigerated to prevent them from becoming rancid.

Add vitamin E to your diet — about 400 IU a day. It appears to work directly on reducing the LDLs and removing free radicals, adverse chemicals formed from eating excessive fats.

Also add up to 800 mcg a day of folic acid, which helps maintain healthy fibrinogen and homocysteine levels. Folic acid is abundant in leafy green vegetables.

High triglycerides increase your risk for heart disease, and drinking more than 300 mg of caffeine a day increases these fats. This translates to three five-ounce cups of percolated coffee, five colas, or two coffees and two colas. Green tea, protective against tumors, contains 40-60 mg of caf-feine per cup. How about one cola or coffee and then drinking green tea?

Aerobic, stress-bearing exercise will reduce your risk for heart disease in addition to a good diet. You need five days of exercise a week doing something aerobic for half an hour. Fast walking, biking, home exercise equipment, and mild jogging are all effective.

A Very Individual Decision

Clearly, there are many aspects to consider when considering ERT. But we don't hear much about are the lesser-known benefits.

In another study, from the University of Southern California, post-menopausal women who received estrogen replacement were 40 percent less likely to develop Alzheimer's disease (or have milder symptoms if they did). The study took place over the course of 11 years and included nearly 9,000 women.

The above studies suggest that women who have bypass surgery or are at a higher risk of developing Alzheimer's disease, may want to give ERT special consideration — especially if their breast cancer risk is low.

Resource Guide

Hormone Level Testing

Aeron Life-Cycles: Offers hormone saliva testing by mail. Results within 5 to 7 working days can then be taken to your doctor. 800-631-7900.

Compounding Pharmacies

In addition to hormone supplements, these pharmacies offer assistance in locating a physician in your area who is knowledgeable in prescribing natural hormone supplements.

Bajamar Women's Healthcare Pharmacy
800-255-8025

California Pharmacy and Compounding Center
800-575-7776

College Pharmacy
800-888-9358

Women's International Pharmacy
800-279-5708

A Few Final Thoughts

There are other symptoms of menopause, including depression and weight gain. By eating a diet high in soy products (and other beans), whole grains, and fresh vegetables, and low in fats, sugars, and caffeine, you will be optimizing your health and guarding against many degenerative diseases that often appear in later years. Eat well and exercise regularly and you won't gain the weight your friends on ERT are gaining. There's no easy solution to menopause, but there's more available to you than just taking a pill and bleeding for the rest of your life. Menopause, when allowed to take place, will pass — giving way to the postmenopausal zest Margaret Mead described in older women in many of the more primitive cultures she studies.

Weigh the pros and cons of estrogen as well as other hormone therapies and make your own decision. Your doctors are your partners, not your parents. It's your body and your life. Take care of it.

Chapter 5

Stop Breast Cancer Before It Happens!

By now our average one-in-nine risk of developing breast cancer has been well-imprinted in the memory of just about every woman in this country.

I prefer to turn the one in nine statistic around. Looking at it from this vantage point, chances are eight in nine that you will never be diagnosed with breast cancer.

What's more, there are many excellent ways to boost your chances of not getting breast cancer (or having a recurrence) — and these simple strategies will be well worth a little extra effort since they will also lower a multitude of other serious health risks.

Eat the Right Stuff

In my opinion, the most alarming news about our breast cancer risk is this: Women who consume Western diets, such as a typical American diet, have the highest rates of breast cancer worldwide. Women who consume traditional Mediterranean diets have an intermediate risk, relative to the rest of the world. And women who consume traditional Asian and Hispanic diets have some of the lowest rates of breast cancer in the world. In fact, the breast cancer rate of American women is eight times higher than that of Korean women and 22 times higher than that of Thai women.

This is no genetic coincidence. Asian and Hispanic women who move to the U.S. and other Western nations, and abandon their traditional diets in favor of a Westernized diet, soon catch up with Western women in terms of breast cancer risk.

Since diet has been strongly linked to breast cancer incidence, your first line of defense against breast cancer should be dietary — adjusting your diet to more closely resemble the breast-cancer fighting characteristics of Asian and Hispanic diets. And at the same time, avoid the breast-cancer promoting foods (such as animal fat and high-sugar foods) found in Western diets.

This translates into an anti-breast cancer diet that consists mostly of whole grain foods, legumes (or beans), vegetables, fresh fruits, and little, if any, meat, poultry, and dairy foods.

The Low-Fat Advantage

The low-fat aspect of this diet helps fight breast cancer by maintaining healthier estrogen levels in your body. Here's how: Increased estrogen is one of the only known risks for breast cancer, which is why estrogen replacement therapy and birth control pill use have been linked to breast cancer. Body fat makes estrogen (even when a woman is postmenopausal), so extra body fat means extra estrogen.

A low-fat diet helps you maintain a healthier weight so there's less fat on your body, and thus less estrogen is produced and stored in it. This explains in part why studies have revealed higher rates of breast cancer — and breast cancer recurrence — among overweight women.

For breast cancer prevention, studies suggest that no more than 15-20 percent of your total calories come from fat, and the lower your intake in this range, the lower your risk will be. Don't try to cheat on this fat intake limit. Studies show animals that consume 25 percent of their calories as fat have the same mammary cancer rates as animals consuming 40 percent of their calories as fat.

It's very important that most of the fats you do consume come from plant or fish, not animal, sources. For salads, marinades, cooking, etc., olive oil (used sparingly) is your best choice. The most healthful olive oil is considered to be "extra virgin," cold-pressed or expeller pressed if available.

Women who eat fish also have lower breast cancer rates than those who don't. Fish oil inhibits the body's production of prostaglandin E2 (PGE2), too much of which can inhibit the immune system's ability to kill breast cancer cells.

Animal studies even suggest a low-fat diet during pregnancy may reduce the breast cancer risk for any female children you have.

It's important to note that this diet includes very little, if any, chicken or eggs, red meat, and milk or other dairy foods. These all contain the saturated animal fats that have been linked to breast (and certain other) cancer when consumed in high amounts.

Don't Forget the Phytoestrogens

Another important dietary prevention step is to include plenty of phytoestrogens (plant estrogens) in your diet. These are estrogens that nature intended us to have — consumed as part of our daily diet. They are natural hormones with just the right strength. Too weak to cause, yet strong enough to protect against, health problems such as breast cancer.

Phytoestrogens are found in whole grains and legumes. The lower breast cancer rates among Asian women may be explained, in part, by the fact that soy foods (such as soy milk, tofu, and miso, which are made from soybeans, a legume) and rice are staples of most Asian diets. Hispanic women consume lots of rice, beans, and tortillas, which are made from corn or wheat. All of these foods are rich in phytoestrogens.

These hormone-like substances may help prevent the growth of hormone-dependent cancers such as breast cancer by behaving like the drug tamoxifen in the body — but with no side effects.

In one recent study, premenopausal women in their 20s were given 60 grams of soy protein a day. The effect on their hormones was similar to that found in women on tamoxifen, a controversial anti-estrogenic drug, which is used to prevent development, as well as recurrence, of breast cancer. The tamoxifen controversy comes from its possible side effects — including an increased incidence of endometrial cancer.

According to Dr. Herman Adlercreutz, a major phytoestrogen researcher, phytoestrogens may also reduce hot flashes and other menopausal symptoms, which are much less prevalent in Japanese women. In other words, phytoestrogens have an effect similar to hormone replacement therapy — without the risks!

Soy is also the only known source of genistein, a phyto-estrogen that has been shown in test tube and animal experiments to block the growth of breast cancer cells, so eating soy foods regularly may protect you against breast cancer.

Soy products may contain as much as 50 percent fat, however, so choose tofu, soy milk, soy cheese, soy mayonnaise (called nayonnaise) and other soy products that are no-fat or low in fat. You can find them in many health food stores. If you buy canned refried beans, choose fat-free. And for tortillas, choose corn or whole wheat.

Other Diet Tips

Here are some other tips for enlisting what you put in your mouth in your fight against breast cancer:

Please pass on the sugar: Several studies have linked high sugar consumption to increased breast cancer risk. This is not surprising when you consider the massive amounts of glucose cancer cells need to thrive — 10 times more than normal cells.

An epidemiologic survey reported in the *Journal of Medical Hypothesis* reviewed breast cancer rates for 21 countries. Based on their findings, the researchers concluded that high sucrose (sugar) intake is a major risk factor for the development of breast cancer in women over 45.

Antioxidants: Women who want to lower their breast cancer risk should also boost the antioxidant content of their meals at every opportunity. Fruits and vegetables are a main source of antioxidants.

In two Swedish studies reported in the *Archives of Internal Medicine*, researchers found a breast cancer decrease with a high intake of the antioxidant beta carotene, the form of vitamin A found in many red, yellow, and orange fruits and vegetables. Green vegetables were also protective.

If you're not big on vegetables, think of new ways you can incorporate them into your diet. Raw baby carrots make sweet afternoon snacks (or dip them into non-fat bean dip for a quick lunch). Grated carrots and yellow summer squash can be added to canned spaghetti sauce and poured over pasta. You can also puree these vegetables and use them in soups or spaghetti sauce — and you won't even taste them. Beta carotene is also found in fruits such as apricots and cantaloupe.

Miso, a fermented soy food used as the base for miso soup, is also full of antioxidants. In a study that appeared in the *Journal of Nutrition Sciences and Vitaminology*, it was reported to prevent a variety of diseases including mammary cancer. This extra protection is attributed to vitamin E, isoflavones, and saponins and other cancer-fighting compounds that are found in fermented food products — but not destroyed during the preparation. To make miso soup, a teaspoon or so of miso (a thick paste), tofu chunks, and slices of green onion are added to a bowl of hot water, without additional cooking. Miso is high in sodium, so eat it, but sparingly.

Another key feature of the Asian diet is green tea — a proven weapon against fat, aging, and cancer. Green tea contains antioxidants called polyphenols. One of these, EGCG, has been shown to decrease mammary tumor size and inhibit mammary tumor formation in animals. Three cups a day are considered to be protective.

Eat plenty of fiber: If you follow the diet described above, you should get plenty of fiber. If you experience constipation, however, upping your fiber intake should take care of the problem and will lower your breast cancer risk as well. Women with two or less bowel movements per week have 4.5 times the risk of precancerous breast changes than women whose frequency is greater than once per day, according to researchers from the University of California at San Francisco.

More Diet Benefits!

The most exciting aspect of this anti-breast-cancer diet is that it can significantly reduce your breast cancer risk — plus your risk for other, even more prevalent, health threats.

Your risk for most other cancers, which claim even more female lives than breast cancer, will also drop significantly on this diet. And your risk of heart disease, which is the leading cause of death among females, will also decrease dramatically.

In fact, a healthy diet is so important that many experts believe *a poor diet is a greater health risk than smoking.*

Environmental Influences

The media bombards us with news about foods that contribute to cancer. It's enough to make you want to throw up your arms in frustration. Please don't. Making changes gradually and over a longer period of time can be surprisingly easy.

Several environmental influences have also been shown to contribute to breast cancer development. Now let's take a look at environmental influences and some additional steps you can take to further reduce your breast cancer risk.

Environmental Estrogens

The higher your estrogen levels, and the longer you are exposed to estrogen, the greater your risk becomes for getting breast cancer. You can't control the number of years between the time you began menstruating and when you started menopause — years when your body produces the most estrogen. But you can lower your exposure to organochlorines — industrial chemicals made from chlorine gas that act like estrogen in your body, increasing your exposure to this hormone.

Each year, 40 million tons of organochlorines are produced. Eighty percent of them are used to make plastics, bleach, solvents, and pesticides. These chemicals don't just disappear. They remain in the environment and are stored in tissues of all living things, moving up the food chain and increasing in numbers as they do.

Here is what a recent issue of *Science* magazine recently reported about certain estrogenic chemicals: The estrogenic potencies of combinations of such chemicals were up to 1,600 times as potent as any chemical alone. This synergistic interaction of chemical mixtures may have profound environmental implications.

Estrogenic chemicals, remember, are chemicals that increase human estrogen levels. This is one of the only known risk factors for developing breast and other reproductive cancers. Estrogenic chemicals are also suspected to play a large role in the declining sperm counts among men, which are on average approximately half as high as they were 100 years ago.

(In the environment, estrogenic chemicals are credited with resulting in abnormal sexual development in reptiles, birds, and male fish. These days a lot of crocodiles in Florida, for example, have undersized penises. Others have genitals that are half-female and half-male. Left unchecked, this type of problem could conceivably interfere with reproduction and eventually lead to extinction of numerous species.)

The findings reported by *Science* were based on only three estrogenic chemicals, the pesticides dieldrin, toxaphene, and endosulfan. Yet the pervasiveness of estrogenic chemicals is astounding. For starters, they have been found in air and water. In plastic packing materials. In construction, upholstery, and carpet materials. In many chemically treated and dyed fabrics. In dry-cleaning supplies. In our tap, bath, and shower water (chlorine). In popular household cleaning products — especially chlorine bleach and other products that increasingly contain chlorine bleach. In many personal care and cosmetic products. In certain pesticides that are widely used to grow the food we eat (produce as well as meat and poultry, which contain pesticide residues from feed). In numerous food additives and preservatives, even food dye. And the prevalence of these chemicals in our environment is growing.

Use of synthetic food dyes for example, has increased five percent per year since 1979. These food dyes are found in lunch meats, hot dogs, snack foods, candies, beverages, and many other foodstuffs. Red Dye No. 4 was taken off the market because it was found to cause cancer. Its cousin, Red Dye No. 3, however, is still widely used and is estrogenic and a known carcinogen. It was even recently proven to promote the growth of breast cancer cells!

In 1993, the *Journal of the National Cancer Institute* published data suggesting that organochlorine residues "are strongly associated with breast cancer risk." A University of Michigan study showed that women with malignant breast tumors had twice as many organo-chlorines in their breast tissue as women the same age and weight without cancer. What was astonishing was that the pesticide levels in their breast tissue were nearly 1,000 times higher than the FDA considers to be safe in food. These researchers believe that most of the women in their study were exposed to organochlorines in their diets.

This is a good reason to eat organic foods. Whenever you can find organic produce, buy it. It may cost a little more, but it's worth it. To cut costs, you might consider growing some of your own food for inexpensive organic produce. A large pot will produce plenty of lettuce or squash or tomatoes if you don't have room for a large garden.

Also, try to eliminate meat and dairy products. If you can't, at least limit them to low-fat or non-fat products since pesticides tend to get stored in the fat cells of animals. Meat and dairy foods that are free of growth hormones and antibiotics are also preferred.

But what else can you do to begin to protect yourself against ongoing assault by estrogenic chemicals? According to Craig Dees, a research chemist with the Molecular Toxicology Group of the Department of Energy's Oak Ridge National Laboratory, who headed up recent research on Red Dye No. 3, the safest approach is to "avoid chemicals period." This requires looking at everything on your table, in your home, and in the world around you, in a new way. What's more, you will discover that chemicals are so prevalent that it is physically impossible to entirely eliminate your exposure to them. Instead, unless you are willing to move away from civilization to a remote, unpolluted, and probably unpopulated area, you will have to settle for second best: minimizing your exposure.

This might include throwing out dozens of toxic household cleaning products and replacing them with a few biodegradable, non-toxic, multiuse products. For starters, Bon Ami (which appropriately means "good friend" in French) is a good cleanser alternative to Ajax and Comet and contains no chlorine. Another solution is to install chlorine-removing water filters in your home.

Ultimately, we need to re-evaluate the necessity of every chemical source in our homes. If this solution sounds too extreme, consider this: higher breast cancer rates are seen with higher usage rates of toxic household cleaning products. (And in general, unless a cleaning product says "non-toxic" on the label, it is toxic.) This news is bad enough, but there's even more you need to know about chemical interactions....

Non-estrogenic chemical compounds can also be life-threatening. New findings now suggest that the mysterious symptoms such as the headaches, fatigue, short attention span, aches, and rashes that have become known as Gulf War Syndrome, may be the result of exposure to complex chemicals mixtures. The U.S. Defense Department still can't explain what caused so many Gulf War veterans to come down with this syndrome, but a study funded by Texas billionaire H. Ross Perot appears to provide some answers.

Perot hired a team of research toxicologists and epidemiologists to do something the U.S. Defense Department has yet to do. They tested simultaneous exposure of two and more of the insecticides and other drugs used by Gulf War vets, on chickens. None of the chemicals caused problems on their own. But when combined, Perot's research team began seeing nervous system damage in the chickens as well as symptoms similar to those suffered by vets with Gulf War Syndrome. The researchers' explanation for the reaction: possibly system overload. One blood enzyme (butyrlycholinesterase), for example, broke down the chemicals. But when an anti-nerve gas agent was introduced into the mix, it monopolized the enzyme and kept it from attacking the insecticide chemicals. If this is in fact what happened to the Gulf War Syndrome vets, we not only lost soldiers over there to friendly fire, but we also injured thousands of others with "friendly" chemicals.

The bottom line on the above findings is this: Until (if ever) further testing is completed, we simply won't know all the risks that chemical interactions may pose for us. We can, however, minimize our exposure to as many chemicals as possible in an effort to avoid these unknown risks.

The Pesticide and Breast Cancer Connection

How Some Pesticides May Contribute To Cancer

The link between pesticides and breast cancer may not be the inherent "toxicity" of these chemicals, but the effect they have on our hormone levels.

Dr. Mary Wolff, of the Mount Sinai School of Medicine, reported in the *Journal of the National Cancer Institute* that one group of pesticides, called organochlorines, may stimulate estrogen production. And a woman's lifetime exposure to estrogen and high levels of the hormone seem to correlate with her risk for breast cancer: the more years your body produces estrogen, the greater your risk may be for developing this disease.

Just look at some commonly observed risks for breast cancer: early menstruation, late menopause, and having no children. What they all have in common is more estrogen.

The earlier you began menstruating, the earlier your body began producing more estrogen. The later you began menopause, the longer your body was exposed to more estrogen. If you had no children, your body was not given an estrogen break that occurs during pregnancy when hormone levels are altered.

Now researchers are looking at another aspect of estrogen production: pesticides that affect hormone production. Certain pesticides increase estrogen production and are called "estrogenic," because as they break down in our bodies they act like estrogen. DDT (our bodies store it as DDE in fat tissues) and PCBs (polychlorinated biphenyls) are two pesticides that act like estrogen.

Although DDT has been outlawed for several years, residues which still exist in the soil will continue to find their way into the foods grown in that soil. Known to be a carcinogen from animal studies, DDT is not broken down in our bodies efficiently. Instead, it stores itself in our fat tissues.

In Dr. Wolff's study, women with breast cancer had their blood tested for residues of DDE. High levels of this pesticide were found in cancer patients' blood. In fact, these women showed a four times greater incidence of breast cancer than women with lower blood concentrations of DDE.

Women Over 50 at Greatest Risk

One reason for the increase in breast cancer in women over 50 may be that these women had the greatest exposure to DDT, which began being used in 1945. If there is a link between pesticides and breast cancer, we can expect this increase in breast cancer to continue for generations.

More than 220 million pounds of chemicals thought to alter our hormones are currently used on 68 different crops each year, according to Environmental Working Group, a non-profit research organization in Washington. These chemicals are sprayed particularly heavy on grapes, lettuce, and tomatoes, although many other crops are treated with these chemicals, as well.

Heavy concentrations of organochlorines can also be found in the meat and dairy products of animals that consumed non-organic feed. (Remember, organochlorines are stored in fat cells, so the higher the fat content of meat and dairy products, potentially the higher the hormone-altering pesticide content).

A preliminary study, which was published in the *Archives of Environmental Health* last year, reported on the levels of chemicals found in breast tissues in women with either breast cancer or non-malignant breast disease (like breast cysts). This study showed higher levels of estrogen-producing pesticides in women with cancer. In fact, the women with breast cancer had more than twice as many PCBs and DDEs in their breast tissue as women the same age and weight without cancer.

How high were the levels of pesticides found in their breast tissues? Nearly 1,000 times higher than the amount the Food and Drug Administration considers to be safe in the foods we eat!

Israelis Find an Answer

While breast cancer rates continued to rise throughout 28 countries in Europe from 1976 to 1986, the breast cancer mortality rates for young women actually dropped in Israel. This is remarkable, because risk factors that are thought to contribute to breast cancer, like an increase of dietary animal fats, actually rose in Israel during this time. Still, researchers determined there was a 20 percent decrease in breast cancer in women under age 65 in this country at a time when the rest of Europe showed an . increase.

This decline was not magic; it appears to have been chemical. Up until 1978, milk and dairy products in Israel had extremely high levels of DDT and other carcinogenic pesticides. In fact, Israelis were known to have high amounts of organochlorines in their body fat and breast milk.

A public outcry in the spring of 1978, however, called for the ban of these pesticides, and the Supreme Court threatened to take action if necessary. As a result, three moderate-strength carcinogens, which increased estrogen production in women and were used in dairy farming, were banned and breast cancer decreased.

Westin and Richter, who headed the Israeli study, commented, "If we assume that DDT and/or BHC (both chlorinated pesticides) are causes of human breast cancer, could their elimination from the diet result in a dramatic drop in breast cancer rates? The evidence available would indicate that the answer is yes."

The Delaney Clause and Beyond

How do we get organochlorines out of our foods? It's not as easy as you might think. The Delaney Clause passed by Congress in 1958, prohibited carcinogens in processed foods. But this law was not well enforced, and Carol Browner, administrator of the Environmental Protection Agency, has asked Congress to update the law. But instead of outlawing these chemicals in all foods as the original bill did, a new bill was written (HR 1627) that allows some cancer-causing pesticide residues to be in foods.

Steps You Can Take to Reduce Pesticide Poisoning

For now, many of our foods continue to be laced with pesticide residue, including pesticides which alter female hormone levels. Here are some steps you can take to reduce your exposure:

● Reduce your consumption of animal fats. Eat very lean meats and fat-free dairy products for the majority of your animal protein intake.

● Have one or two days a week when your protein comes from vegetable sources (grains and beans make a complete protein when eaten together) to further reduce your animal fat intake.

● Grow some of your vegetables. Lettuce can be grown in a pot on a patio, and sprouts can be grown in jars on your kitchen counter.

● Buy organic produce whenever possible, especially grapes, raisins, and lettuce. (Pavich packages organic raisins in 15 oz. tins that will last a year in the refrigerator. Fax them at 805-725-5690 for ordering information.)

● Become more politically active. Support the Delaney Clause. Write your congressman and ask that it be strengthened to phase out all carcinogenic pesticides that are used on food processed or fresh.

There are plenty of ways to reduce your breast cancer risk by avoiding exposure to pesticides. It's simply a matter of just doing it.

Chlorine in Water and Breast Cancer

A recent review of chlorine and its effect on cancer from Physicians Committee for Responsible Medicine points out the connection between chlorination of drinking water and carcinogens (cancer-causing agents). Chlorinated drinking water has been found to contain chemicals called trihalomethans (THMs) which are carcinogenic. Interestingly, the water which was tested did not contain THMS before it was chlorinated. One type of chlorine, organochlorine, found in pesticides and insecticides, has been strongly linked to breast cancer because it acts like estrogen in the human body, and increased estrogen is one of the only known risks for breast cancer.

Is it possible to eliminate the chlorine from our diet when it's in all the water around us? Yes, but you can't stop there. Even the chlorine in your shower water can migrate through your skin and affect your health. A good chlorine removing shower filter is something that's a must for every household. If you can't find one, call 800-728-2288 and ask for some information on their chlorine-removing shower head.

These are simple and relatively inexpensive ways of reducing the negative effects of chlorine. The reason chlorine is added to city water systems is to reduce the spread of infectious diseases which can be transported through water.

Hormones in Milk and Breast Cancer

Can bovine hormones in milk contribute to breast cancer?

Very possibly, says Dr. Samuel S. Epstein, professor of occupational and environmental medicine at the University of Illinois School of Public Health.

No, say such groups as the FDA, National Institutes of Health, and the American Dietetic Association.

Why this discrepancy? Because BST (a hormone called bovine somatotropin) in itself is inactive in humans, destroyed during pasteurization, and can't get through the intestinal walls because it's broken down in the digestive tract.

Meanwhile, consumer groups argue about the pros and cons of genetic engineering; dairy producers are seriously considering giving BST to cows because it greatly increases their production of milk; and women are confused about what to buy for their families, especially if they have small children. Is it worth looking for hormone-free dairy products or are they really safe?

It's not BST that's the problem, argues Dr. Epstein, but rather a substance called IGF-1 (insulin-like growth factor-1). Unlike BST, IGF-1 is not destroyed by pasteurization and is absorbed through the intestinal walls. In babies and young children whose digestive systems are not yet fully developed, IGF-1 may very well be absorbed. We just don't know because all of the existing studies have been done on mature rats — not on infant rats, and not on humans of any age.

The problem with IGF-1 is that it causes normal breast tissue to multiply and divide rapidly. Dr. Epstein believes it is highly likely that this eventually causes healthy breast tissue to turn into breast cancer. IGF-1 also gives human breast cancer cells the ability to spread to other organs in the body.

When you give young children milk which contains BST, you may be increasing the sensitivity of their breasts not only to breast cancer through IGF-1, but also to the estrogen-like effects of pesticides found in non-organic foods. And increased estrogens can contribute to breast cancer. Hormone-free dairy products and organic foods may be a little more trouble to find and slightly higher in price, but in the long run, they may your family's best safeguard against future incidents of cancer.

Can Iron Supplements Cause Breast Cancer?

Many women believe that their fatigue can be helped by taking iron supplements. If they feel extremely tired, they may take two or three iron pills. After all, they can't hurt, can they?

Perhaps they can.

Once thought to be completely safe, iron has now been found to cause adverse effects in laboratory animals. The American Institute for Cancer Research, in Washington, D.C., has recently published the results of a study on iron and breast cancer in rats. When the rats were given ten times the normal dosage of iron, there was a significant increase in breast cancer.

Some oncologists have already begun to caution their patients with breast cancer to avoid taking any multivitamins that contain iron, pending further research. While it is still too early to know what effects too much iron in the diet can have on women who have an increased risk for breast cancer, like a family history of the disease, it is known that iron can cause free radicals, substances that can damage cells.

High iron stores have also been associated with cardiovascular disease, a growing problem in postmenopausal women who lack the protective effects of estrogen on their heart.

Does this mean you should not take iron supplements at all? That depends. Certainly, if you menstruate heavily, are pregnant, are breast feeding, or are a strict vegetarian, iron may be a helpful or necessary addition to your diet. To be sure, ask your doctor for a blood test which will show whether or not you have too much stored iron. If you do, you may want to eliminate iron from your supplements.

Most women get enough, but not too much, iron in a well-balanced diet by eating a little meat, fish, or poultry along with a food containing vitamin C (potatoes, citrus, tomatoes) to enhance absorption. The iron in vegetables is not easily absorbed, but you can boost its absorption by cooking acidic foods, like tomato sauce or vegetables sauteed with a little lemon juice, in cast-iron pots or pans.

If you're feeling tired, don't assume your fatigue is due to a lack of iron. It could be a low-grade infection, a virus, a blood sugar imbalance, or due to non-iron dietary imbalances. Get a diagnosis from your doctor or health provider before reaching for extra iron. It could cause more problems than it solves.

Other Dietary Considerations

In addition to following the diet discussed earlier and eating organic foods when available, consider making further changes in your consumption of alcohol and the use of nutritional supplements. Here's why:

Alcohol: A review in the *New England Journal of Medicine* on alcohol and breast cancer focused on three separate studies that all showed a 60 percent increase in breast cancer in women who had one or more drinks a day. The review does not indicate whether these drinks were beer, wine, or hard liquor. Nor does it take into account dietary intake. However, if you are at a particularly high risk for breast cancer, daily drinking may not be wise for you.

Some research suggests that wine (especially red) may be safer to drink than beer or hard liquor. This has been attributed to certain nutrients (such as polyphenols and antioxidants) found in red wine.

The Alcohol-Breast Cancer Connection

Estradiol is a sex hormone implicated in breast cancer. Estradiol levels are higher in postmenopausal women who drink alcoholic beverages regularly and socially. An article in the *Journal of the American Medical Association* (*JAMA*) reports on a study where women who were on estrogen replacement therapy (ERT) had their estradiol levels checked after drinking alcohol or a placebo.

After drinking alcohol, their estradiol levels increased three times in an hour. It took six hours for their hormone levels to return to their original levels.

Women who were not on ERT, who drank either alcoholic beverages or the placebo, did not have variations in their estradiol levels. The authors suggest these results indicated that women on ERT who drink alcohol regularly may be significantly increasing their risk for getting breast cancer. Since the holidays are upon us, we wanted you to have this information immediately.

Ginsburg, E.S., et al. "Effects of alcohol ingestion on oestrogens in postmenopausal women," *JAMA*, 176(21), 1747-1751 (1996).

Conflicting information on the link between alcohol and breast cancer risk, however, comes from Europe. The death rate from breast cancer in Spain, Greece, and Portugal is less than half that of the U.S. (Plus, the overall cancer rates for Greek, Spanish, and Portuguese women are also exceptionally low.) Yet wine consumption in these countries is four times higher than that of the U.S. The reason for the lower rates of breast cancer in these other countries is explained in part by other dietary differences. For example, U.S. sugar consumption is twice that of Spain, Greece, and Portugal. In 1988, the average American consumed 1/3 pound of sugar per day! And high sugar intake is a major risk factor for the development of breast cancer in women over 45.

Still, the alcohol in any beverage can increase estrogen levels and, in turn, boost breast cancer risk. Alcohol also weakens the immune system, making it harder for the body to fight against a cancer threat. In spite of the nutritive value, wine is no substitute for the excellent nutrition you should be getting from other sources.

Smoking: A study by the American Cancer Society indicates that a woman's risk of dying from breast cancer is 25 percent higher if she is a smoker. And that percent rises proportionally to the number of cigarettes smoked per day as well as the total number of years smoking. There is a 75 percent higher risk for women who smoke more than two packs a day.

Nutritional Supplements: Supplements do not replace healthy food; they give your body additional support. The following nutrients have specifically been associated with lowering a woman's risk for breast cancer.

Garlic: While it's actually an herb, garlic does more than make foods taste good and keep away vampires. It is thought to be a potent anti-carcinogen when eaten regularly. If you like it, use it freely. If your breath smells, you should consider taking garlic tablets, or use Breath Asure capsules. They work!

Vitamin C: A review published in the *Journal of the National Cancer Institute* stated that taking only 380 mg of vitamin C a day would lower breast cancer in this country by 16 percent. Fresh fruits and vegetables contain large amounts of vitamin C. If you like, you can add 500 mg in supplement form as well.

Iron: This mineral should be avoided by women at high risk for breast cancer, unless you have a severe iron deficiency. Studies show that lower iron stores were associated with fewer incidents of breast tumors than high iron. Nutritional supplements are available without iron.

Selenium: An inverse relationship has been seen between dietary selenium and breast cancer. Since selenium is a trace mineral that may be low in the soil where fruits, vegetables, and grains are grown, adding selenium in supplemental form could be wise. No more than 200 mcg is suggested (high amounts may be toxic).

Vitamin D: This vitamin, manufactured in your body from exposure to sunlight, may not be necessary if you live in a sunny climate and spend time outdoors. But if you don't, you may want to make certain any dietary supplement you take contains vitamin D. Research has shown that there is less breast cancer in the sunnier regions of both the U.S. and Russia.

Vitamins A & E: Studies abound linking diets high in beta-carotene (the natural plant form of vitamin A) and vitamin E (found in nuts, seeds, and oils) to cancer prevention. They do not address breast cancer specifically, but a diet and supplements emphasizing antioxidants is your best defense. Other antioxidants you may hear about include CoQ10 (co-enzyme Q10), pycnogenol, and n-acetylcysteine. While they may be

---

The Link Between CoQ10 and Cancer

Coenzyme Q10 (CoQ10) is a vitamin (vitamin Q10) that, along with vitamin B_6, has been found to be low in people with cancer. CoQ10 is made from tyrosine, an amino acid found in proteins like meats and beans. But to make CoQ10, the body needs a number of vitamins, and without the coenzyme form of vitamin B_6 — one of the necessary vitamins — there can be dysfunctions to the DNA, which lead to mutations and cancer. Most vitamin formulas with B_6 contain pyridoxine HCL. The coenzyme form of B_6 is called Pyridoxyl-5-phosphate (P-5-P).

One more fact about CoQ10: it requires fatty acids to be taken along with it or it can't be absorbed well. Some CoQ10 products have no fatty acids added to them. If they don't, you need to take them with a meal that contains some fats. Other products have fatty acids added, and are well absorbed at any time. If you have difficulty finding either P-5-P or CoQ10 with fatty acids in your health food store, and want to try them, you can call Advanced Medical Nutrition Inc. (AMNI) at 800-356-4791 and ask for Donna. She's familiar with the products they carry that we especially like.

Folkers, K. "Relevance of the biosynthesis of coenzyme Q10 and of the four bases of DNA as a rationale for the molecular causes of cancer and a therapy," *Biochem Biophys Res*, 224(2), 358-361(1996); *Intl Clin Nutr Rev*, July 1997.

excellent, you would do well to eat the diet we've described with lots of garlic, and a good multivitamin/mineral supplement.

Do not be misled by the one-a-day type vitamins that claim to provide 100 percent of various Recommended Daily Allowances. These are barely enough to prevent serious malnutrition diseases, such as scurvy. Your best bet is the newer mega multivitamin/mineral formulas, which have a daily dose of six capsules, taken at three time intervals throughout the day for maximum absorption. One brand we like, Optimox, offers pre- and postmenopausal formulas and can be ordered by calling 1-800-722-9040. Another is Maximum by Healthy Resolve, which can ordered by calling 1-800-728-2288.

Organochlorines Around Us

Food isn't the only vehicle for organochlorines to find their way into our bodies. Another major culprit is tap water, which is chlorinated in order to kill unfriendly bacteria. But this comes with a trade-off: The water that makes its way into your home contains organochlorines and has been strongly linked to an increased incidence of breast cancer. Chlorine can be removed from tap water, however, with a seven-stage filter and from shower water (which is absorbed through the skin) with a Hydro Spray shower filter (call 800-728-2288 for more information).

Another way to reduce the amount of estrogenic chemicals in your environment is to use biodegradable and nontoxic household cleaning products whenever possible for washing dishes, clothes, windows, floors, and counters, etc. Also, when you can, choose environmentally friendly interior furnishings such as wool area rugs over hardwood flooring and natural fiber linens, drapes, and clothes. Synthetic materials, especially when new, contain chemicals which are emitted into the air, where they can be inhaled.

Finally, we've yet to find a study on this but are suspicious that a deodorant and breast cancer link may exist. Approximately 50 percent of breast cancers occur in the upper-outer quadrant of the breast — closest to where deodorant is applied — while only six percent of breast cancers develop in the lower-inner quadrant — farthest away from where deodorant is applied. The skin will absorb a certain amount of anything that is put on it. Furthermore, applying deodorant after shaving may be especially risky, because tiny skin nicks can act as an open door to any carcinogenic chemicals contained in the deodorant.

My favorite deodorant is baking soda, or sodium bicarbonate. Like the popular (but pricey) deodorant stones, it is a salt and therein lies it's effectiveness. It kills odor-causing bacteria. It's incredibly versatile, too: It can be mixed with corn starch for a smoother-feeling powder. It can also be mixed with your favorite moisturizing cream, and then you have a cream deodorant.

I've asked a lot of women about any safe deodorant alternatives they might use. Here's what they've told me:

One woman from Petaluma, California, uses a vitamin C solution she makes by mixing 1,000 mg of vitamin C crystals in four oz. of water. She applies the solution, then pats on a little cornstarch. Another reader from Marysville, Kansas, wrote that she's been using Desitin brand diaper rash ointment, which is made from zinc oxide and cod liver oil, and really likes it. Generic brands containing the same ingredients would work equally well. She just dabs on a little after bathing and is odor-free for 24 hours.

But the most popular alternative turned out to be baking soda. Like the popular (albeit pricey) deodorant stones, it is a salt and therein lies its effectiveness in keeping you dry and odor-free. It kills odor-causing bacteria. The only drawback is it can sting a little if applied immediately after shaving — from the salt coming in contact with shaving nicks. Still, I've been using it for a few months now and this just might be my deodorant for life. It's incredibly versatile, too: It can be mixed with corn starch for a smoother-feeling powder. It can also be mixed with your favorite moisturizing cream, and then you have a cream deodorant.

Debra Lynn Dadd, author of *Home Safe Home* ($18.95 from Tarcher/ Putman), likes it best, too. She writes, "I have been using it for 17 years, and nobody has ever complained. In fact, I have recommended it to a number of people who have suffered for many years with unconquerable body odor, and they say it's the only thing that has ever worked for them." In addition to deodorizing the underarm, baking soda helps eliminate refrigerator, freezer, even cat litter-box odors. It's also a great cleaner for teeth, bathroom fixtures, and much more.

For feminine hygiene, vitamin C solution alone, can be used on the vaginal area. This is an especially good tip since using talc-containing powder in the vaginal area has been linked to an increased risk of ovarian cancer. If you want to use a powder, use cornstarch. (Ditto for baby bottoms.)

In general, most commercial feminine hygiene products contain hazardous ingredients that are best avoided. Even mild soaps can irritate this especially sensitive area and upset the natural balance of vaginal flora. In fact, contrary to what advertisers would like you to believe, you shouldn't have to use anything special on this area. A daily water rinse while bathing should provide sufficient odor control. If not, consult your physician to check for an infection or other problem.

Perhaps best of all, all of the above safe deodorant alternatives are extremely inexpensive. A two-pound box of baking soda costs around $1.40, while a two- to three-ounce container of a commercial deodorant preparation costs around $3 to $4. That's a little less than four and a half cents an ounce for baking soda (which you probably already have in your kitchen) vs. around $1.40 an ounce for the commercial stuff, which is often dangerous.

Nonantiperspirant deodorants may contain the bacteria-killing ingredient triclosan, which can cause liver damage when absorbed through the skin. Aluminum-containing deodorants may contribute to brain and other disorders. And antiperspirants and deodorants have historically been hazardous. In a recent 10-year period, more than eight different ingredients were banned by the FDA or voluntarily removed from products because they posed a threat to users.

Of course, one of the things that makes commercial deodorants so popular is their convenient packaging. Simply pick one up, remove the top, and spray or roll on. But you can make your own deodorant and have convenience, too. Liquids, such as the vitamin C solution can be stored in little spray bottles, perhaps an attractive perfume atomizer. Creams can be stored in little cosmetic or other jars. (I found a pretty gold-topped, glass Avon jar at a yard sale, washed it well, and now it's one of the highlights of my bathroom counter.)

Finally, the perfect place to store a powder is in a baby powder sprinkle container or dusting powder container, complete with the application puff. Just be sure to clean any container or puff well before use to remove old talc residues.

Sometimes the best solutions are also the least expensive.

For even greater peace of mind, start replacing other personal care products, such as moisturizing lotion and soap, with environmentally friendly formulas as well. These formulas tend not only to be environmentally friendly, but also user friendly — i.e., safer for you to use on *yourself*.

A final environmental factor that is still in question as a breast cancer risk contributor is electromagnetic fields. It is suspected that electricity, and lights at night, reduce levels of the hormone melatonin, which in turn, allows estrogen levels to rise.

According to a study recently reported in the Journal of the National Cancer Institute, women who work at certain electrical jobs had a 30 percent higher incidence of death from breast cancer than those in non-electrical jobs. The link was strongest in telephone installers, repairers and line workers. No increased risk was found in telephone operators, data keyers, computer operators and programmers, or air traffic controllers. But more research is needed in this area to more accurately evaluate risks.

Until more is known, a common-sense approach may be in order: Don't live or work near major power lines, don't sleep under an electric blanket, turn off your computer when it's not in use, don't stand in front of an electric stove or microwave oven for extended periods of time, etc.

Implants and Breast Cancer Risk

In the first comprehensive review of the scientific literature, internationally recognized cancer expert Samuel Epstein, MD, has concluded that implants pose significant risks of breast cancer. The study documenting Epstein's findings appeared in the *International Journal of Occupational Medicine and Toxicology.*

In addition to a detailed analysis of current literature, the review includes confidential industry and government documents on the carcinogenicity of silicone and polyurethane breast implants.

"Risks of breast cancer have been ignored in the current controversy over implants," stated Dr. Epstein, chair of the Cancer Prevention Coalition and pathology expert at the School of Public Health, University of Illinois-Chicago. "Evidence on the carcinogenicity of implants, particularly polyurethane, is strong. Recent epidemiological studies claimed as proof of safety are grossly flawed. Such studies would have even given a clean bill of health to asbestos."

Dr. Epstein continued, "Both industry and the Food and Drug Administration (FDA) have suppressed evidence on the cancer risk of silicone breast implants. The FDA has still failed to act on the recommendation by their own leading scientists to send Medical Alerts to women with silicone implants warning them of their cancer risks."

Based on his report, Dr. Epstein renews the call for a medical alert. He also urges a long-term surveillance program for women with polyurethane implants.

Hormone Supplements

You increase your lifetime exposures to estrogen when you take birth control pills or are on hormone replacement therapy (HRT), whether the hormones are manufactured by pharmaceutical companies or are natural. A review in the *Lancet* indicated that most studies of young women with breast cancer showed an increased risk that was associated with using birth control pills before the age of 25. And a *New England Journal of Medicine* study showed a "fairly strong" association between long-term exposure to birth control pills and an increased risk for breast cancer.

Another study from the *New England Journal of Medicine* (this one by Harvard researchers) discovered a 32 percent higher overall breast cancer risk for women taking estrogen supplements. Women whose supplements contained estrogen and progestin had an overall 41 percent higher risk. And women between the ages of 60 and 64 who had taken hormones for five years or more had a whopping 71 percent higher risk! These findings were based on the health histories of 69,000 women between 1978 and 1992.

The good news about HRT is that increased risk appears to dissipate after estrogen supplements are stopped.

Contrary to what hormone supplement manufacturers would like you to believe, the widely advertised health benefits of lower heart disease and osteoporosis risk with HRT are not standing up to long-term scrutiny. There are safer and more effective ways to reduce these risks, but HRT is not panning out to be one of them. In fact, one study that is currently in progress as of this writing recently made preliminary results available. It has found higher heart disease rates among women on HRT, even though their cholesterol levels tended to be lower.

Asian women rarely experience menopause symptoms and they have much lower rates of heart disease and osteoporosis, yet rarely use HRT. Researchers say Asian women have high levels of the hormone estriol in their bodies.

A limited number of estriol studies have suggested that estriol reduces breast cancer risk, as well as the risk of recurrence. There are many unanswered questions about estriol, however, because of a lack of research. Plus there are many other safe, proven ways to reduce your risk of breast cancer without estriol.

Still, if your breast cancer risk is unusually high, estriol supplements may be a reasonable option to pursue — along with other *proven* breast cancer risk-reduction strategies. Guy Abraham, MD and research gynecologist in Torrance, California, recommends trying di-estrogen. It contains the two forms of estrogen that have not been linked to breast cancer — estriol and estradiol. For more information on this compounded estrogen, call the Women's International Pharmacy in Madison, Wisconsin, at 800-279-5708.

Finally, last year the FDA approved yet another form of hormone supplementation for us all to take: Bovine growth hormone is now being given to cows by most dairies to increase milk production. This hormone causes an increased level of insulin-like growth factor called IFG-1, which causes normal breast tissue to multiply rapidly. It could cause healthy breast tissue to turn into breast cancer. IFG-1 also allows breast cancer cells in humans to spread to other organs in the body. If you are using dairy products, make certain they do not contain bovine growth hormones.

Other events in a woman's reproductive life that affect hormones may also influence breast cancer risk. These include full-term pregnancy, abortion, and lactation.

Each full-term pregnancy a woman has appears to reduce breast cancer risk. Researchers believe this is due to reduced estrogen levels during pregnancy. On the other hand, delaying a first pregnancy until age 35 or older appears to increase risk. To complicate matters further, an abortion was found by one study to increase a woman's breast cancer risk by as much as 50 percent. Yet naturally occurring miscarriages appeared to have no affect. Additional studies are needed to more accurately identify risk in this area.

Finally, lactation, because it also suppresses estrogen levels, also lowers breast cancer risk. A study from the University of Wisconsin at Madison found that women who nursed their babies for several months lowered their risk even more. The World Health Organization currently recommends nursing through the first two years, and the average age of weaning worldwide is 4.25 years. In general, the longer a woman nurses, the greater the health benefits for both she and her child.

Any woman who thinks she needs to wean her baby early in order to return to work should seriously consider expressing milk for those times when she is away from her baby. Also, there's the option of part-time nursing — nursing the baby when the mother is available such as in the morning and evenings before and after work, and reserving formula for only those times when the mother is at work.

Proximity to Nuclear Plants Increases Risk

Recent evidence links nuclear reactors to rises in breast cancer rates. Internationally, only four of 16 industrial countries studied — New Zealand, Australia, Hong Kong, and Israel — showed declines in breast cancer mortality between 1971 and 1986, while rates in all others rose. Of the four industrial countries that showed declines, none had large commercial nuclear reactors operating in or near their borders during this period, while all the others did.

Regional U.S. statistics also support this link between nuclear reactors and breast cancer incidence. The effect is greatest in highly populated areas located near reactors. For example, Suffolk and Nassau Counties on Long Island: Between 1970-72 and 1987-89, breast cancer mortality rates for Suffolk — which is located approximately 10 miles across Long Island

Breast Cancer Clusters

If you live in Hawaii, you have a 32 percent lower risk of dying of breast cancer than the national average of women. If you live in Washington, D.C., your risk is 28 percent higher than the national average. In fact, a report from the National Cancer Institute has found that women who live on the east coast from New York City to Philadelphia are living in an area where breast cancer incidents are higher than in the rest of the country. It's called a cancer cluster. Smaller clusters on the east coast include northeast New Jersey, central New Jersey, Philadelphia and Long Island, N.Y. On the west coast, the San Francisco area has a very high incidence of breast cancer.

What does this mean to you if you live in any of these areas? We think it means you may want to take extra steps to reduce your risk for breast cancer. Here are a few suggestions. Put a chlorine-removing filter on your shower to reduce your exposure to this carcinogenic material that is absorbed through the skin (call 800-728-2288 for more information). Eat more organic produce to reduce your exposure to organochlorines, chemicals that act like estrogen in your body. Eat more soy products to increase the beneficial plant estrogens (phytoestrogens). Do regular breast self-exams and check in with your doctor regularly for any follow-up exams.

Sound from the Millstone nuclear plant near New London, Connecticut — which began operating in 1970 — jumped 39 percent.

Researchers believe this phenomenon is the result of low-level radioactive contamination making its way from reactors into nearby water, then into locally grown produce and other food products such as milk and meat, and then into consumers. To protect yourself, don't live near a reactor or consume water or other food products from near a reactor site.

Better Than a Mammogram

One of the most common reasons women give for not examining their breasts regularly is, "I don't know what I'm looking for," according to Dr. Sharon Olson, an osteopath in northern California.

Dr. Olson's response is, "Don't look for anything. Instead, just get familiar — very familiar — with what's there. Only then," says Dr. Olson, "will you be in the best possible position to detect important changes right away."

Those two last words, "right away," are especially important. Because in spite of widespread use of mammography and regular exams by doctors, two-thirds of all breast cancers are still discovered by women themselves. So if you do develop breast cancer, you will be most likely to find it. By finding it sooner, rather than later, you may also be able to give yourself the advantages that come with early detection — starting with the option of less disfiguring surgery.

Still, many of us have yet to establish regular, meaningful self-exams into our normal routines. But that's about to change. Dr. Olson recently shared her unique breast self-exam techniques with me. After reading about them, I think you'll agree, this is one of the most thoughtful and comprehensive approaches around. One you can get excited about, stick with, and even share with others.

Dr. Sharon Olson's Best Breast Exam Tips

1. Timing. Dr. Olson recommends that menstruating women exam their breasts on the 1st or 2nd day of their periods. Monthly hormone cycling makes this the time when most benign lumps will disappear.

If you do not have periods but still have your ovaries, examine your breasts throughout the month to find out when they are the least lumpy. Then designate this as your regular exam day. It may fluctuate a bit from month to month since not all women have 30 to 31-day hormone cycles. Sometimes a lunar calendar (for example, every full moon) will be more accurate. To establish a lunar schedule, check a lunar calendar the day your breasts are least lumpy and then examine your breasts every time the moon is in that phase.

If you are postmenopausal or don't have your ovaries, Dr. Olson suggests using either the full moon or the new moon as your regular exam day.

During pregnancy, always continue self-exams. Keep in mind that your breasts are preparing for nursing. During the first trimester, your breasts might feel like premenstrual breasts. This improves with the second

More on Mammograms

There is still a controversy over mammograms. Who needs them, how often, and are they as beneficial as mainstream groups suggest? This is a decision each woman must make for herself, and one which is highly influenced by family history, and length of estrogen production (the longer you menstruate — years, not days per month — the higher your risk, it is suspected, for breast cancer). The National Women's Health Network has a few additional comments on mammograms.

First, remember that a clear mammogram does not mean you have no tumors. Although the American Cancer Society says that mammograms won't miss finding tumors, this is not true, especially in women with dense breast tissues. In fact, mammograms miss 10 percent of the tumors in women over 50, and nearly 25 percent in women in their 40s. At best, mammograms are only part of a breast cancer prevention program.

Do regular breast self-exams. The breast exams, along with mammograms if you choose, offer a much better screening than mammograms alone. Get to know your breasts and how they feel. Touching your breasts regularly is not taboo. It is smart preventive medicine.

Whenever possible, have any previous mammogram films sent to the radiologist(s) for comparison.

Pearson, Cynthia. "Mammography controversy," *The Network News*, March/ April 1997.

and third trimester. During lactation, it's best to examine breasts after nursing, when they are emptiest.

If you have breast implants, examine those, too. You need to know how they, and the adjacent tissue, feel.

Finally, if you have an extra nipple, and/or extra breast tissue, examine that, too. In utero, we all have two milk ridges with many nipples, similar to those of cats and dogs. These usually regress before birth. If they don't, however, they may also have breast tissue and may develop cancer. Sometimes extra breast tissue will be present without an extra nipple. One clue that it is present is if it responds in similar ways to hormonal changes as your other breasts, such as premenstrual tenderness.

2. Visual Inspection. Although most of us think an exam is about feeling for lumps, Dr. Olson emphasizes it's also important to inspect our breasts visually.

To do so, she recommends standing in front of a mirror first with your arms up, second with the arms at your sides, third, leaning forward so your breasts fall away from the chest wall, and fourth with your hands behind your head or on your hips and your pectoral muscles (the muscle behind your breast) contracted. In all four positions, study the contours, shading and symmetry. Also look for minor, but most likely harmless, variations between the breasts. Perhaps one hangs lower. Perhaps one breast or nipple is larger than the other.

Note the appearance of blood vessels that can be seen under the skin. Memorize these distinctions. Make notes if you're a note person. Areas of concern include: lumps you can see, puckering, if upon leaning over, breasts don't fall symmetrically or a breast doesn't pull away from the chest, increased vascularity (blood vessels) in one breast.

3. Tactile Inspection. Repeat the first three positions above, but this time, feel your breasts. Remember, you are not feeling for lumps as much as you are familiarizing yourself with how your breasts feel. Again, the idea is only when you know what's normal can you detect what's abnormal. Use a regular pattern to feel your breasts, such as circular from the inside out or outside in. Soaping up your breasts can make it easier to feel various tissue variations and distinctions. When you are in the leaning over position, feel behind your breasts and along the chest wall behind them.

When doing this, you should notice a ridge at the lower edge of the breast. It's called the inframammary fold. If it's tender or irritated, don't wear underwire bras or do anything else that might irritate it.

Areas of concern include: swollen lymph nodes in the armpit area and any lump that is hard and does not move freely within breast tissue. Such a lump may seem stuck, like a little crab with extended legs that are holding onto the surrounding tissue.

About Nipple Discharge: Studies have found that most women's nipples will express discharge when stimulated. This is usually milky or colostrum-type discharge that is normal. Areas of concern include: discharge that expresses with or without stimulation, and is crusty, bloody, green, or black.

Once you master this routine, it should take approximately three to five minutes, longer for lumpier breasts.

4. Documentation. For the ultimate in accuracy, Dr. Olson suggests keeping a breast health folder. It can include a breast map, a rough sketch of each breast in which you draw various points of interest such as a lump or lumpy area. In the margins, make descriptive notes such as "date, lump at 11 o'clock, two inches out from nipple, feels like hard lemon seed, moves freely inside tissue." Once a point of interest is mapped, each exam thereafter will, of course, include checking for any changes in the characteristics you noted. This will take a lot of guess work out of your exams. Your breast health folder should also include copies of all mammogram and ultrasound reports.

To further demystify self-exams, it helps to know what's actually inside our breasts. They are much more than simply masses of extra flesh. In addition to being sexually responsive, breasts produce milk. This requires breast tissue to be somewhat complex.

Breast tissue includes lobules (little sacks that make and store milk), ducts (pipes that bring milk to the nipple), plus arteries, veins and nerves, and finally, connective tissue to hold everything together. Breast tissue itself feels firm and rubbery. Yet breasts themselves tend to be soft because the breast tissue is sandwiched between layers of fat. The major muscle in the area, the pectoralis, is located behind the breast. Behind it are the ribs, which can feel hard and lumpy.

It also helps to know that breast tissue doesn't line up behind the nipple in a perfect circle shape. Instead, most is located toward the armpit and upper breast.

As our discussion was coming to a close, Dr. Olson emphasized that what's most important in self-exams is to pay attention to what our hands are telling us. In the course of her work as an osteopath (a doctor who manipulates bones and other body parts) her hands have become especially sensitive and she is convinced that cancer tissue emits different energy than healthy tissue. Furthermore, this difference can be sensed subconsciously. In fact, she doesn't think it's mere coincidence that most breast cancers are discovered by women. "We can usually sense on some level that something's changed, something's happened," and this can lead to discovering a lump. She did so one day when she put her cold hands under her arms to get warm.

Start Making Changes Now!

After reading this report on breast cancer causes and preventives, you may feel a bit overwhelmed by the dozens of prevention strategies. And it can be overwhelming if you envision implementing everything at once. Instead, remember that prevention is a long-term proposition. More important than doing everything at once is to try taking one step at a time.

The opportunities to do so will often present themselves in the course of your normal activities. For example, the next time you go grocery shopping, put salmon instead of beef steaks in your shopping cart. Or the next time you're buying personal care items, choose chemical-free, environmentally friendly formulas. The more prevention strategies you manage to implement, the lower your breast cancer risk will drop.

If you are persistent, after a while many prevention strategies will be at work for you — with little or no extra effort or sacrifice.

Fibrocystic Breast Disease

The Myth of Fibrocystic Breast Disease

Ask your family physician or gynecologist what fibrocystic breast disease is, and he or she may rattle off a list of symptoms to you that include lumpy breasts, nipple discharge, pain, swelling, and tenderness.

Ask a pathologist (a doctor who examines tissue biopsies) to describe fibrocystic breast disease, and you're likely to hear a detailed list of about 15 microscopic conditions that can be present in breast tissue.

Ask a radiologist (one who reads mammograms) about this disease and you're likely to get yet a third definition that revolves around the characteristic of extra dense breast tissue.

A Meaningless Diagnosis

Even if the experts could accurately define fibrocystic breast disease, for all intents and purposes, it is a meaningless diagnosis.

The 15 microscopic conditions that pathologists believe cause fibrocystic disease are actually common pathological changes that take place as a normal result of the aging process. And the breast tissue density that radiologists claim causes fibrocystic breast disease is actually a normal condition of youth — the breasts of younger women tend to contain comparatively less fat tissue and more breast tissue, which is denser.

As for the more general symptoms of lumpiness, nipple discharge, pain, swelling and tenderness; the latter are common premenstrual symptoms. What most doctors don't tell you is that lumpiness and nipple discharge are common in many women and have not yet been proven to be precursors to any negative medical condition.

Of all the conditions listed above, only one has been linked to the development of breast cancer. It is a rare pathological condition called *atypical hyperplasia*. If you have this, and a family history of breast cancer, you probably have an increased breast cancer risk.

The Real Dangers of Fibrocystic Breast Disease

According to Dr. Susan Love, author of *Dr. Susan Love's Breast Book*, the term "'Fibrocystic disease' is as fanciful as anything Lewis Carroll ever invented. It's not only fanciful, however; it's dangerous. It causes a number of problems for those women who 'carry the diagnosis.'"

For starters, it can prevent you from being accepted for medical insurance coverage. And if a company does insure you, it may exclude your breasts from coverage. That means if you do have real breast problems, you'll have to rely on your own financial resources for medical treatment.

Next, the belief that you have a disease can be detrimental to your mental health, for example, if it causes you to worry. And unproven "treatments" like eliminating caffeine from your diet or taking vitamin E supplements are a wasted effort.

Finally, more radical medical treatments can be catastrophic. Some doctors actually recommend mastectomy to prevent the possibility that a fibrocystic breast will develop cancer — which is about as intelligent as the solution of removing all breasts in order to prevent breast cancer.

Cancer Link Unfounded

Like premenstrual syndrome, fibrocystic breast disease is a fairly recent medical phenomenon around which much confusion has developed. Most of the early research on fibrocystic breast disease took place in the '30s and '40s and focused mainly on women who had breast biopsies. An increased risk of breast cancer for women with so-called fibrocystic was never actually proven. It was mere speculation.

Some of these studies put the cart before the horse. They found "fibrocystic breast disease" in cancerous breasts that had been removed. It was therefore assumed that the "disease" caused the cancer when in actuality the cancer may well have developed independent of the "disease."

Other studies asked women who had breast cancer if they'd had previous biopsies. It then compared them to women who didn't have cancer, sought medical advice about the condition of their breasts, and in some cases had a biopsy. These studies then equated having biopsies with having fibrocystic breast disease. Again, no cancer link was established.

A final group of early studies showed that women diagnosed as having fibrocystic breast disease appeared to develop breast cancer at twice the rate of the general female population. It didn't take into account what pathological characteristics the biopsy showed, however. What's more, it didn't establish a link between having a biopsy on a particular breast and then that breast later developing cancer. In many cases, subjects had the right breast biopsied, then later developed cancer in the left breast, or vice versa.

Yet, in spite of the inconclusiveness of these early studies, almost all subsequent writing about fibrocystic breast disease was based on their unfounded conclusions.

Harmlessness Proven, Yet Myth Continues

Finally, in 1985, Dr. David Page of Vanderbilt University conducted an extensive study of over 10,000 biopsies. He discovered that none of the microorganisms associated with fibrocystic breast disease had any connection to cancer — with one exception. He established a link between the presence of *atypical hyperplasia* (which, by the way, is very rare) and an increased breast cancer risk.

A year later, in 1986, the College of American Pathologists made a formal announcement stating that fibrocystic breast disease does not increase the risk of developing cancer. Still, the myth that fibrocystic breast disease is a precursor to cancer lives on.

Questions and Answers

Q. Why do I never see any data on cancer survival rates past five years?

A. Cancer survival rates are measured by the five-year standard because for most cancers, survival rates tend to level off after five years.

The main exception to this general rule is breast cancer, for which survival rates continue to decline. According to the American Cancer Society, the overall five-year breast cancer survival rate, regardless of initial diagnosis (localized, regional or distant spread), is 73 percent; the overall 10-year survival rate is 63 percent; and the overall 15-year survival rate is 56 percent.

Since most women still pursue only conventional surgery, chemotherapy, and/or radiation treatment for breast cancer, boosting these survival rates higher is a very realistic possibility. Studies show that less conventional treatments such as improving nutrition and joining support groups are also effective in combatting breast cancer. And even Dr. Susan Love, one of the nation's foremost authorities on breast cancer, encourages breast cancer patients to investigate alternative treatments. It would be interesting to see survival statistics on conventional vs. alternative vs. combined conventional and alternative treatment, but none are yet available.

Q. Why should I try to reduce my disease risks when so many disease-causing genes are being discovered?

A. The presence of a defective gene does not automatically imply that a person will develop a particular disease — such as obesity or breast cancer — rather, *gene expression* can be strongly influenced by external factors.

Recent advances in gene research do not take into account the far more important factors in disease causation, such as nutrition and lifestyle.

Dr. T. Colin Campbell, a Cornell University nutritional biochemist, says, "More important than knowing which genes cause which disease is knowing how to influence those genes by dietary and lifestyle practices. So even if you suspect you may have a disease-prone gene, you may be able to suppress its expression with good health habits.

Unfortunately, failure to recognize that a gene's expression can be prevented through dietary and lifestyle practices can lead to an attitude of fatalism, the idea that genes alone determine health. And the results can be truly tragic.

Every once in a while we hear of young women who have had perfectly healthy breasts removed because of fear of a family history of breast cancer — without considering dietary and lifestyle changes as the powerful disease-fighting alternatives they truly are. For example, soy beans and foods made from them (tofu, etc.) contain genistein. It is very similar structurally to estradiol, binds to estrogen receptor sites, and acts like tamoxifen in fighting estrogen-sensitive breast cancer development and recurrence.

In addition, genistein inhibits new blood vessel growth, in turn further inhibiting tumor growth. Researchers believe these are key reasons why breast cancer development and recurrence rates are significantly lower in many Asian countries than here. Not because of genetics, but because of much higher soy consumption.

By ignoring proven ways to influence our health, much of the recent gene research has told only part of the story. Perhaps a better way to view a defective gene is as already having one strike against you — this doesn't mean you will definitely strike out. Follow good diet and lifestyle practices and you may avert a strike-out with a bad gene. Plus, you may also spare yourself countless other health problems.

Q. Does a high level of stress increase breast cancer risk?

A. We know of no studies that have addressed this question, but believe it is certainly one of the most important of all. We do know that women with breast cancer who join support groups as part of their treatment have longer average survival rates than women who don't. One of the main functions of these support groups is stress reduction. Numerous studies have also established a significant link between high stress levels and numerous other diseases, including cancer in general and heart disease. This is because stress significantly weakens the immune system — which includes our body's ability to prevent cancer development. In view of these facts, there's an excellent possibility that women with lower stress levels also have lower breast cancer rates. More importantly, stress reduction is one of the most important steps you can take to prevent disease in general.

Other Cancer Threats

Colon Cancer: More Widespread Than Breast Cancer, Yet Easier to Avoid

Statistics show slightly more women than men are expected to lose their lives to colorectal cancer in 1997. Plus, colorectal cancer has a much higher mortality rate than even breast cancer. In fact, "deaths from colorectal cancer are second only to deaths caused by lung cancer, the number one cause of male and female cancer deaths in the nation," says Dr. John J. Lynch, associate medical director of the Washington Cancer Institute at Washington Hospital Center.

Rosemary and Breast Cancer

We know that the results from animal studies do not always translate into similar results for humans, but an interesting study published in the *Journal of Nutrition* showed that the herb rosemary kept normal cells from mutating into cancer cells in the breast tissue of rats. One reason for this, the authors of the study believe, could be an antioxidant found in rosemary called rosmanol.

Rosemary contains a number of other chemicals that may contribute to this anti-tumor protection. But don't think you can sprinkle a little rosemary on your chicken or add it to your vinegar and eat whatever you like. Rats who were on a low-fat diet with rosemary had fewer tumors than rats on a high-fat diet. And for now, we don't know how much rosemary would be helpful to add to your diet. But using it a little more freely in your cooking sounds like a good idea for added antioxidant protection if you like it's flavor.

Sakamoto, Kazuko, PhD, et al, Penn State Univ., *Journal of Nutrition*, May 1996.

Still, many people aren't aware of the prevalence and deadliness of colorectal cancer. Perhaps in large part because many people are uncomfortable talking about it. This embarrassment, however, is literally killing us. Like breast cancer, colorectal cancer can be prevented with a healthy diet and regular exercise. In addition, regular screening can result in early detection which increases chances for survival. But only 37 percent of colorectal cancers are discovered at an early, localized stage compared to an 85 percent early detection rate for breast cancer.

This bleak outlook would change, however, if we would follow the new screening guidelines of the American Cancer Society. For men and women 50 years old or more, the new guidelines recommend asymptomatic people of average risk for colorectal cancer get a fecal occult blood test (hemoccult) annually to check for any signs of cancer or pre-cancerous polyps. Simply removing any benign polyps eliminates the possibility of them becoming cancerous.

In addition, the ACS recommends the same population have a digital rectal exam and a flexible sigmoidoscopy every five years to check the lower bowel or instead, have a total colon examination by colonoscopy every ten years or double-contrast barium enema every five to ten years. A New England Journal of Medicine study by J. V. Selby, shows flexible sigmoidoscopy screenings alone could reduce colorectal cancer deaths by up to 60 percent. But statistics show only 7 percent of Americans have ever had the procedure. (Yes, we know it's unpleasant. But it could help you avoid advanced-stage colorectal cancer treatment down the road, which would be much worse.)

Ovarian Cancer Risks

Too much sun significantly increases the risk of skin cancer. Yet too little sun can increase other health risks, including breast and intestinal cancer risks. Now a new study has linked a lack of sun to increased risk of ovarian cancer. Apparently women between the ages of 45 and 54 who live in the northern U.S. were five times more likely to die from ovarian cancer than women in sunnier, southern states, according to findings by researchers at the University of California at San Diego. They believe these increased risks are due to lower vitamin D intake from less sun exposure. Vitamin D has also been linked to lower rates of osteoporosis since it helps the body absorb calcium into the bones. If you live in an area that doesn't get much sun, you might consider vitamin D supplements, especially during the winter.

In another study, this one by researchers at Boston's Brigham and Women's Hospital, tricyclic depressants such as Elavil, and benzodiazepine tranquilizers such as Valium and Halcion were found to increase the risk of ovarian cancer twofold. Women who used these drugs before age 50 had an increased risk of up to 3.5 times higher. This was a preliminary study, so more research on this will likely be underway soon.

Fight Cancer With Green Tea

The next time St. Patrick's Day comes around we'd like to suggest you try an alternative beverage to green beer — green tea. We further strongly recommend it as a year-round alternative to coffee. Green tea, a drink made from the unfermented buds and first two leaves of the tea bush, *Camellia sinensis*, is a drink we've talked about in the past, and for good reason.

Green tea contains antioxidants called polyphenols that destroy free radicals — chemicals that harm healthy cells — and drinking this tea may even help prevent and shrink tumors. In addition, green tea contains a substance called epigallocatechin gallate, which is believed to protect against cancer.

Some researchers found that women who drank green tea regularly reduced their risk for pancreatic cancer by 47 percent, colon cancer by 33 percent, and rectal cancer by 43 percent! Polyphenols and other substances in green tea also show an inhibiting effect against cancer of the stomach, liver, skin, and lung.

The recent interest in green tea's disease-fighting ability stems from a state in central Japan known as Shizouka Prefecture, a tea-producing region. Health officials there noticed that residents had an exceptionally low incidence of cancer, and after ruling out every other factor, concluded that the low cancer rates were a benefit of extra high levels of green tea consumption — about 10 small Japanese tea cupfuls daily.

The Shizoukans also use the tea leaves only once, unlike other Japanese who often brew several pots of tea from the same leaves. The single-brew practice enables Shizoukans to consume more healthful nutrients per cup of tea.

Black tea, which is just made of fermented green tea leaves, also contains antioxidants, but has six times less. This is the result of chemical changes caused by the processing of black tea. A cup of green tea is packed with healthy stuff, as more than 35 percent of the weight of green tea leaves are comprised of these beneficial polyphenols. Green tea is also a good source of folic acid, which offers powerful protection against heart disease by breaking down harmful homocysteine.

Researchers also believe the health benefits of green tea may be more broad-based, offering general protection against numerous health threats. It appears to help lower blood pressure and cholesterol levels, help stabilize blood sugar, and kill decay-causing bacteria. Indeed, Japanese men, in spite high smoking rates, have the lowest rate of heart disease in the world (even lower than French men), plus a surprisingly low rate of lung cancer.

The polyphenols in green tea also seem to suppress excessive accumulation of fat and decrease fat in obese people. It seems to be most effective when you drink a cup of green tea before you exercise. Green tea does contains caffeine, just like coffee, but it has much less (40-60 mg compared with 75-110 mg in coffee). While the amount of caffeine consumed by moderate to heavy coffee drinkers has been associated with health problems like osteoporosis, gall bladder pain, heartburn, and ulcers, green tea has not.

We recommend drinking two to three cups of green tea daily. This is the amount that studies have associated with health benefits. And instead of just drinking green tea on St. Patrick's day, we suggest drinking at least two to three cups of green tea daily for a week or more. If you regularly drink coffee, black tea, or soda, try drinking green tea instead. You will have no withdrawal symptoms, because green tea contains caffeine. In addition to adding a healthy, nutrient-dense beverage to your diet, this will give you a chance to see whether coffee, black tea, or soda are adversely affecting your health. We strongly suspect that there are many more adverse affects than have been documented to date, including coffee adversely affecting some cases of varicose veins.

If you want or need to avoid caffeine entirely, there is a simple method you can use to eliminate most of the caffeine in green tea. Take a tea bag or the loose tea in a teapot or tea infusor and steep it in boiling water for 30 seconds. Remove the tea from your teapot or cup and throw away the liquid. Using the same tea bag or loose tea, make another cup or pot, allowing the beverage to steep a full minute or more. Since most caffeine is released in hot water during the first 30 seconds, you are left now with the benefits of green tea with little or no caffeine. St. Patrick's Day or any day, remember to think green and to drink green. Green tea, that is!

Chapter 6

Unnecessary Surgeries and Drugs

I've seen it so many times: A patient goes into surgery thinking that a miracle was about to be performed, only to be disappointed when the "miracle" is much less than expected. While many forms of modern surgery are truly miraculous, there are countless procedures that have *not* been proven to be completely necessary or beneficial. And yet, we insist upon putting ourselves through torture.

That's where this chapter comes into the picture. Many of us go through needless operations or take unwarranted drugs because we don't know any better. Hopefully, the following information will help you avoid unnecessary surgeries and drugs.

Hysterectomy

How a Hysterectomy Affects Your Sex Life

Each year, approximately 665,000 American women have hysterectomies — and the average age of the patients is just under 43 years.

For the majority of women who undergo this procedure, sexual behavior will only be affected during the recovery period. If you've yet to consider how a hysterectomy will impact your sex life, here's a brief review of what might be in store.

After Surgery

Most hysterectomy patients are instructed to wait at least six weeks before resuming intercourse. By this time, sufficient healing has taken place to have intercourse.

In the meantime, however, it is usually advised that a woman engage in other, less physically demanding forms of sexual expression. These can include hugging, kissing, cuddling, and various means of stimulating one's partner, which don't cause the recovering patient discomfort. Around two weeks after surgery, clitoral stimulation to orgasm without intercourse can begin.

Vaginal tenderness may continue up to 12 weeks after surgery. Still, as a general rule, it's okay to resume intercourse around the six week mark. If you experience some discomfort, take advantage of positions that minimize the trouble.

Depending on the specifics of a woman's surgery and other individual factors, timetables for resuming various levels of sexual activity may vary. It is important for the patient to discuss these issues with her physician. And in the event satisfactory answers are not offered, a second opinion is in order. Oftentimes nurses can provide valuable information.

Most women who have hysterectomies, around 83 percent according to one study, report that the quality of their sex lives is as good or better after their surgeries than it was before.

When Problems Arise

Although a large percent of hysterectomy patients experience no decline in sex life quality, with 665,000 such surgeries a year, the remaining 17 percent adds up to over 113,000 women annually whose sex lives are adversely affected.

But the trouble isn't just with patients who experience a direct negative impact from the surgery. A 1985 study revealed that after a hysterectomy, two out of 12 husbands found their wives less sexually desirable.

When sex lives do go awry after a hysterectomy, obstacles can often be overcome by the patient herself or with professional help. The key is to take action as soon as a problem presents itself. Most problems are usually the result of one, or a combination, of the following:

● **Decreased Desire for Sex:** Twenty to 30 percent of all hysterectomies include removal of the ovaries which are a major source of testosterone and estrogen. In animal studies, this loss results in decreased sexual desire. In many women, estrogen replacement therapy is effective in restoring the woman's sex drive.

In other cases, a decreased desire for sex can be caused by psychological factors. These most commonly include feelings of grief, and sometimes depression. These feelings are usually temporary and normal. They result from the patient experiencing loss as a result of the surgery: Loss of sexual identity, loss of menstrual rhythmicity, and loss of reproductive ability. In many instances these feelings resolve themselves as the woman confronts them — working through a grieving period and also realizing that her feminine identify is founded on more lasting elements such as personality and accomplishments. Otherwise, outside counseling can be helpful in overcoming more stubborn feelings of loss.

● **Altered Anatomy:** Loss of the uterus can also affect sexual response. During arousal and orgasm, the uterus enlarges slightly and elevates within the pelvis, which in turn increases the amount of space in the vaginal canal and results in a physical urge for intercourse. Once the uterus is gone this phenomenon ceases to occur and is missed by some women.

During deep penile thrusting, it is also common for a woman to feel the uterus move internally. This sensation, as well, is no longer possible. Also, uterine contractions, which are a characteristic of orgasm, cease to occur.

In the event the absence of any of these uterine sensations interferes with a woman's sexual response, she is advised to refocus on other stimulating sensations to assist in arousal.

● **Vaginal Dryness:** Another common detractor from sexual pleasure after a hysterectomy (as well as menopause) is vaginal dryness. Natural lubrication normally takes place as a result of increased blood circulation around the vaginal walls during arousal. After a hysterectomy, however, lubrication may not be forthcoming. This can occur as the result of loss of estrogen (if ovaries were removed), decreased sexual desire, or postoperative discomfort. The easiest way to overcome this scenario is to use a water-based lubricant.

● **Tissue Damage:** Some women experience decreased sexual response as the result of scar tissue that forms in the vagina after a hysterectomy. This scar tissue is not as sensitive and doesn't engorge and stretch as well as other genital tissue during arousal and climax.

● **Nerve Damage:** Hysterectomies that involve more than the removal of the uterus and ovaries can also result in nerve damage. For this reason, many women experience postoperative numbness. Oftentimes this numbness disappears within several weeks, after initial healing has taken place. In the event of permanent nerve damage, many women still retain the ability to have an orgasm. To do so, however, some women must shift the focus of their arousal to new aspects of sexual stimulation.

● **Fear of Painful Intercourse:** In some women, postoperative tenderness, vaginal dryness and other changes can lead to a fear of painful intercourse. This can result in a condition called vaginismus in which the vagina literally shuts down: vaginal muscles become tense, tighten up and make it difficult if not impossible to insert a penis. The best solution, of course, is to overcome the primary cause. For example, try a lubricant if vaginal dryness seems to be a problem.

The most important thing for a hysterectomy patient to remember is that after the recovery period, chances are her sex life will be as good or better than before. If a problem does arise, it is likely that it can be overcome. Perhaps with one of the simple strategies mentioned above or with professional help.

Q. I have uterine fibroids and my doctor says the only sure cure is hysterectomy. Is this a good idea?

A. Although hysterectomy may be the only sure cure for fibroids, it isn't necessarily a good idea.

Physicians frequently recommend hysterectomy as a treatment for fibroids — especially for women who do not want more children. In fact, uterine fibroids are the most commonly listed reason for hysterectomy. But that doesn't mean that a hysterectomy is the best solution. There are a number of worthwhile alternatives to consider trying first.

The better course of action may be no treatment. Fibroids are benign masses and therefore, are perfectly harmless in and of themselves. They are also very common and occur in about 40 percent of all women. So if you have been feeling that there is something uniquely wrong with you, there isn't. You are a member of a very large minority. Most of these women have smaller fibroids and are usually symptom-free. So if the fibroids aren't bothering you, there's no reason to bother yourself with a course of treatment.

Fibroids can cause problems, however, and may require treatment as a result. These problems include heavy bleeding that may cause obstruction, severe pain, or harmful interference with other organs. Still, hysterectomy is not inevitable and should be used only as a last resort. Here are some other treatments you may want to pursue initially.

First, you should know that the growth of fibroids can be stimulated by pregnancy or taking birth control pills, so if yours have recently grown following either of these two scenarios, the situation may easily remedy itself after pregnancy or if you discontinue the pills. The fibroids may then shrink once your hormone levels adjust back to normal. Menopause will also deactivate fibroid growth. So if you suspect you are approaching this transition, again, you may want to sit tight and do nothing.

In some cases, it may also be possible to shrink fibroids through diet. Strategies include cutting down on animal fat, and increasing your intake of fiber, vitamins A, E, C with bioflavonoids, zinc, copper, and iodine. Avoiding commercial meat, dairy, and egg products, to which hormones are added, may help as well.

Hormone therapy can assist in shrinking fibroids, but only temporarily. Hormone therapy must be discontinued after six months, after which the fibroids tend to grow back.

There are a number of non-hysterectomy surgery options, too. Occasionally, a D and C procedure will work. Plus, there are other surgical procedures to remove fibroids and still leave the uterus intact.

These include myomectomy and hysteroscopic resection. Still, approximately 10 percent of the time, new fibroids will grow after the surgery.

In the case of the final option, hysterectomy, it is advisable to see a doctor other than your own for an objective second opinion (and perhaps even a third). Then make your own decision. And decide to have a hysterectomy only if *you* are convinced that it is the best choice.

What Women Don't — and Do — Tell Each Other About Hysterectomy
by Genevieve Carminati*

It was probably within the first year after I was hysterectomized, or shortly past then, that I received a phone call from my distressed older sister. I was probably only 26, which would have made her only 27 years old. She told me that the latest fertility specialist she had consulted, a

* Genevieve Carminati is a counselor and board member of the HERS (Hysterectomy Educational Resources and Services) Foundation. She has written extensively concerning the personal and political aspects of hysterectomy.

woman gynecologist, had alarmed her with a frightening diagnosis. "You have a large tumor in your cervix," the doctor had warned. "You need a hysterectomy right away."

I am ashamed to admit that an indescribable and scary excitement that bordered on delight began to spread through my chest, my throat. I was, though worried about my sister, practically beaming as I stood in my kitchen listening to her frantic voice. "Look," I advised, "you'd better listen to that doctor. You don't want to take any chances with something so serious."

But she wouldn't buy any of it.

I couldn't understand why at the time I felt so disappointed in her. But why should I want that for someone I loved so dearly? It wasn't as if I didn't know what it would mean for her; I had only to look at what a horror it had been, and was, for me. Did I want her to have to endure what I was experiencing since having my sex organs excised; the fatigue, the insomnia, the panic attacks and anxiety, the pain, the loss of sexual feeling, and on and on?

Several years later at a HERS Foundation conference I attended, women asked questions and shared information and experiences in an open forum. One obviously distraught woman stood up and asked the group, "Why didn't my friends tell me the truth about what would happen to me if I went through with this surgery? Why didn't they tell me the truth that the surgery would destroy my life and leave me with a whole new set of medical problems that will never go away! I feel as if my friends were as responsible for what happened as the doctor who wielded the knife! How can women lie to other women this way?"

A sad, tired, and angry woman rose in the crowd. "Why didn't your friends tell you? I'll tell you why. For the same reason that my friends didn't tell me — and the same reason I won't tell my friends the truth. When women ask me what it's been like for me since my hysterectomy, I smile and tell them, 'Fine. Great. Best decision I ever made. Have one. You'll feel better.' And why? Why would I do such a cruel and deceptive thing? Because I want these women to be like me. I don't want them to be healthy while I have to live my life — *the rest of my entire life* — in a state of pain and regret."

Misery loves company, I realize now, explains only a part of why women don't always tell each other what they know about hysterectomy. The whole system is set up to keep women from talking about their experiences. We "know," though we may have no idea where we picked up this knowledge, that any woman who has trouble of any kind following a hysterectomy is just "crazy." Most physicians let us know individually prior to our surgery that any post-hysterectomy problems we encounter will be "all in our heads," that well adjusted women do fine after the surgery; hysterical women have problems. We are set up.

So we stay silent, and we convince ourselves that other things are to blame for our post-hysterectomy problems. This prevents us from talking to our doctors and having them judge us crazy.

Which brings up another reason why women aren't always honest about their post-hysterectomy experiences: Women don't necessarily recognize that what they are experiencing is a result of being hysterectomized. When a friend or relative asks how a woman is feeling since her hysterectomy, and that woman knows she isn't bleeding anymore and isn't worried anymore about the condition for which she had the surgery, she may answer, "Great! Never better!"

Is she suffering from loss of sexual feeling? Perhaps, but she figures sex just becomes less enjoyable as we get older, doesn't it? Is she more tired than ever? Well, yes, she can barely get through the workday in order to drag herself home and to bed for the remainder of the day, but that's probably because she doesn't get enough exercise, she may think, or, well, she's not 25 anymore, right? Maybe she has begun to suffer from bone and joint pain since the surgery, but has been told that she is developing arthritis, and even men get that. Or perhaps her marriage is in a distressed state, but well, she convinces herself, nothing is guaranteed to last forever, is it?

Maybe the women we ask to tell us how they're doing since their hysterectomy simply don't know how to answer us. Maybe they don't know how they're doing because they were never made aware of what they could expect as a result of this surgery and how this sur-gery could change their lives, their bodies, their minds, their spirits.

Maybe women think they are telling us the truth when they say, "Never better! Never felt better in my life!" because they don't know that what we are asking them is how do they really feel, totally. Not if their incisions have healed well. Knowing what I know now, even knowing what I knew then, I can't imagine how I'd have been able to endure the responsibility of being the woman who finally convinced her beloved sister to be hysterectomized.

Elective Hysterectomies Are

Five Times Riskier

Women who opt for hysterectomies to treat benign ovarian tumors or cysts run a five times greater risk of developing complications than women who simply have the noncancerous growths removed, according to a recently published University of California, Los Angeles study.

Complications from these elective surgeries included infections, bowel obstruction and blood clots. One woman in the study died of blood clot complications, according to Joseph Gambone, lead author of the study and an associate professor of medicine at UCLA.

Such results should come as no surprise, says Dr. Dan Matz, an obstetrician-gynecologist and past director at the Northridge Hospital Medical Center. "If you do more surgery, you can expect more complications." The study included 100 women who had hysterectomies to treat benign ovarian tumors or cysts, of whom 28 suffered complications. And 100 women who had only the benign masses removed, of whom only five suffered complications.

In addition, women in the incidental hysterectomy group lost twice as much blood and remained hospitalized an average of three days longer.

Still, up to 45,000 hysterectomies annually (10 percent of the U.S. total) are performed in association with removing benign masses, said Gambone. Although the uterus is uninvolved, it is removed anyway for the purpose of eliminating the future possibility of uterine cancer development.

"Should you remove the uterus with no medical reason, just because you are already inside the pelvis? My personal response is no," added Matz.

Another study of almost 1,000 cases of ovarian tumors with low malignancy potential suggests that removal of both ovaries, plus the uterus, when an ovarian tumor is discovered results in nearly as many complications and deaths from the treatment itself as from the tumors, says Cornelia Trimble, MD, of the Johns Hopkins School of Medicine. Therefore, when the tumor is limited to one ovary, she also recommends less radical treatment — removing the affected ovary or only the tumor — and no further treatment.

New Treatment Avoids Hysterectomy for Fibroids

Fibroid tumors are found in over 30 percent of women between the ages of 35 and 55, and more than half of the 750,000 to 800,000 hysterectomies performed each year in the U. S. are for fibroids.

Many fibroids are asymptomatic, or symptoms are mild enough that no treatment is needed. Others, however, cause pain, pressure, abnormal bleeding, urinary and bowel problems, and pain during intercourse. Does this mean a hysterectomy is in order?

Absolutely not, says Dr. Ernst Bartsich, associate professor of obstetrics/gynecology at the Department of Obstetrics and Gynecology at the New York Hospital-Cornell Medical Center. It offers a new technique called myolyosis, an outpatient procedure that preserves the uterus and a woman's ability to have children.

"Today, there is a long way to go before arriving at a decision to have a total hysterectomy for fibroids," he says. He points out that a routine hysterectomy for fibroid tumors of the uterus is an unacceptable practice. In addition to myolyosis, other surgical options to hysterectomy include submucous resection, a viable treatment for many small fibroids; myomectomy, a major surgical procedure that does leave the uterus intact in most cases; and supercervical hysterectomy, a hysterectomy in which the cervix is left intact.

Of course, it's always best to avoid surgery entirely when possible, and often it is with fibroids. We know there is a connection between estrogen and fibroids, because these benign tumors stop growing and often shrink at menopause when our estrogen levels drop. Lifestyle changes to reduce estrogen levels may shrink fibroids sufficiently to avoid surgery.

Lifestyle improvement may also help, such as a better-quality diet and stress-reduction. For even more information on alternative remedies, we recommend Dr. Susan Lark's book *Fibroid Tumors and Endometriosis* (priced at $16.95, to order, call 1-800-841-2665).

"Every woman's situation is unique," says Dr. Bartsich. "It's important for each woman to get a complete evaluation and carefully review all the options before deciding what treatment is best for her." We agree, a uterus is too important to lose in all but the most dire of circumstances.

Plastic Surgery

A nose job may leave a patient with more than a pleasing profile. But did you know that it may also leave a person sexually disabled for life! WHAT??? Apparently, there is a tiny organ in the nose called the vomeronasal which contains sensory cells that interact with pheromones. In the course of remodeling a nose, a surgeon may unwittingly remove it. In experiments with young mice, this has resulted in significantly delayed adolescence, failure of ovaries to mature, and lifetime failure to mate. That's just one example of the dangers that lurk ahead in the world of plastic surgery.

Plastic Surgery's Most Dangerous Procedures

"It seems as if new plastic surgery procedures crop up like weeds," says Dr. William Rosenblatt, a New York cosmetic surgeon and former president of the New York County Medical Society. "Some are excellent, but some represent meaningless hype generated by surgeons who, in competing for patients, want to attach their name to a unique surgery or surgical technique. And some are genuinely dangerous. Here is a case of 'consumer beware.'"

Dr. Rosenblatt advises would-be plastic surgery patients that "there are a host of 'hot' new procedures touted by the media that are either too new, too useless, or frankly too dangerous. The problem is that patients often don't know the difference between hype and sound advice — nor are they expected to — and it is far too easy for a surgeon trying to promote himself to take advantage of that." In light of this, Dr. Rosenblatt analyzes the following examples of procedures he considers high on his "think twice" list:

Autologous Breast Augmentation

Touted as breast augmentation without implants, this is a double procedure that entails both liposuction of a given area (usually the hips, thighs, or abdomen) and reinjection of suctioned fat into the breasts. Surgeons have used the present silicone implant scare to perpetuate the alleged safety of this procedure.

The Problem: "Every aspect of this procedure presents problems," says Dr. Rosenblatt. "Fat, once transplanted, is eventually reabsorbed by the body." In autologous breast augmentation, this occurs in a matter of months, and the procedure must be repeated over and over again to be effective. More important is that as the fat re-absorbs, it leaves calcification. This occurs as a result of the autologous fat transplant and indicates a pre-cancerous lesion. Because of this, a biopsy, which is costly and stressful, is always indicated.

Endoscopic Procedure to Reduce Frown Lines

Deep vertical creases between the eyebrows give patients an 'angry' or 'depressed' look. These creases, located in the corrugator muscle, are often the first signs of aging on a young face and occur as early as the 20s. Classically, the only way a plastic surgeon could get to these muscles in order to resect them to improve or flatten the creases was through brow lift surgery. Brow lift features a long incision in the hairline and the elevation of forehead skin in order to reach this muscle group.

Now, a new technique utilizes an endoscope, an instrument used to view and subsequently treat the body surgically through small incisions (in this case using three small stab wounds at the hairline), to resect the muscle. This rids patients of the unwanted creases, takes about an hour, and is performed on an outpatient basis.

The Problem: "While this procedure is not dangerous," says Rosenblatt, "it may or may not be very effective and plays on long-standing public opinion that a brow lift, with a longer incision, is a serious or debilitating surgical procedure. Untrue. A brow lift incision is hidden in the scalp. It is invisible and heals quickly and usually without complication. Following a brow lift, patients normally return to activities within a week."

Also, brow lift surgery offers many bonuses that the endoscopic procedure doesn't: In addition to erasing the crease in the corrugator muscle, a brow lift will raise a drooping brow line, tighten upper eyelids, and improve deep horizontal forehead creases and crow's feet. The endoscopic procedure is designed only to resect corrugator muscle and, because of the tiny tunnels the instrument provides, the surgeon may or may not even be able to adequately resect the muscle. On cost and time basis, the endoscopic procedure and a brow lift are parallel. This is especially important for the patient who believes, wrongly, that a brow lift is similar to a face lift and can take up to four hours to perform: The surgery takes about an hour.

Endoscopic Breast Augmentation

Like the frown line surgery, the plus here is that the procedure inserts saline breast implants without the classic scars under the breast, around the nipple, or under the arm. Instead of a direct approach, a wider endoscope is inserted into the navel, and empty plastic implant sacs are tunneled up to the breasts. The implants are then filled with saline solution to increase breast volume to the desired size.

The Problem: "The problem here is control in terms of even and appropriate placement of the implants," says Dr. Rosenblatt. "Whenever a surgeon is working from a distant location — approaching the breast through the naval or abdomen, there is always risk of uneven results. This surgery is promoted to alleviate scars on, under, or around the breasts, but direct incisions for implants are usually only two inches long and are nearly invisible within six months to a year after surgery. Why risk asymmetrical placement of the implants when such a small scar is at stake?"

In addition, patients should be aware that all endoscopic procedures in plastic surgery are relatively new. Complete data on their effectiveness and safety will not be available for several years.

Autologous/Non-Autologous Combined Injectable Substances

These new injectable substances, which come by many names, combine non-autologous collagen or fibril with a patient's own blood or fat in an effort to prevent rejection by the body and to achieve more long-lasting results. They have been used to soften deep facial wrinkles and creases, to augment lips, and to augment areas of the nose in patients who have suffered nasal injury or deformity or in whom primary rhinoplasty has overcorrected the septum or nasal tip.

The Problem: "Once again, this is more of a gimmick than a serious advance in cosmetic surgery," says Rosenblatt. "The fact of the matter is that rejection can't be prevented. And that's not really an issue because all patients who receive injectable substances should be tested twice and again on a yearly basis for allergic reaction before proceeding with the procedure."

The real issue here is that combining injectable substances with the body's own blood or fat does not contribute to longer lasting results. Liquid substances are always reabsorbed by the body.

Lip Augmentation

There are many procedures to augment lips. Among them are collagen injection, Gore-Tex implants (yes — the same stuff that's in your ski jacket — it's been used successfully in repairing human heart valves for years), lip advancement, and autologous lip implant or transplant. Lots of choices. And lots of hassles if you choose wrong.

The Problems (and Solutions): "Collagen is a big problem," says Rosenblatt. "It was the first plastic surgical application for lips during the mid- to late-1980s and remains a popular procedure. But it's outdated and over- popularized. Collagen doesn't work well in the lips. It doesn't last long because we use our lips so much that the collagen tends to flatten in a month or two. Collagen was not designed for use in areas as large or as active as the upper or lower lip. Gore-Tex is also troublesome — it never feels truly natural and tissue can harden around it." That's the bad news.

The better news for lip augmentation is lip advancement, a surgical procedure that advances top or bottom lips through an incision along the vermillion border of the lip and the subsequent removal of a strip of skin above it, creating a larger or fuller lip. A second option in lip augmentation is autologous implant or transplant. During this procedure, the surgeon places a strip of skin harvested from behind the ear or in another inconspicuous place under the skin of the lips. The rich blood supply to the lips and mouth keeps the transplanted skin functional, and skin is usually not reabsorbed by the body.

Laser Surgery —
The Worst Case of Plastic Surgery Hype

Lasers, lasers everywhere and not a single one of them works better than conventional surgical instruments in plastic surgery. "With the possible exception of hemangiomas or blood vessel anomalies, the use of lasers in plastic surgery is the ultimate example of hype," says Rosenblatt.

"The public is taught to think of lasers as a magic bullet, but in cosmetic surgery this just isn't true. A laser is a beam of light that serves the same purpose as a scalpel. It is no safer or riskier than conventional surgical instruments, and lasers, like scalpels, are only as effective as the surgeon using them."

On that note, Dr. Rosenblatt advises patients to observe the golden rule of cosmetic surgery: "If it sounds too good to be true, chances are, it probably is."

Breast Enlargement by Hypnosis Brings Charges

And finally, a practitioner who offers breast enlargement by hypnosis has been accused of false advertising by the Kentucky attorney general. Steve Marek operates a counseling service in Lexington and claims that some women suppress their breast growth during puberty. By regressing them back to puberty and asking them to release their repression, theoretically, their breasts may enlarge. The lawsuit charges that there is no medical evidence to support Marek's claim, and asks $2,000 for each willful violation of the state's Consumer Protection Act. There are also reports of this scam taking place in California and Florida.

The FDA's Dirty Drug Secrets

Imagine a large-scale disaster. One in which 140,000 American lives are lost in a single year. What could possibly cause such a massive slaughter? A hurricane? An earthquake? A terrorist attack?

Actually, none of the above. The answer is prescription drugs. And it's only a small picture of the real destruction being caused by these FDA-approved medications.

In addition to 140,000 deaths annually, prescription drugs cause an estimated one million injuries severe enough to require hospitalization each year, and another estimated two million injuries that occur during hospital care. These statistics translate into a lifetime risk of 1.3 in 5 of being severely injured by a prescription drug. And these are conservative estimates.

Worst of all, it appears that most prescription drug injuries and deaths are completely preventable. A 1997 study of over 2,000 hospital patients in Salt Lake City found that 50 percent of adverse drug reactions among hospital patients could have been prevented. A 1987 study found that 72 percent of preventable hospitalizations involved prescription drugs. Another study found that 75 percent of those who died due to complications from antibiotic use (yes, antibiotics can kill) should never have been prescribed antibiotics at all. It's also highly possible that the majority who suffer drug-related injuries and deaths are female, since approximately 75 of all doctor office visits are made by women.

Most consumers are surprised to discover how little safety testing is actually required prior to a drug's approval. In his book, *Deadly Medicine*, Thomas J. Moore describes the highly limited and inadequate testing process for one class of drugs, Class I antiarrhythmic drugs, in great detail. It's a real page-turner and reads like a suspense novel, complete with rigging of small-scale pre-approval testing and high-ranking scientists who were working for both drug companies and the FDA, and oftentimes as researchers and medical school professors as well. Unfortunately, this story isn't fiction. It's incredibly well-documented.

In the end, larger, post-approval study results suggest that the six largest-selling Class 1 drugs had caused between 40,000 and 70,000 accidental deaths during 1989 and 1990 alone. Throughout the years, it is clear that hundreds of thousands died prematurely, an estimate in which two insiders, marquee professors* Raymond Leon Woosley, Jr., MD, PhD and Joel Morganroth, MD, concurred in interviews. Still, most of these drugs continue to be available.

---

*Marquee Professors are medical school doctors who are authorities in the field; their names are on medical journal articles and textbook chapters; and they often sit on important FDA or other committees. Drug companies use them as consultants and to promote their drugs. Morganroth, for example, was affiliated with Hahnemann University and the University of Pennsylvania, is the founder of the National Cardiovascular Research Center, and from 1986 to 1988 did consulting work for drug companies Hoffman-LaRoche, Wyeth Laboratories, Merck, Burroughs Wellcome, Schering-Plough, Merrill-Dow, DuPont, Squibb, Upjohn, Sterling-Winthrop, ICI Pharmaceuticals, Bristol-Myers, and 3M. In the same three-year period, he published 69 medical articles, often combining drug company and scientific work. Woosley, at the time of the study was a Vanderbilt University professor, FDA advisory committee member, and had also worked with most of the major drug companies.

The findings of the Cardiac Arrhythmia Suppression Trial (or CAST), resulted in one of the drugs, Tambocor (made by 3M), being taken off the market by the FDA. Another drug, Enkaid, was voluntarily withdrawn by maker Bristol-Myers. Although CAST findings made news headlines, the media never learned of the extent of the disaster and the story fell quietly by the wayside. A congressional hearing on how the Tambocor disaster was allowed to happen ended when the chairman, Representative Ted Weiss, died. No other member of Congress stepped in to take his place. A follow-up trial to CAST, called CAST II, was abruptly terminated early-on, after more than nearly six times as many patients taking Ethmozine (supposed to be the most benign drug of the class) had died as those taking a placebo. The FDA never insisted that maker DuPont disclose this finding to doctors. Shortly thereafter, DuPont sold Ethmozine to another company, Berlex. Today, Ethmozine and many other Class I antiarrhythmic drugs (used for arrhythmia or irregular heart beating) are still available and widely prescribed in spite of a lack of further testing to confirm whether they actually prevent or promote cardiac arrest.

Trading One Health Problem for Others, Including Cancer

There is virtually no such thing as a risk-free prescription drug. Of the 50 top-sellers, seven can cause addiction, 18 are highly toxic, 18 have known cancer risks, and 25 have known cardiac (heart) risks.

Of the 3,200 FDA-approved prescription drugs, 42 percent cause cancer in animals. Only 211 produced no birth or other defects when tested in rabbits and rats. And only six of these are considered safe for use during pregnancy (based on evidence from human studies) — five are thyroid hormone replacement drugs and the sixth is a prescription form of folic acid. Cholesterol-lowering and cancer chemotherapy drugs are especially carcinogenic, with 83 and 87 percent respectively causing cancer when tested in animals.

What do all these statistics mean to you? According to drug safety expert Thomas J. Moore, author of *Deadly Medicine* and *Prescription for Disaster*, "prescription drugs ought to be ranked second only to cigarette smoking as a cancer hazard." He further states, "there is no such thing as a safe drug."

Skeptics like to shoot down the cancer risk of prescription drugs by claiming that animal testing uses doses much higher than humans would be taking. Not necessarily. Salmon calcitonin, used long-term for osteoporosis prevention, causes cancer in rats and mice at lower doses. This suggests that an important consideration in deciding whether to use a prescription drug, is whether you will be taking it short- or long-term. In general, the longer a known carcinogen is used, the higher the risk of cancer. Ditto for the risk of other adverse effects.

For maximum safety, however, always evaluate drugs on an individual basis. The deadliness of various prescription drugs differs tremendously. For example, the standard dosage for the popular antihistamine Hismanal is one tablet daily. One extra tablet, however, can cause deadly cardiac arrest.

Here are some other popular drugs that aren't nearly as safe as widespread use might lead you to believe:

Anti-Arrhythmics (drugs for irregular heartbeats). Research suggests most class 1 drugs in this category cause more deadly cardiac arrests than they prevent. A safer option might be up to 1,000 mg daily of magnesium, which helps regulate heartbeats.

Anti-inflammatories. These include aspirin, ibuprofen, and Naprosyn. It's estimated that their long-term use results in roughly 70,000 hospitalizations annually, mostly due to damage caused to the stomach lining. Alternatives include magnesium and vitamin B_6 supplements for headache relief.

Estrogen Supplements. A Harvard study of 65,000 nurses found a 71 percent higher incidence of breast cancer among women aged 60 to 65 who'd taken supplemental estrogen for five or more years. That's a lot of risk to take for a drug category that has yet to be solidly proven to prevent heart disease and offers only second-rate protection against osteoporosis. Safer options include a healthy lifestyle and more phytoestrogens (plant source estrogens), such as soy foods. For more information on hormone supplements, see chpater 4.

Calcium Channel Blockers (including Procardia and Cardizem). The FDA based approval of these drugs on their short-term ability to lower blood pressure. With long term use, however, study after study of persons taking various calcium channel blockers has produced a large number of unexplained deaths and other medical problems. Safer alternatives include weight loss, stress reduction, and magnesium supplements (up to 1,000 mg/day).

Ritalin. Nearly 10 percent of school-age boys (and a lower percent of girls) take Ritalin because they have been deemed hyperactive (in medical jargon, attention deficit disorder or ADD). Short-term testing shows Ritalin calms disruptive children and results in better attention and retention. Long-term safety testing, however, is lacking. It has been shown to cause cancer in animals and addiction in adults. Limited study to date also indicates that Ritalin can cause both temporary and irreversible brain damage in children. If you know a child taking Ritalin, urge the parents to contact the Developmental Delay Registry at 301-654-0944, for other treatment options.

Serotonin Reuptake Inhibitors. These include Prozac and its close chemical relatives, Paxil and Zoloft. Initially, manufacturer Eli Lilly claimed that Prozac was nearly free of side effects. However, during a 10-year period, FDA reports associated it with more serious adverse reactions, hospitalizations, and deaths than any other drug. Non-drug solutions include amino acid therapy and nutritional therapies, as outlined in *Potatoes Not Prozac* by Kathleen Desmaisons, ($23 from Simon & Schuster).

There Are Many Others

If a drug you are taking is not reviewed above, don't assume it's safe. Read about the adverse side effects in the *Physicians Desk Reference* (your doctor and local library should have one) and in the drug's patient package insert, available from your pharmacist. Although what you read may tempt you to stop taking a prescribed drug, it is not advisable (and can even be dangerous) to do so on your own. Instead, consult with your doctor and get a second opinion from a doctor who specializes in non-drug therapies. To find such a doctor in your area, call the American Holistic Health Association at 714-779-6152.

Empty Reassurances and a Lack of Overall Safety

Perhaps one of the most disturbing aspects of prescription drug use is what happens when one comes into question. There is a well-documented pattern of doing nothing and/or reassuring patients that a harmful drug is perfectly safe to take. For example, in 1989, when the National Institutes of Health released evidence that widely used class 1 antiarrhythmic drugs were killing more patients than they saved, 75 percent of cardiologists weren't willing to warn patients to whom they had already prescribed the drugs. Worse yet, 21 percent of cardiologists surveyed continued prescribing these deadly drugs. By now, well over 100,000 have likely died needlessly from taking these drugs.

Who's to Blame?

Even when the public is well aware of a potential catastrophe, there is a disturbing lack of caution. Back in 1983, the recent discovery of the HIV virus created alarm among hemophiliacs, (or "bleeders"). They take clot-promoting drugs made from human blood. The National Hemophilia Foundation (NHF) issued an advisory to the nation's 14,000 hemophiliacs that stated: "The NHF AIDS task force ... urges hemophiliacs to maintain use of clotting factor...." In less than 21 months, over 7,000 of these individuals were infected with HIV!

There's also a disturbing lack of safety monitoring throughout the entire system. For starters, drug recalls occur weekly. Plus, the government doesn't track prescription drug injuries or even deaths. Instead, the secondary cause of death is recorded. For example, among the above mentioned hemophiliacs who have died, the cause of death was usually recorded as AIDS-related deaths, not deaths caused by an HIV-infected clotting factor.

The first step for most people on their way to a prescription drug injury or death, however, is taken when walking into the doctor's office. One survey discovered that, although all drugs have risks of harmful reactions or side effects, 60 percent of patients received a prescription that wouldn't benefit them. *A Harvard study found that 46 percent of the time, this happened because patients demanded drugs.* Around 25 percent of the doctors in the same study admitted prescribing drugs for a sort of placebo effect, because it "had a positive psychological effect on the patients and their families." This Harvard study concluded that about 75 percent of doctors intentionally gave ineffective drugs to appease or trick patients, while around 25 percent of doctors were misinformed about the drugs they were prescribing.

There are dispensing mistakes as well. Another study found that over 30 percent of pharmacies filled two prescriptions with potentially lethal interactions.

Finally, there's you, the patient. Most believe their prescriptions are perfectly safe. But a 1994 FDA survey found that more than 70 percent of patients reported their doctor telling them nothing about the potential harmful effects of prescribed drugs — when all but a few of the thousands on the market do have risks.

Many consumers assume that our highly regulated medical system will quickly identify drugs that do more harm than good. Not necessarily. Once on the market, adverse reactions to a drug (or a combination of drugs) frequently go unreported by doctors, even though such reports are the FDA's main means of learning about adverse reactions. Fewer than a third of doctors are even familiar with the FDA's form for making official reports. "Most doctors don't know the system exists," says Dr. Brian L Strom, who heads up the department of biostatistics and epidemiology at the University of Pennsylvania.

In addition, many adverse reactions simply go unnoticed by doctors. In the case of Class I antiarrhythmic drugs, they are supposed to prevent cardiac arrest in high-risk patients. So when these patients have a cardiac arrest, most doctors assume that it would have happened anyway.

In the case of fen-phen and Redux, "No one had initially thought to examine patients' hearts because animal studies had never revealed heart abnormalities and heart valve defects are not normally associated with drug use," said Dr. Michael A. Friedman, the acting commissioner of the FDA. Even then, human chemistry is very different than that of mice and other animals, so we need our medical decision makers to remember that animal testing can't always predict our response. Also, until recently, the diet drugs were used only short-term, so data on the safety of the newer trend of long-term use was not yet available.

Will prescription drugs be safer in the future? A new bill on Food and Drug Administration modernization is expected to pass both the House and the Senate, and be approved by the White House soon. It will allow even faster approval of new medicines for AIDS, cancer, and other diseases. This, of course, might also mean even less safety testing prior to making new drugs available.

What Can You Do to Protect Yourself?

As always, ask your doctor about studies showing the safety and effectiveness of any drug you're considering taking. Look for data that applies to your gender, age group, and length of time you anticipate taking the drug and other considerations that might affect how you respond to the drug.

Also look for bottom-line results, such as a lower incidence of death. A surrogate endpoint, such as lower blood pressure, lower cholesterol, or less arrhythmia, doesn't always decrease the risk of death. In the case of Class I Antiarrhythmic Drugs, the only two drugs that were comprehensively studied decreased arrhythmia (a risk factor for cardiac arrest), but also increased the incidence of deadly cardiac arrests. Ask your doctor to share with you the known side effects of a drug (or look them up yourself at the local library), as reported in the *Physicians Desk Reference*. Then weigh these risks against the potential benefit, while keeping in mind that many drugs have unknown and even unreported side effects.

In the final analysis, you may come to the same conclusion as we have around here: It's usually best to try safer alternative treatments first, and prescription drugs only as a last resort. This includes replacing as many prescription drugs as you can with natural, safer alternatives, such as reducing calcium intake and increasing magnesium intake to regulate irregular heart beating. This strategy of natural treatments first, may save you from suffering adverse drug side effects as well as adverse drug interactions.

The best way to protect yourself against the numerous safety shortfalls is to just say no to prescription (and over-the-counter) drugs whenever possible.

Proceeding With Caution

The purpose of this article is not to alarm you, but alert you to the fact that prescription drug use poses serious, and often needless, risk of injury and death.

The solution is not to become an extremist and swear off drugs. But rather, to exercise maximum caution before proceeding. This should include a thorough review of the actual health risk present, a proposed drug therapy's specific health benefits and risks, and the potential benefits and risks of safer alternative therapies. Other considerations should include the fact that many conditions will eventually clear on their own. And many will experience the placebo effect. In fact, approximately 30 percent of patients improve with phony sugar pills.

Some drugs have dramatic life-saving effects, such as insulin, without which persons with juvenile-onset diabetes die within weeks. Most drugs, however, have much less dramatic health benefits — with many drugs benefitting fewer than one percent of users when prescribed appropriately. Oftentimes, when all things are fully considered, non-drug treatments suddenly emerge as the sanest, soundest, and most obvious choices.

Here are just a few of the many drugs you need to be extremely cautious with while using:

Reevaluating Premarin
by Alan R. Gaby, MD*

Many postmenopausal women are advised to take Premarin to treat menopausal hot flashes and other menopausal symptoms and to prevent osteoporosis and heart disease. Although the safety and effectiveness of estrogen replacement therapy has been vigorously debated, one factor has been generally overlooked; namely, the treatment of mares that are involved in the manufacturing of Premarin.

Premarin, as the name indicates, is derived from the urine of pregnant mares (PREgnant MARes' urINe). According to the package insert, Premarin is derived "exclusively from natural sources." However, the way the horses are treated in the production process is anything but "natural." To produce the drug, horses are impregnated, then fitted with a rubber collection device so that all of their urine can be collected. According to the group People for the Ethical Treatment of Animals (PETA), the mares are then forced to stand on concrete floors in stalls measuring just eight feet long and three and a half to five feet wide for most of their 11-month pregnancies. Allowing the mares to roam about in the pasture might result in the loss of precious urine, which is worth $17 a gallon to Wyeth-Ayerst Laboratories, the makers of Premarin.

For more than six months, the restrictive stalls prevent the mares from taking more than one step in any direction. The physical confinement also makes it impossible for them to turn around or even to lie down properly. This type of treatment sometimes causes the mares to become crippled, and deaths have been reported. No doubt, there are other more subtle, but still traumatic, consequences of this imprisonment. Shortly after

---

Reprinted from the *Townsend Letter for Doctors*. Dr. Gaby is the author of *Preventing and Reversing Osteoporosis* (Prima, 1994).

giving birth the mares are reimpregnated, separated from their foals, and put back on the production line. As far as the offspring are concerned, the majority are sold to feedlots, where they are fattened and then slaughtered; others are killed immediately or kept as replacements for worn-out mares.

In the past there were few alternatives to Premarin. Today, however, synthetic 17-beta estradiol is available in the form of tablets, transdermal patches, and vaginal creams. Less carcinogenic forms of estrogen such as estriol or triple estrogen (80 percent estriol, 10 percent each of estrone and estradiol, invented by Jonathan Wright, MD) are available through compounding pharmacists. These formulations resemble the estrogen secreted by the human ovary more closely than the conjugated estrogens derived from horse urine. In addition, these forms of estrogen do not carry the energetic fingerprint of animal cruelty.

Estrogen replacement therapy may not be necessary as often as most doctors believe. Natural progesterone and DHEA, both secreted by the ovary, may turn out to be more effective than estrogen for osteoporosis prevention. In addition, claims that estrogen replacement prevents heart disease are based entirely on questionable retrospective studies and may turn out to be incorrect. Furthermore, the possibility that estrogen causes breast cancer must be kept in mind, although estriol and triple estrogen are probably less likely to be carcinogenic.

Although estrogen replacement therapy is of great benefit to some women, others who are taking estrogen probably do not need it. On medical grounds, the advisability of taking estrogen should be reevaluated for many women. If estrogen treatment is indicated, a formulation should be chosen that does not cause unnecessary cruelty to animals. There is no need for estrogen replacement therapy to be accompanied by the guilt of torturing innocent animals.

Tamoxifen or Soy?

Tamoxifen is an anti-estrogenic drug used to protect women who are at high risk for breast cancer, since it is believed that long-time exposure to estrogen increases a woman's risk for this disease. However, like all medications, tamoxifen has side effects. In doses of 20 mg/day it increases the risk of endometrial cancer by five times. It has been shown to cause liver tumors in rats, suggesting that we look at its effects on the livers of women.

Women at high risk for breast cancer who opt not to take tamoxifen have another option: soy protein. A recent study showed that premenopausal women in their 20s were given 60 grams of soy protein a day. The effects on their hormones and duration of their menstrual cycle was similar to those found with women on tamoxifen. Additionally, Japanese and Chinese women who eat a high soy diet have a low rate of breast cancer.

The Laxative Habit

Recently, we received a heartbreaking letter from a subscriber about her sister who has had a lifelong habit of abusing laxatives. With the recent news that one of the ingredients of several popular laxatives, phenolphthalein, is carcinogenic, her sister was worried about getting cancer. (These products, including Ex-Lax, Evacu-U-lax, and Feen-a-mint, have since been reformulated.)

The sister has used laxatives for so many years that she can't have bowel movements without them. Many older persons, concerned with maintaining bowel regularity, also become laxative dependent. We are worried about more health problems than cancer from relying on laxatives.

Why Women Use Laxatives

Some women use laxatives as a form of weight control. They think, erroneously, that by eliminating wastes in their colon they can keep their weight down. All they are doing is getting rid of the body's wastes more quickly. For women who have abdominal bloating, laxatives are tempting. They can often reduce bloating by reducing the bulk in their intestines. But bloating is often a sign of poor digestion. Perhaps digestive enzymes (either pancreatic or plant enzymes found in health food stores) would eliminate their bloating.

Some women use laxatives because they help them feel "empty and clean" inside, rather than full. One recent client of mine who abused laxatives was reluctant to stop them because she didn't want to feel full. She reduced her meal portions, took enzymes for a few weeks, and felt better without her laxatives than with them.

Then there are women who use laxatives because they're constipated. Often, constipation is a sign of a magnesium deficiency, and the only side effect of taking a lot of magnesium is soft, sometimes even runny, stools. We'll talk about using magnesium later. Constipation can also come from not eating enough fiber or not drinking enough water. Both are needed to bulk up and soften the stools so they can be easily eliminated. Exercise is another component if you're constipated. It's one way of tonifying all your muscles, including your intestines. Without tone, the intestines don't contract and push stools along to be eliminated.

Why the Laxative Habit Is Harmful

There are various kinds of laxatives, each having different properties. Some produce bulk, allowing the stools to become larger. As the stools touch the walls of the intestines, pressure builds up and they can be more easily passed — if there is tone in the intestinal muscles. Some laxatives are lubricants, which soften the stools. But the majority of the most popular laxatives — both over-the-counter and herbal — are irritants and stimulants. These act like sandpaper inside the colon, or repeatedly stimulate the nerves inside the colon. Taken occasionally, they should not cause any harm. Taken regularly, they irritate the lining of the intestines or cause a dependency on the stimulation. All laxatives reduce the natural tone in the muscles of the intestines and cause people to depend on them in order to have bowel movements.

Which Laxatives Do What?

Bulking agents like Metamucil and psyllium seed husks help the stools retain water. This, in turn, helps them get larger and often softer. But you need to drink plenty of water along with them. These bulk-forming laxatives can contribute to obstructions in the esophagus as well as the small and large intestines if the stools don't pass completely.

Many bulking agents contain sugar, which can cause an imbalance of friendly to unfriendly bacteria in your intestines (sugar feeds the bad guys). These bad bacteria, or pathogens, can contribute to gas and bloating.

Lubricants like mineral oil soften the stools, but they also can decrease your absorption of important oil-soluble nutrients, like vitamins

A and E, and essential fatty acids. Large doses of mineral oil can also cause anal leakage, anal itching, and hemorrhoids.

Irritants and stimulants have a direct effect on the walls of the intestines, stimulating the nerves and blood vessels. Irritants act like sandpaper and can eventually reduce the sensitivity of these nerves, causing the intestines to lose their tone. Without tone, the muscles of the intestines can't contract on their own and help expel the stool without help.

Irritating laxatives include glycerin suppositories, castor oil, and two herbs — cascara sagrada and senna. Natural herbal laxatives are no safer than others. Any laxatives that are used regularly, which cause irritation or stimulate the nerves in the intestines, can cause problems.

Safer Alternatives

Magnesium, especially magnesium citrate and oxide, helps attract water to the intestines, building pressure and allowing solid wastes to soften and be expelled more naturally. Overuse of magnesium, especially magnesium sulfate, could affect your fluid and electrolyte (sodium, potassium, chloride) levels. A number of alternative physicians believe the majority of people are magnesium-deficient.

Magnesium is found in nuts and legumes, as well as in whole grains. It is also a mineral our bodies need more of when we're under stress. We suggest taking enough magnesium to soften the stools, but not more than 1,000 mg daily, and only as much as you need for regular bowel movements. Be sure to drink plenty of fluids when you take magnesium.

Two kinds of fiber help with normal elimination — soluble and insoluble. Insoluble fiber, like wheat bran and the fiber found in celery, act like sandpaper. Don't overdo it. The idea is not to substitute Metamucil with wheat bran. Add soluble fiber, like rice bran (found in brown rice), oat bran (from oatmeal), and the skin on all beans, and you reduce the irritation in the intestines as well as increase the bulk of your stools. This means eating plenty of vegetables, beans (take Beano or other enzymes if they give you gas), whole grains (like brown rice and oats), and some fresh fruit with its skin.

Exercise helps you move all your muscles. As you move by walking, dancing, or swimming, even the muscles in your small and large intestines move. You want to tone your muscles, and this means more than firming up your biceps and triceps. It means bringing the ability to contract and relax back into your intestines after frequent laxative use. Get into the exercise habit, and work on your abdominal muscles to help firm out the outside of your tummy. Inside are your intestines. When you work your abdominals, you're toning your colon.

Psychological intervention is sometimes necessary for breaking a laxative habit, especially if it's related to body image, poor self-esteem, or other psychological issues. In such cases, laxative abuse is part of an eating disorder and requires developing a new outlook as well as new habits.

It seems harmless to use laxatives, but it's not. And bloating, gas, constipation, or infrequent bowel movements are often a sign that something's wrong. Look for the problem, then look for a natural solution. Modifying your diet, regular exercise, drinking more water, and perhaps taking digestive enzymes is the safest way to eliminate the problems caused by laxative abuse.

Colloidal Minerals: A Marketing Scam That Could Hurt You

Millions of dollars of nutritional supplements are sold each year by pharmaceutical companies and companies that manufacture or package vitamins, minerals, and herbs. The competition is fierce and we have become the victims of numerous unsubstantiated claims.

Take a look at a new form of supplement — colloidal minerals. There is not a single study to support the claims being made about them that Alexander Schauss, PhD, could find after searching through 40 years of databases containing almost 30 million papers.

Many claims about the benefits of nutritional supplements are based on scientific studies published in peer-reviewed medical and nutritional journals. Some studies are conducted on laboratory animals, others on people. While studies on people are best, we should at least be able to find some to back up the statements shouting the benefits of a supplement.

What Are Colloidal Minerals?

Simply put, colloidal minerals are minerals found in clay, then are freed from the clay when it's mixed with water. The kind and amount of minerals depends on what is in the type of clay it comes from.

Montmorillonite, bentonite, kaolinite, and vermiculite (used by gardeners as a growing medium) are forms of clay from which colloidal minerals are taken. These clays also contain aluminum silicates, and large amounts of aluminum have been linked to Alzheimer's disease in numerous scientific studies.

Some colloidal minerals have from 1,800 to 4,400 parts per million of aluminum. Foods usually have less than 10. Can taking colloidal minerals over a long period of time contribute to Alzheimer's? No one knows. There are no studies showing it's safe to use them. If the claims about colloidal minerals being very highly absorbed are true, they could flood the body with toxic levels of aluminum! Magnesium protects the brain from getting too much aluminum, but colloidal minerals high in aluminum are low in magnesium.

Unsubstantiated Claims Can Be Harmful

Higher absorption? According to Dr. Schauss, "When an element is soluble, it is usually more absorbable than when it is insoluble. Calling the product colloidal makes the product insoluble by definition. If it were a soluble solution, it could not be colloidal."

Still, vendors of colloidal minerals are saying they have superior absorption to other mineral forms — 10 to 12 times greater than minerals in tablets or capsules. Some claim their colloidal minerals are 95 percent absorbed. But there is not one study to back up these claims. If colloidal minerals really were absorbed as well as the people who sell them say, you could be getting toxic amounts of them into your body.

Colloidal minerals are also said to be better absorbed because they are negatively charged. This is physically impossible, as doctors and physiologists well know, because the small intestine walls through which nutrients are absorbed are negatively charged. Try this experiment with two magnets. Put the negative side of one against the negative side of another. The two sides are repelled. If, indeed, colloidal minerals were negatively charged, the walls of the small intestines would keep them from being absorbed.

Colloidal minerals are "organic." Some companies even claim their colloidal minerals are superior to others because they are organic. But minerals, by definition, are inorganic. Can your body absorb them? Sure. Especially if you're low on that particular mineral. Your body comes equipped with a sophisticated process in your intestines that allows you to absorb inorganic minerals from the foods you eat and the water you drink.

All that "organic" colloidal minerals means is that the clay from which they come may contain some humus, which is organic material. This is another marketing ploy to fool you into thinking this product is superior.

What About the Dangers of Iodine?

If these claims weren't enough, colloidal minerals may also cause radiation contamination. Clay is highly absorptive, which is why montmorillonite is used in some intestinal cleansers. It is especially good in absorbing all forms of iodine. We know from studies in the 1960s that clay-humus soils absorb high levels of radioactive iodine from nuclear fallout. And nuclear testing is being done throughout the world. Some clays are old enough to have absorbed radioactive iodine-131 from decades past. Are the colloidal minerals being sold high in radioactive iodine-131? There are no laboratory analyses we know of that tell us. If they are, how long would it take before any long-term negative effects occurred? No one knows.

How Can These Claims Be Made?

You are probably not a doctor, scientist, or physiologist. Neither are the health food store personnel or sales people in multi-level marketing companies who sell colloidal minerals. And many doctors and health practitioners are too busy or lax to look for the substantiation behind claims of various products. Besides, some people swear by them.

Anecdotal stories boost the sales of products like colloidal minerals. Some people feel terrific after they take them. Why? There are several possible reasons. The first is called "the placebo effect." This is a phenomena — backed up with scientific studies — that says you can get positive results from a food, drug, nutritional supplement, hands-on healing, etc. for up to 30 days if you believe it will work. The placebo effect doesn't last forever.

But many stories told to health practitioners and passed along from person to person are due to this phenomena. If anything you're doing is working for you for one month, but not after that time, it may be due to the placebo effect, not the effectiveness of the substance or course of treatment you're taking.

Another reason some people may feel good after taking colloidal minerals is that people who need minerals will get some absorbed from this source. They will also get them from mineral-rich foods. When your body needs minerals you will absorb more of them from your foods and supplements than if your mineral levels are not low. This doesn't mean that colloidal minerals are either superior or safe, however.

How to Know if Colloidal Minerals *Are* Superior?

In time, many statements we find to be true today may be found false tomorrow. Or vice versa. Perhaps we will discover that colloidal minerals have something in them that makes them better than other forms of minerals.

For now, a manufacturer or distributor of colloidal minerals would need to show you and me a certificate of analysis from an independent laboratory stating that the product they're selling contains the minerals they say it has, along with the amounts of aluminum and radioactive iodine-131. Anecdotes and testimonials are not enough in an area where there is so little known, and where a product could be much more dangerous to take than beneficial.

Consulting Clinical & Microbiological Laboratory (CCML) is an independent lab in Portland, Oregon that tests the ability of colloidal minerals to inhibit the growth of various microorganisms. In one study, they tested five colloidal silver products. One showed no ability to stop the growth of microorganisms and, in fact, *was contaminated itself.* Other products varied greatly in their effectiveness. If you're going to take mineral supplements, take those that are citrates, chelates, or picolinates. At least they're safe.

Calcium Channel Blockers, Cancer, and What the Studies Really Say

It's easy to get swept away by media blitz, hype, and inaccuracy — especially when it comes to health matters. In fact, there is often more misinformation surrounding medical studies and natural remedies than truth. Part of the reason for this is that sensationalism sells. Another is that pharmaceutical companies spend billions of dollars advertising their products (historically more than is spent on research and development), and the media is often swayed by these massive advertising dollars.

Still another reason is that we just don't know as much about health matters as we'd like to. Even good medical studies have more holes in them than Swiss cheese, and holes don't sell newspapers, magazines, or advertisements for radio and TV shows. Take the recent study that proclaimed that calcium channel blockers cause cancer in older people.

Calcium channel blockers (CCB) are medications used to reduce contractions of the heart muscle. They are used for people with irregular heartbeat and angina. And they are the most widely prescribed medicine for high blood pressure. A recent observational study published in the *Lancet* showed that CCB increase a variety of cancers in people over 71 by interfering with signals given by calcium to cancer cells that limit their growth. The study also showed that people who took CCB had more heart disease and diabetes than those who did not. They were on more medications for heart disease and were hospitalized more often than people who didn't take these drugs.

So, this means calcium channel blockers are bad, right? Maybe, but not necessarily. Remember, this was an observational study, not a randomized, double-blind study. Doctors observed a number of connections that may be attributed to CCB and may not.

For instance, if you reduce the risk of getting one specific illness — especially if you're over the age of 70 — you increase the risk of getting another one. All the people who took CCB who did not get heart disease were more likely to get another big disease like cancer. Perhaps this was due, in some people, to the CCB. Perhaps it was just the next illness these people had been coming down with for many years. Knock out the heart disease and a slow-growing cancer you might otherwise never see gets the time it needs to grow. Maybe CCB do promote cancer, but the current tests for carcinogenicity might not be sophisticated enough to recognize these promoters.

What are some other limitations of this particular study? It was done on older people, so we don't know what CCB do in people who are younger. And because more people who took CCB were admitted to hospitals, they were in a setting where cancers could more easily have been detected than in people who didn't get more thorough examinations. The CCB that were used are called short-acting. Already there are other calcium channel blockers with slow-release formulations that may not cause the same problems.

From this and previous studies on CCB, we still don't know how harmful they are in relation to their usefulness. We do know that all drugs have some adverse reactions, and CCB may not be as safe or useful as many doctors believe. Large, clinical trial studies that could give us this information will not be completed for four more years. Meanwhile, we need to make decisions. Until there are large, random, double-blind studies, we still won't know. And as good as any study is, there are always gaps that cause us to stand back and say, "We don't know for sure."

Still other studies have linked CCB to an increased risk of angina, strokes, fatal heart attacks, and bleeding from the stomach and intestinal tract.

So pharmaceutical companies that make CCB and other medications will keep funding studies to show their drugs are more helpful than harmful. Meanwhile, the media repeatedly magnifies the risks attached to more natural, less expensive solutions — like magnesium.

Remember, the action of CCB is to keep calcium from getting into the smooth muscles of the heart and causing inappropriate contractions. Magnesium does that, too. Magnesium is a mineral that specifically relaxes muscles. It has become one of the first medications to be given to someone after they have had a heart attack. Why not use it preventively, instead of or prior to trying CCB? This would be especially prudent in view of the fact that the large majority of American women (and men) are magnesium deficient.

Just how harmful is magnesium in larger doses? Melvyn R. Werbach, MD, in his gigantic reference book, *Nutritional Influences on Illness, Second Edition* (Third Line Press, Tarzana, CA, 1996) shows no references at all for the harmful effects of magnesium.

Still, the media lashes out in spite of no good studies showing magnesium to be harmful. One doctor with a radio show who professes to be knowledgeable about nutrition pulled out a poorly designed and executed study on the dangers of magnesium. There are always poor studies to support any position. It is not the media's role to present inflammatory statements against either drugs or natural alternatives.

Do Your Homework

When looking at the harmful effects of any medication, first look to see if the studies were observational or random. Did doctors observe something about the cause and effect of drugs and a disease, or were some of the people in the study given the drug and others a placebo without anyone knowing which until the study was over?

Were the studies done on men, women, or both? Results will often vary. The way our bodies respond to medications and nutrients can be gender-specific. Studies done on men may not apply to you. What was the age of the participants? Are you in this age group? Would the results found tend to apply to you or your grandparents?

If you were going to get the worst side effect the study talks about, would that be okay? If not, what other options exist for you? You may find that vitamins, minerals, herbs, and other more natural substances have also been found to be beneficial, and with fewer side effects. As long as we really don't know enough about anything we put into our bodies, why not try more natural approaches first, where carcinogenicity and serious side effects are less frequently an issue?

You also have the ability to discuss other options with your doctor or health practitioner and take a combined approach. A change in diet and exercise, a few vitamins and minerals, and very low doses of a medication may work for you in place of high doses of numerous drugs.

Listening to the media, or taking the word of your doctor who may be highly influenced by the free samples and biased literature passed out by pharmaceutical companies may be the quickest, easiest way for you (as well as your doctor) to deal with a health problem. But you're stuck with the results they give you, and some may not be what you expect.

Do your homework and make the decision that gives the least harmful side effects. In the long run, it's worth the effort. Treatments that emphasize improved nutrition and exercise may even help prevent the development of other health problems.

Will Zocor Help You Be There?

by Alison Lapinski, RPh*

Lower your risk of death from heart disease by 42 percent. That's the big health benefit being proclaimed by the high-priced advertising campaign for the drug Zocor. The ads themselves play on one of the issues nearest and dearest our hearts: our grandchildren. They show pictures of older people playing with children under the headline, "It's your future. Be there."

This campaign includes fancy promotion banquets for doctors and pharmacists like me, four-page ads in *Reader's Digest* and other expensive magazine space, even prime-time television commercials. And it's working. Zocor is today's best-selling cholesterol drug, maybe the best-selling drug in the country. I'm well aware of this, because roughly half the prescriptions I fill these days are for Zocor.

But will it really help you be there as the ads suggest? Don't bet on it.

As a skeptical pharmacist, I've already attended Zocor banquets in my area. They're always at the most lavish restaurants; always with an open bar. The last one I attended included giant shrimp appetizers and lobster entrees. This meal consisted of nearly all high-cholesterol, high-fat foods, complete with creamy dips and plenty of butter for the lobster and bread. Yet only one of the doctors complained. He had already had a heart attack and wouldn't touch anything except green salad and red wine.

Perhaps the most interesting aspect of this dinner, though, was that Zocor's maker, Merck, is still urging doctors to prescribe Zocor for women, as if the seven-study review from last fall's *Annals of Surgery* never appeared! (The study found no correlation between high cholesterol and heart disease among women.) None of the doctors objected to this either.

The Side Effects of Zocor Aren't Pretty Either

Zocor or simvastatin lowers cholesterol by inhibiting the enzyme HMG-COA reductase, which our bodies need to make fat into cholesterol. By inhibiting this enzyme, the amounts of total cholesterol, LDL, and

Alison Lapinski is a pharmacist in Joliet, Illinois, and a consumer advocate for safer pharmaceutical choices.

triglycerides are reduced, while HDL increases. That would be great if that was the end of it. It's not! It's just the beginning....

Our bodies need cholesterol to make estrogen, progesterone, testosterone, DHEA, and other important hormones. By lowering cholesterol levels, Zocor also has the potential to lower our hormones to dangerously low levels. The package insert that comes with Zocor (which consumers receive on request only) reveals that Merck is fully aware of this. I know because the insert advises that women who are pregnant, breast-feeding, or thinking about becoming pregnant shouldn't take Zocor. Tinkering with the hormones of reproductive-age women can have serious consequences such as infertility, pregnancy complications, and can even result in nutritionally deficient breast milk. Yet the large majority of women who are taking Zocor are postmenopausal. What about their hormone balances?

As a pharmacist, I fill many prescriptions for women who take both Zocor and hormone supplements. Zocor may be creating the need for this extra estrogen and progestin. Yet there are scores of hormones in our bodies. What about the others? Without adequate cholesterol supplies, the body can't make enough of them, either.

I also have some serious concerns about the study, one single study, which Merck is using as the sole support for the Zocor health claims:

● First, the study was too short. Just 5.4 years, while Merck advocates life-time use of Zocor.

● Second, the study wasn't about people with only high cholesterol, whom Merck is targeting in its advertising. This was a study of 4,444 Scandinavian men and women with histories of high cholesterol and heart disease.

● Third, the study focused on mostly men. Of the 827 women who participated in the study, 420 took a placebo and only 407 took Zocor. That's too small of a group to make me comfortable about the findings. Especially in view of the serious side effects that were discovered.

● And fourth, the study wasn't just about the beneficial effects of using Zocor alone. It combined using Zocor and a low cholesterol diet. We don't really know how many of the 42 percent fewer deaths from heart disease were due to Zocor and how many were due to the diet.

Will Zocor Do for You What It Did for Them?

In view of these considerations, before someone starts (or continues) taking Zocor, I recommend taking a few minutes to answer these questions:

1. Are you male? If you aren't, it's highly doubtful lowering your cholesterol will lower your risk of death from heart disease.

2. Like the people in the study, can you stick with a low-cholesterol diet?

3. Is lowering your cholesterol worth risking the side effects of this drug? The study reported that side effects included cerebrovascular disorders, muscle weakness, trauma, elevated liver enzymes, suicide, and gastrointestinal system cancers. The latter three can indicate an impaired immune system. Not very promising. And side effects are bad enough that they caused six percent of the study participants (over 1 in 20) to drop out.

4. What are my other options? You already know a lot of them, such as more dietary fiber, garlic supplements, two to three cups of green tea daily, and our favorite mineral, magnesium — up to 1,000 mg a day.

The Italian and Meditation Solutions

Now here's the little-known Italian solution we use around here: Drink eight ounces of low-fat soy milk every day. We call it the Italian solution because it's based on a study by soy and cholesterol expert C. R. Sitori, from the University of Milan. He had patients like our husbands, whose cholesterol stayed high in spite of standard low-fat diets, replace animal protein in their diets with soy protein. After just three weeks, the patients showed an average 21 percent decrease in total cholesterol — about what you can expect with Zocor.

If you want to use soy protein like the study, you'll find it at a health food store and can add one to three tablespoons a day to a food or beverage. The taste is fairly bland so you'll hardly notice it. Plus, the only known side effects of soy foods are positive — such as extra protection against cancer. To know whether the Italian solution is working for you, get two home cholesterol test kits and check your level before you start, then three weeks later.

There's also the meditation solution. Years ago, a physiologist from the University of California at Los Angeles named R. Keith Wallace discovered that people who had been practicing TM (transcendental meditation) for at least 10 years experienced 80 percent less heart disease than those who didn't. No drug can come near to making this kind of claim. And even meditating daily for a few months will reduce stress levels and thus benefit your heart.

For maximum benefit combine several natural therapies. If you think drinking soy milk or eating soy protein powder or other soy foods and drinking green tea is silly, maybe you didn't know that Japanese men who consume these have the lowest heart-disease rate in the world. Lower than French men. Also, remember to consult with your doctor before discontinuing any medication, including Zocor.

Now here's one last thought: It's easy to get swept away in the cholesterol craze. And it's good to be health conscious. But we also need to keep our wits about us and remember that high cholesterol is not a death sentence. It is only one of many factors that increase the risk of heart disease. Other factors such as obesity, smoking, poor eating habits, high stress, and lack of exercise also affect our risk. And there's good news about these risk factors. They can be changed to lower our overall risk of dying from heart disease — without taking Zocor.

Chapter 7

Sex, Hygiene, and a Woman's Health

Once-a-Year Pap Smear Too Frequent?

Intervals between pap smears can be as long as five years and still have minimal effect on increasing a woman's health risks, according to researchers at Erasmus University in the Netherlands. In a recent study, they discovered that women between the ages of 35 and 64 who have a pap smear once every five years still reduce their risk of dying from cervical cancer by about 90 percent. Since the introduction of the Pap smear, cervical cancer mortality rates in the U.S. have declined from 14 to 4 per 100,000 women.

Pap smear frequency is a highly debated issue.

Until recently, gynecologists recommended them annually, while the American Cancer Society took a strong position that every three to five years was sufficient.

Then in 1985, the American College of Obstetricians and Gynecologists organized a task force to review Pap smear screening guidelines. The task force came up with a new recommendation. It suggests that a woman who has had three normal consecutive annual Pap smears can decrease the frequency according to "the discretion of her physician."

The American Cancer Society endorses this new stance. However, it was part of the task force. So it appears that the new position is a compromise between the previously diverse recommendations of gynecologists and the American Cancer Society.

Still, many gynecologists continue to recommend annual Pap smears for all their patients. This continues in spite of the fact that it has been shown that cervical dysplasia and cervical cancer are related to sexually transmitted diseases. Therefore, if a woman has had several years of negative tests, and is in a monogamous relationship, it is highly unlikely that she will develop either of these two diseases which are detected by Pap smears.

History of the Pap Smear

The Pap smear is named after the individual who discovered and popularized it, Dr. George N. Papanicolaou, who was born in the late 1800s on the Greek island of Euboea.

He attended the University of Athens at age 15, but was most interested in the humanities and playing the violin. It was only to please his domineering physician father that Papanicolaou went to medical school. He also received a PhD in Zoology. His thesis was about sex differentiation among water fleas.

Impulse Leads Papanicolaou to Pursue Research in U.S.

The early part of Dr. Papanicolaou's life was guided by impulse. After completing his formal education, Dr. Papanicolaou returned to Greece to pursue a career as a researcher. Instead, he promptly married and left for France, for a honeymoon and to find a job.

Soon, however, the Balkan war of 1912 to 1913 broke out and the couple returned to Greece. Dr. Papanicolaou served as a physician and met American volunteers who told him of plentiful opportunities in the United States. Without further investigation, Dr. Papanicolaou decided they should move to America. His father-in-law bought boat tickets for the pair — and the Papanicolaou's soon arrived at Ellis Island, in late 1913, with barely the $260 required to meet immigration requirements.

The only job Papanicolaou was able to find was selling carpets at Gimbels. His second day on the job, however, he ran into a fellow passenger from the trip to America. He was so embarrassed to be discovered selling rugs that he quickly quit and got hired in a laboratory at the New York Hospital.

Animal Rights Concerns Lead to First Pap Smears

By 1916, Dr. Papanicolaou was working as a researcher on a project that studied female guinea pig eggs. To collect the eggs, however, the guinea pigs had to be sacrificed. In addition, only eggs at a certain stage of development could be used, so many of the guinea pigs were destroyed unnecessarily.

To avoid this needless destruction of laboratory guinea pigs, Dr. Papanicolaou set out to study the menstrual cycle of guinea pigs in order to more accurately determine when would be the best time for egg gathering. He began introducing a nasal speculum into the vaginas of the guinea pigs, and eventually began scraping cells from the vaginas for microscopic examination. These were the "first" Pap smears.

In 1920, Dr. Papanicolaou began studying cell scrapings from the vagina and cervix in humans. He observed the irregularity of cervical cancer cells, began collecting data, and in 1928 he made a presentation of his results at a medical conference. His report was poorly received, however. The prevailing viewpoint at the time was that biopsy and tissue examination, rather than individual cell analysis, were the only ways to detect cancer cells.

Book and Personal Dedication
Finally Popularize Pap Smears

Not until the late '30s did Dr. Papanicolaou resume his cervical cancer studies. In 1942, a book entitled *Diagnosis of Uterine Cancer by the Vaginal Smear* was published. It featured highly detailed drawings of the various cells encountered on Pap smears. For the remainder of their lives, Dr. and Mrs. Papanicolaou worked teaching the new technique to other physicians and laboratory personnel — paving the way for worldwide availability of the Pap smear.

Dr. Papanicolaou received numerous awards and honors. In 1960, he was nominated for the Nobel Prize in Medicine. That same year, the Papanicolaou Cancer Research Institute in Miami was opened. After his death in 1962, two postage stamps were dedicated to him: one in 1973 in Greece and one in 1978 in the U.S.

Since 1941, the Pap smear has helped reduce the cervical cancer mortality rate from 14 per 100,000 females to a current rate of four per 100,000.

Beware of Douching Dangers

In view of the widespread prevalence and popularity of feminine hygiene products, it's especially easy to take the healthfulness and safety of douching for granted.

Numerous studies, however, suggest that douching on a regular basis is not nearly as safe as might be expected. An increased risk of ectopic (tubal) pregnancy, pelvic inflammatory disease (PID), and cervical cancer have all been linked to douching.

Health Risks of Douching

A study from 1990 that was published in the *New England Journal of Medicine* reported that women who douched three or more times a month had a 3 ½ times greater risk of developing pelvic inflammatory disease.

Another study, published by the *American Journal of Epidemiology*, linked douching to cervical cancer. This study examined the douching habits of nearly 750 women and found that those who douched more than once a week had nearly five times the risk of developing cervical cancer — regardless of the type of douching solution that was used. Researchers suspected that ingredients found in the douche solutions disrupted vaginal secretions and bacteria that normally protect against invasion by cancer causing microbes.

It is known for a fact that frequent douching (as well as the use of vaginal deodorants) can alter the acidic and alkaline balance of the vagina, and this can increase susceptibility to infections including sexually transmitted diseases. What's more, in the event that a douche bag or bottle is not thoroughly cleaned between uses, it can grow hostile bacteria. An unsuspecting doucher can then infect herself.

Benefits of Douching

Women who are prone to vaginal infections may be able to prevent them with *occasional* douching, and a plain water solution is often sufficient. Otherwise, a homemade solution of one or two tablespoons of vinegar in one quart of water, or a baking soda and water solution can be used. Herbal and other natural douche solutions can be used to treat vaginitis and other common vaginal conditions.

How To Douche

Precautions to take when douching include the following
- Use lukewarm water — barely warm enough for comfort.
- Clear the nozzle of air before inserting it into the vagina.
- Use low pressure when introducing the solution into the vagina. Douching is a simple rinsing procedure. High-pressure douching can accidentally force solution into the uterus and abdominal cavity.
- Never douche during pregnancy.

Myths About Douching

Some women believe that douching after intercourse can prevent the contraction of sexually transmitted diseases but, in most cases, it does not.

Nor can douching prevent conception. Even if a woman immediately races to the bathroom, some sperm will already have made their way into the uterus. Douching will then propel additional sperm into the uterus even as it rinses others out of the vaginal canal.

Douching is not necessary for good personal hygiene since the vagina naturally cleanses itself.

Sex: The Truth About the G Spot
Where did it go? Did it ever really exist?
Or were we duped?

If you've never experienced one of those highly acclaimed G spot orgasms, you're not alone. In fact, the majority of women haven't. What's more, you may not be missing out on much. A review of key literature that led up to the popularization of the G spot, as we know it today, suggests that it's more a matter of fiction than fact.

Back in 1950, an article appeared in the *International Journal of Sexology* titled "The Role of (the) Urethra in Female Orgasm." In the article, a gynecologist named Ernest Grafenberg described a sensitive spot along the urethra, which is imbedded in the front wall of the vagina. (The urethra is the passageway through which urine is voided from the bladder.)

At times, Grafenberg noted, this spot gushed clear transparent fluid from the urethra. Furthermore, he described the spot as one of "innumerable [erogenous] spots [which] are distributed all over the body, from where sexual satisfaction can be elicited." Nothing unique about that!

Media Puts Super Orgasm Spin on G Spot

Over 30 years later, in 1981, the stage was set for the G spot to gain its current notoriety as a producer of super orgasms. Three articles appeared in the *Journal of Sex Research* which related female orgasm with ejaculation to "the G Spot." The first article was merely a collection of anecdotes. The second was a study based on a single woman's G spot orgasm experience. The third article was based on reports from 47 women and included a description of how to find a G spot, noting that it was often necessary to press deeply into the tissue of the front vaginal wall to reach it.

The authors failed to note one very important point, however: The same spot they were describing was also the sensitive urethra spot that Grafenberg first described — in fact, it was called G spot after him. Therefore, it was debatable whether the spot in question was a point of true sexual stimulation, or rather a point at which the urinary system could be stimulated. Deep tissue manipulation might have actually stimulated the urinary system to the point of urine loss since the urethra is imbedded in the vaginal wall at the G spot location.

Suddenly the G spot was in the national spotlight as the giver of the ultimate orgasm. Within months, articles about the incredible G spot orgasms appeared in the *Philadelphia Inquirer, Omni*, and other major national publications. In September 1981, Beverly Whipple, one of the authors of the third article, appeared on the "Donahue" show. Whether the G spot was special or not to begin with, it was now — now that it was identified as the source of the ultimate female orgasm, complete with ejaculation!

G Spot Experts Ignore
Negative Research Results

G-spot experts wasted no time in further fueling the public's interest in it. Just a year later, Beverly Whipple, along with two other colleagues, authored a new book called *The G Spot and Other Recent Discoveries About Human Sexuality*. Shortly before this book was published, though, a fourth study was reported at a meeting of the Society of Sex Therapy and Research.

This study failed to confirm the existence of a unique spot which stimulated female ejaculation. It was also demonstrated that when a minority of female study participants did manage to stimulate a certain spot to the point of "ejaculation," the only fluid to be produced was urine. This study was conveniently *not* included in the book. So what scanty and questionable scientific evidence the authors of *The G Spot* did present to support its existence went undisputed.

During the next few years, the G spot enjoyed a tidal wave of primary media attention. And for women who couldn't manage to have G spot orgasms on their own, numerous special G spot vibrators were developed.

Yet the G spot failed to live up to its reputation with the general female public, as well as in numerous subsequent scientific studies. In one study which appeared in the *Journal of Sex and Marital Therapy* in 1984, only ten out of 27 women managed to produce G spot "ejaculation." Five of these women described the sensation they experienced as "almost agreeable sensations," but not sensations of sexual arousal or orgasm. And one participant repeatedly stressed that her "ejaculation" did not represent a sexual climax, but rather, something else.

But what else? Was the G spot an area that produced a true sexual orgasm? Or was it merely an area near the urethra that, when stimulated, produced an involuntary loss of urine?

Interest in G Spot Fades Away

Today, the popularity of the G spot seems to have fallen by the wayside. This has most likely happened because it has not lived up to the high expectations we were led to believe about it.

Many sexologists now regard the G spot as an extreme attempt to conform female sexuality to the male norm of ejaculation with orgasm. Others view it as a classic example of how incredibly effective the promise of heightened female sexual experience can be in producing television viewership and selling books, newspapers, magazines, and sex aids.

As for those of us who've yet to achieve the ultimate orgasm that the G spot is reputed to produce, we might not be missing out on much, if anything.

Birth Control

On the Pill? Change Your Diet!

Millions of women today use birth control pills for contraception, and other purposes as well. "The Pill," as it is commonly known, is also recommended by many doctors to reduce the risk of pelvic inflammatory disease (PID), reduce menstrual cramps, regulate women's menstrual cycles, and manage endometriosis (an often painful condition which occurs when some of the tissues that line the uterus get outside the uterus or attach to the ovaries or fallopian tubes).

While you may have heard reports, both pro and con, on the pill's effects, you probably haven't heard much about how it changes your need for certain nutrients. And it does. Whenever you take a medication over a long period of time (more than two to four weeks), you should consider the possibility that it is having an effect on your body's chemistry. If it uses up more vitamins or minerals you can simply adjust your diet to compensate. If you do nothing, you run the risk of having side effects somewhere down the line.

You may not create a disease or illness, but unnecessary water retention, breast tenderness, premenstrual depression, increased colds and flus, or fatigue can lower the quality of your life. Many doctors do not concern themselves with the slight deficiencies that can occur from using oral contraceptives. They are looking for illness or disease. But you can maximize your wellness by paying attention to your diet and making a few important changes.

Taking the pill regularly depletes your body of a number of B vitamins: B_6, B_{12}, biotin, and folic acid, as well as the mineral zinc. Vitamin C has been found to be lower in women who use oral contraceptives. Vitamin E, which helps prevent blood clots, is especially important, since taking the pill can result in your body having more estrogen than it needs — and women who have extra estrogen may be more prone to forming blood clots.

While taking oral contraceptives does not always lead to major nutrient deficiencies, you may find some symptoms associated with a lowered dose of these vitamins and minerals disappear when you modify your diet.

Here are the vitamin and mineral deficiencies to watch out for when taking the pill:

● **B$_6$** The pill uses up some of the B$_6$ in your body, and this depletion can lead to premenstrual depression, water retention, menstrual changes, and nausea. Meats and fish, whole grains like brown rice and whole wheat bread, and brewer's yeast, are all high in vitamin B$_6$.

● **B$_{12}$** Vitamin B$_{12}$ is also depleted when you take the pill, and this is a vitamin that is not particularly easy to absorb. Lean meats and fish are the best source for this nutrient which is found in very small quantities in vegetarian diets. If you are taking oral contraceptives, you may want to take a multivitamin or B-complex that includes B$_{12}$, rather than rely on diet alone. Since vitamin B$_{12}$ is absorbed in the large intestines, anyone on birth control pills who experiences intestinal problems like inflammatory bowel disease or excessive chronic gas should be checked by a physician for a B$_{12}$ deficiency.

● **Biotin** is another B vitamin often found low in women on the pill. Deficiency symptoms include fatigue (are you more tired now than before you began taking the pill?), dry hair or excessive hair loss, depression, and eczema. To compensate, include good quantities of brown rice and brewer's yeast in your diet. Egg yolks, high in fats, are also high in biotin.

● **Folic acid** deficiency can lead to anemia and is also associated with birth defects in the fetuses of pregnant women. Medical research suggests your folic acid levels should be normal before you become pregnant to prevent serious problems (such as neural tube defects) in a developing fetus. So if you're taking the pill and want to get pregnant eventually, keep your folic acid levels high now as well as later. Folic acid was named after the word "folate" which means leaf. It's found in dark green leafy vegetables and brewer's yeast. Because folic acid is more stable in dark, cool places and is destroyed easily at high temperatures, keep your veggies refrigerated until you're ready to use them, and cook them lightly using a medium flame.

● **Vitamin C** is plentiful in most fruits and vegetables. Citrus fruits, broccoli, kale, brussels sprouts, bell peppers of all colors, and potatoes are all particularly high in vitamin C. Since your body does not store vitamin C, which protects against colds and flu as well as infections, you want good amounts of this vitamin in your diet every day.

● **Vitamin E** is a fat-soluble vitamin that can help keep your estrogen levels normal and help prevent those blood clots that can come from having excessive estrogen. It also helps prevent miscarriages and increases fertility, which is important to consider if you eventually want to have children. The best sources for vitamin E are raw nuts and seeds, and vegetable oils. Use all oils sparingly in your diet, but concentrate on including almonds, filberts, and safflower oil — highest in this important vitamin.

● **Zinc** is a mineral which is depleted by the pill. A deficiency can be a contributing factor to fatigue, decreased alertness, and increased infections. Some foods high in zinc include grains like brown rice and bran flakes, chicken, turkey, and pumpkin seeds.

But the pill does not just create deficiencies, it also increases the absorption of calcium. This means you don't have to worry about getting enough calcium in your diet. Especially if you eat whole grains, broccoli, tofu (soy bean curd), and salmon. Or dairy foods, such as milk and yogurt, of course.

Antibiotics May Cause Birth Control Pills to Fail

Birth control pills work by elevating a woman's hormone levels. After antibiotics are used, however, women sometimes suffer from breakthrough bleeding. This is a sign of low circulating female hormone levels which can cause a lapse in the effectiveness of birth control pills.

Normally, helpful bacteria in your intestines act as "recycling centers" for hormones which the body has used, and subsequently dumped into your small and large intestines. About 60 percent of circulating female hormones end up here. Then, if conditions are normal, intestinal bacteria break these hormones down into pieces which the body can reuse.

Unfortunately, antibiotics are known to destroy certain helpful bacteria that are responsible for this recycling process. When the population of these bacteria is reduced, recycling rates drop and greater amounts of female hormones are lost through excretion. The end result: women taking birth control pills may end up with undesirably low hormone levels which may promote conception instead of prevent it.

An increased risk of osteoporosis is another possible consequence of the reduction of hormone recycling, since estrogen supports bone density.

You can take action, however, to minimize the disruptive effect that antibiotics can have on your body's hormone recycling process.

It would seem that one way to do this would be to eat plain, unsweetened yogurt or to drink acidophilus milk in order to replenish your population of helpful bacteria. However, your large intestines, where most of the estrogen recycling takes place, require different varieties of microorganisms.

Therefore, if you are on the birth control pill, and have taken antibiotics or have been on chemotherapy, you may want to replenish your body's stores of these hormone recycling bacteria: acidophilus, bifidobacteria, and bulgaricum.

Because these bacteria are living organisms, the highest quality supplements are usually found in the refrigerated sections of health food stores (in powder or capsule form), where the temperature is low enough to keep these bacteria alive and healthy.

Stop Birth Control Pills Before Surgery

Johns Hopkins University gynecologist Jean Anderson says that women who take the pill and know they will be having surgery should switch to another type of contraception four to six weeks prior to the surgery. Apparently, women who take the pill may be at increased risk of forming dangerous blood clots because of the role estrogen plays in blood clotting.

Menses

How to Avoid Menstrual Cramps

If you have menstrual cramps and your doctor can't find anything wrong, you have more options than taking painkiller medication. In fact, the ones you take that are advertised to eliminate menstrual cramps may actually be contributing to the cramps you have next month.

The pain associated with menstrual cramps, also known as primary dysmenorrhea, varies from individual to individual and from day to day. It can be sharp pains or a dull ache and they can be steady or come in waves. The cramps usually appear in association with the beginning of menstruation, and generally last for a day or two. Some women are bedridden every month with menstrual cramps. Others take a lot of over-the-counter medication to alleviate them. Neither situation is necessary.

When you understand their cause, you can correct cramps at their source, rather than treat the pain which is merely a symptom.

Primary cramps are caused by an excess of certain chemicals that regulate our cell functions. These chemicals are called prostaglandins and are produced during ovulation and continue to be made until menstruation begins.

The particular prostaglandins responsible for primary menstrual cramps are called PGE2, PGF1, and PGF2, and are manufactured in your body from arachidonic acid. Arachidonic acid is a substance found in animal fats and some cooking fats like margarine. Women with severe menstrual cramps have much higher levels of PGE2 than women without them.

The Body's Solution to Cramps

Your body produces another type of prostaglandin, however, which is helpful to your system: PGE1. This chemical reduces inflammation, helps lower cholesterol levels, and relaxes smooth muscles like the uterus. If you have eliminated most or all fats from your diet in an effort to stay slim, you may be increasing your risk for menstrual cramps. By eliminating even vegetable oils in salad dressings — oils that can help your body make PGE1 — you could be causing a problem that otherwise might not exist.

To prevent cramping, your body needs to stop manufacturing so much PGE2, inhibit existing PGE2, and make more PGE1. But this is difficult to do if you're taking aspirin and/or Midol (aspirin with a muscle relaxant and caffeine). These over-the-counter medications will make you feel better, but they are prostaglandin inhibitors. They block your body's production of all kinds of prostaglandins, even the helpful ones.

A better solution would be to make more PGE1 and decrease one of the contributors to cramp-inducing PGE2 by eating less animal fats of all kinds. This means eating less butter, cream cheese, sour cream, ice cream, full-fat milk, and yogurt, and less beef.

PGE1 is manufactured from the essential fatty acids found in unheated or cold-pressed vegetable oils (sometimes marked "expeller-pressed"). It is also found in abundance in oil of evening primrose capsules, a supplement found in health food stores and some pharmacies.

Other sources of these essential fatty acids which are less expensive are borage seed oil capsules and flax seed oil. Flax seed oil is one of the best sources, but it gets rancid quickly. Therefore, keep it refrigerated and use it within a few weeks. Some women put flax seed oil on their salads or over popcorn, or just take a spoonful once or twice a day. Remember, essential fatty acids are found in unheated oils. Do not cook with flax seed oil or heat it in any way. If you do, you're destroying the substance your body needs. Many women find the capsules of either borage or evening primrose (taken two in the morning and two before bed) are easier to take.

Another way to inhibit production of PGE2 is with vitamin E, which will also reduce inflammation and will increase the blood supply through the veins. If all else fails, rather than taking aspirin in any form, try herb teas like chamomile, mint, ginger, black cohosh, blue cohosh, or crampbark. They help reduce menstrual cramps by relaxing muscles like your uterus.

Food and Cramps

Dairy products may contribute to menstrual cramps because they contain arachidonic acid and also because they are high in calcium, a mineral that causes muscles to contract. Another mineral, magnesium, found in whole grains, beans, and nuts has the reverse effect: it causes muscles to relax. So you may want to decrease your intake of calcium and increase magnesium, both in your diet and supplements.

While most vitamin and mineral supplements contain twice as much calcium as magnesium, a few have equal amounts. Read labels carefully and choose one with high magnesium and not-so-high calcium. One of the first PMS formulas, Optivite, manufactured by Optimox in Torrance, California, has twice as much magnesium as calcium. It has relieved cramps in numerous cases as well as eliminated other premenstrual symptoms.

To further minimize menstrual cramps, begin eating less beef and more chicken and fish. Include one or two meatless days into your weekly menu to help eliminate foods that contain arachidonic acid entirely. Here are a few main course suggestions that are also high in magnesium:
- pasta with marinara sauce and vegetables
- stir-fried Chinese vegetables with garlic and ginger
  over brown rice or noodles (vegetable lo mein)
- Bean, split pea, lentil, or minestrone soup with
  salad and a whole grain roll
- vegetarian chili with brown rice and steamed
  vegetables or a salad

Check With Your Doctor

We've discussed menstrual cramps, or primary dysmenorrhea, and what you can do about them. It's important, however, to realize that your cramps may be secondary cramps (or secondary dysmenorrhea). That means they are an indication that another medical problem exists, like endometriosis fibroid tumors, pelvic inflammatory disease (PID), or an irritation coming from an IUD. These cramps may feel the same as primary menstrual cramps; however, in some cases other symptoms accompany secondary dysmenorrhea, such as painful intercourse or painful bowel movements, which may signal endometriosis.

A change in diet could still be helpful, but if you have menstrual cramps, be sure to have a gynecological examination before you do anything else to determine which type you have and what other approaches may help alleviate them.

History of Menarche

Contemporary teenage girls may be less prepared for sexual maturity than in years past as menarche has changed from a rite of passage to an adolescent hygienic crisis requiring a host of sanitary products, according to a Cornell University historian and expert on women's studies.

"To some extent, the rite of passage for American girls has been transformed from a mother-daughter dialogue to a commercial activity of purchasing sanitary products," says Joan Jacobs Brumberg, professor of women's studies at Cornell and an expert on the history of American women and the social history of American medicine.

"I suggest that as the sanitary products industry commercialized menarche, it paved the way for commercialization of other areas of the body as well, and mothers and teenage daughters talked less about the female body and sexuality at menarche. Rather, the dialogue seems to have shifted to talking — and arguing — about "good grooming" and purchases of items such as high heels, lipsticks, training bras, and other products of the fashion system.

"Yet, menarche for modern girls today has little to do with adult sexuality or adult status," Brumberg points out in her analysis of menarche in America, published in the *Journal of the History of Sexuality*. The analysis includes excerpts from girls' diaries about menarche, which is part of a larger study Brumberg directs on girls' diaries.

Industrialization and public advertising, however, have helped demystify menarche by bringing women's bodies more into the public realm, Brumberg argues. And although menarche in America has no flamboyant rituals of initiation or exclusion, that does not mean it is culturally neutral. The way society openly discusses menstruation and teaches young girls to manage the hygienic aspects of menstruation may be considered modern rituals, says Brumberg.

Whereas girls in the past rarely talked about menarche in their diaries, and when they did it was couched in euphemisms, modern girls write with anticipation, excitement, and even joy about their first periods and comment on the social recognition it garners from peers.

In colonial times, young women learned from their mothers and other adult women that menarche was the "bellwether of female fertility." By the Victorian era, however, "knowledge about menstruation was considered the first step on the slippery slope to loss of innocence," Brumberg says, and girls were increasingly "protected" from the message.

In the mid-1880s, about 25 percent of girls were unprepared for their first periods. By 1895, some 60 percent of high school girls were ignorant about their impending periods.

Concurrently, girls were menstruating younger than ever. In 1780, the average age at menarche was about 17; by 1877, about 15; by 1948, almost 13; today, it is 12.5.

By the 20th century, the "medicalization of menarche" and the belief that mothers were not adequately preparing their daughters for menarche led many middle-class girls and mothers to turn to books for information about puberty while working-class mothers expected girls to learn from friends, sisters, and fellow workers.

"After World War I and its venereal disease outbreaks, the nation embarked on a crusade to promote moral health in which all aspects of sexuality were sanitized, including menarche and menstruation," Brumberg notes. The sanitary products industry grew increasingly larger and by the 1930s and 1940s, filled the information void by providing corporate-sponsored pamphlets. Millions of girls learned about "desexualized" menstruation from these booklets and even a Walt Disney animated film that was seen by about 93 million American young women.

Question and Answer

Q. My periods have always been irregular — starting every 32 to 40 days. Is this something I should be concerned about?

A. Actually, it sounds like your periods are quite regular since they predictably come every 32 to 40 days. The widespread notion that menses should occur every 28 days is based on an average cycle length, not reality. Unfortunately, this 28-day average has caused a lot of confusion about what constitutes true menstrual regularity.

So what is regular? In one study based on nearly 2,500 women between the ages of 15 and 44, the Center for Population Research in Washington, D.C. found that over 75 percent of the women had average cycle lengths between 25 and 31 days. Furthermore, the study found that nearly 90 percent of the women did not have perfectly timed periods. Rather, cycle length varied from month to month by seven or more days.

In general, a very short cycle is defined as less than 24 days, while a very long cycle spans more than 45 days.

Another study has shown that average menstrual cycle length varies according to a woman's gynecologic age: During the first four years of menstruation, the average number of days between cycles drops from 35 to 29.8 days; after 28 years of menstruation it averages around 27 days; and among women who have been menstruating for 40 years, there is an average of 44 days between cycles. The most regular women are 36 years old, 98 percent of whom have cycles that vary between 20 and 43 days, with a standard deviation of 9.9 days.

Other factors can affect cycle length as well. For example it has been found that within the 90-day period following an illness, surgery, or accident, the number of cycles frequently decreases.

Sexual activity also impacts regularity — with women who spend more time with men having greater regularity than women who have sporadic sexual relations or are celibate.

And in one study, researchers at the Monell Chemical Senses center discovered that exposure to certain elements in male and female perspiration can affect menstrual cycles. This explains, at least in part, why women who spend extended amounts of time together, such as female co-workers, sometimes develop a common cycle.

Q. Since the birth of my last child, intercourse has been very painful for me. I have consulted my gynecologist twice about this and he can't seem to find anything wrong with me. Is it possible that something is being overlooked?

A. Painful intercourse after childbirth is most commonly caused by obstetric injury sustained during childbirth (even in the case of a seemingly normal delivery). This can include an improperly performed episiotomy. These types of injuries can oftentimes be corrected. They can be difficult to diagnose, however, because many doctors are simply not trained to recognize them.

If possible, try to find a doctor in your area who is knowledgeable about obstetric injury treatment. If you aren't successful, you might call the office of Dr. Sam Momtazee, assistant professor at Washington University School of Medicine, for further guidance in finding effective care. Dr. Momtazee specializes in the treatment of painful intercourse and believes that between five and ten percent of all women in this country needlessly suffer from it.

Is Candida Keeping You Sick?

If you've been struggling with a chronic illness for years and have tried everything — allopathic medicine and alternative medicine — but still can't get well, you may have overlooked a secondary imbalance that's keeping you sick. You may have an overgrowth of a yeast called Candida.

It's important to understand that you will never "get rid of" Candida. It's one of more than three hundred bacteria that coexist in our digestive and vaginal tracts, keeping one another in balance. You can, however, reduce the colonies of pathogenic, or "bad" bacteria, like Candida, when there are too many of them.

Some women are familiar with Candida as being a cottage-cheese-like vaginal discharge accompanied by itching and irritation. This form of overgrowth often comes from taking antibiotics that kill off the friendly intestinal and vaginal bacteria, which keep Candida from overmultiplying. It is also common in women with diabetes. Vaginal Candida is rarely a long-term problem. It is often controlled with vaginal suppositories or anti-fungal medications, both natural and allopathic, along with eliminating it's favorite food, sugar, for a few days.

It is estimated that 90 percent of Americans have either a minor or major overgrowth of Candida, which often prevent them from clearing up numerous health problems. These include digestive disorders like bloating and gas, chronic fatigue, chemical sensitivities, difficulty concentrating, eczema, headaches, migraines, panic attacks, sore throats, weight gain, and many more.

Yeast or Fungus?

Candida begins in the digestive tract as a yeast. When it grows out of control, it is able to change from a yeast into a fungus, just like a caterpillar changes into a butterfly. As a yeast, it is encapsulated in the intestines, unable to push its way through the intestinal lining. But as a fungus, its long, root-like structures can break through the intestines, get into the blood stream, and cause allergies and other problems. This is called systemic Candida, and is most often found in people with severe, chronic health problems. Withholding food from the fungus is only one

Is It Yeast? Or Something Worse?

With the increasing popularity of over-the-counter yeast infection medications, many women automatically turn to these products when they suspect an infection. Oftentimes, however, the problem isn't yeast. Frequently, it's infectious vaginitis, which is more widespread than yeast infections and accounts for more than 10 million physician visits each year.

Knowing whether you have yeast or vaginitis is important. A common and potentially serious form of vaginitis is bacterial vaginosis (BV), which has been linked to an increased risk of pelvic inflammatory disease, cervicitis, pregnancy complications, preterm birth, postoperative infection, abnormal cytology, and more. Common symptoms include vaginal discharge and a fishy odor, but nearly half of the women with BV report no noticeable outward symptoms. The best way to be sure you don't have it is to ask your gynecologist to test for it at your next visit.

step in its control. It also may be necessary to take an antifungal medication — either pharmaceutical or natural — to kill off some of the overgrowth.

Now, there's one additional factor to consider with systemic Candida overgrowth: the immune system. Usually, our white blood cells recognize the foreign substances in Candida called antigens and kill some of them off. Dr. William Crook believes some people with Candida overgrowth may have a genetic weakness in their immune response to this organism. Others may simply have an immune system that's been suppressed over the years through illness. This is why, with systemic Candida, the immune system needs a great deal of support.

One type of support is to eliminate foods to which a person is allergic, since these foods also produce antigens that require more white cells to kill them off. It's a vicious cycle.

Confusion Over Candida Treatment

Candida was first brought to our attention by two doctors who specialized in allergies, Drs. Orian Truss and William Crook, in the early 1980s. Their patients — who had systemic Candida — were put on extremely restrictive diets: nothing with yeast in it (this eliminated most breads and baked goods, as well as foods with vinegar), no sugar of any kind, no wheat or dairy, and almost no carbohydrates. Few people could stay on this diet long enough to effect changes.

What few people realized was why Drs. Truss and Crook devised such restrictive and difficult-to-follow diets. It came out of their specialty as allergists. And in their individual practices, Dr. Truss and Dr. Crook noticed that their allergy patients with chronic illnesses seemed to remain sick because of an overgrowth of Candida.

Remember now, these were people who had allergies severe enough for them to seek out experts in the field. And these two eminent doctors found that if their patients stopped feeding the yeast and took anti-fungal medications, they still didn't get better because their allergies suppressed their immune system. Their bodies couldn't establish enough friendly bacteria to keep the disease-causing bacteria under control. So Drs. Truss and Crook took their allergy patients off the foods they were most allergic to: molds and fungi (like mushrooms, vinegar, and foods with yeast), dairy products, and wheat.

At the same time, they lowered carbohydrates and eliminated sugar, because these foods fed the Candida. They also put their patients on anti-fungal medications like nystatin and nyzerol. Patients who tried alternative medicine were put on another anti-fungal like garlic or caprylic acid. But many of these medical and alternative treatments didn't work because Candida albicans is a wily critter. Try to kill it and it mutates. By the late 1980s, there were hundreds of species of Candida, and many were resistant to the anti-yeast and anti-fungal medications.

Alternative health practitioners heard about Drs. Truss and Crook's work with Candida, and began diagnosing this overgrowth in almost all of their patients. They used some of the same protocol with the exception of medications. Garlic, caprylic acid, or other "natural" anti-fungals were used instead of prescription drugs. So was the restrictive diet. Some patients got better, many more didn't. Instead, they grew more discouraged and more frustrated. What was missing?

The diets most people were put on to control Candida were often unnecessarily restrictive, causing people to "cheat" and feed their Candida, rather than kill it off. And not many practitioners addressed the issue of probiotics — friendly bacteria — which naturally keep Candida from flourishing.

Identifying Candida and the Treatment That Will Work for You

For some people, just knowing that Candida may be contributing to ongoing illness is enough. Others may want a laboratory test that says, "Yes, this is a problem for you." We know of one excellent laboratory, Great Smokies, that does a Comprehensive Digestive Stool Analysis that's extremely accurate. This Great Smokies panel is a combination of 18 tests that identify bacterial and yeast overgrowths and even show which treatments, allopathic and natural, will work for your specific overgrowth problem.

If you have taken nystatin, nyzerol, fluconozol, or other anti-fungals and still have your original problems, your Candida overgrowth may be one that responds to garlic or caprylic acid instead. And, of course, the reverse is true as well. You may need pharmaceuticals to control your Candida. Garlic may just not work against your particular strain.

Your doctor can contact Great Smokies Diagnostic Laboratory (800-522-4762) for the necessary information and kits. This comprehensive analysis, which evaluates digestion, absorption, intestinal functions, and microbial flora, as well as giving therapeutic information on what will correct these imbalances, costs around $200. Ask your doctor to get the prepaid customer price for you. If you pay when you send in your sample, and do your own insurance form filing, the price can be considerably lower.

A Comprehensive Approach That Works

There are many causes of candida overgrowth. The most common being of an overgrowth of candida albicans in either its yeast or fungal form seems to be the overuse of antibiotics. Antibiotics kill off large colonies of beneficial bacteria in the intestinal tract that keep candida in check. Allowed to spread, Candida mutates from a yeast into a fungus, producing toxic by-products that cause allergy symptoms and digestive tract disorders.

Additionally, these medications create antibiotic-resistant strains of microbes that make it virtually impossible to restore the body's intestinal flora to its original, healthy, balanced state.

Self-Inflicted Vaginal Infections

An increase in the use of spermicides and feminine hygiene products may be contributing to a rise in vaginal infections, according to Dr. Jack Sobel, professor of internal medicine, obstetrics and gynecology at Wayne State University. Vaginal infections account for more than 10 million physician office visits each year.

Dr. Sobel relates the phenomenon to a changing era in which American women are purchasing increasing amounts of non-prescription feminine products. "In the 1960s and '70s, most women were on the birth control pill," he said. "But in the '90s, with the increased use of spermicides relative to the use of condoms and diaphragms, as well as douching, feminine deodorants, tampons, and sanitary pads that are chemically treated, I suspect these products are disturbing a woman's normal vaginal flora and adding to the increase in vaginal infections."

It is not, however, only antibiotic use that is contributing to candida overgrowth. Some antifungals are having the same effect. In an article published last year in the *American Journal of Medicine*, Victor Yu predicted we will be seeing more candida problems with strains other than the most common candida albicans. Already, in four teaching hospitals in the U.S., other strains of candida are appearing that seem to be resistant to fluconazole, one of the most popular new antifungal medications. Resistance to fluconazole has, in the past, been seen only in cases of thrush in AIDS patients. Now it is being seen in other patients, as well.

Poor digestion is another factor in candida overgrowth, since the presence of hydrochloric acid in the stomach helps kill off many types of unwanted fungi. As we get older, our stomachs naturally produce less hydrochloric acid. Some people have almost none. Others neutralize or inactivate their hydrochloric acid when they take antacids such as TUMS and Rolaids. In addition to not being able to digest your food properly, colonies of candida and other fungi can proliferate when your body is not producing sufficient gastric juices. Numerous degenerative diseases like arthritis, lupus, and other autoimmune diseases have connections to fungal overgrowth.

Any change in hormone balance can also contribute to an overgrowth of candida, including pregnancy, the use of birth control pills, and hormone replacement therapy. A diet high in sugars, especially lactose (milk sugar), contributes to high amounts of candida, since all fungi thrive on sugars. This includes alcoholic beverages, which need to be eliminated completely for a while.

Reducing Candida Overgrowth With Diet

Diet is a key in controlling candida. There's no way around it. If you continue to eat foods high in sugar, it doesn't matter what else you do. You won't get well. All the antifungals in the world won't help you. You can't kill off a yeast while you're feeding it and expect to get better. Candida overgrowth is stimulated by feeding the yeast or fungus. You simply have to starve it. This means eating a diet higher in protein (fish, chicken, tofu, beans) and lower in all sugars and starches. A diet high in carbohydrates, such as starchy vegetables, grains, pasta, bread, fruit and fruit juice, and refined sugars, is not a healthy diet for someone who has an overgrowth of any yeast or fungus. Concentrate on eating lots of vegetables and protein with small amounts of fruit. People often need to be on this diet for three to six months to get results.

Because a suppressed immune system makes it difficult to control a fungal infection, you'll also want to boost yours by eliminating any foods to which you are allergic or sensitive. These may be "good" foods that impair your immune system. This means they're not good for you at this time. If you get sleepy after eating corn products (tortillas, corn chips, polenta), eliminate corn from your diet temporarily. If chicken makes you feel mentally foggy or tired, don't eat chicken for now. You're better off with a limited diet that allows you to get better than with eating a wide variety of foods that prevent you from healing.

Medications and Supplements That Work

S. Colet Lahorz, RN, author of *Conquering Yeast Infections: The Non-Drug Solution,* is a nurse and acupuncturist in Minnesota who has found a comprehensive solution to candida overgrowth. She includes a four-part colon cleansing program using Caprol, an antifungal oil; bentonite, a fine clay used as an intestinal cleanser; psyllium, as additional fiber; and implanting acidophilus. We believe her approach in thoroughly cleansing the colon and repopulating it with beneficial bacteria is a key to controlling this overgrowth.

Lahorz has her patients on the colon cleansing program twice a day for three months. In our experience, a lengthy program is essential in getting the results you're looking for. Just eating better and taking a little acidophilus for a few weeks won't accomplish anything.

For repopulation, we would suggest using Natren brand probiotics (friendly bacteria). It's one of the strongest we have ever seen and it's available in most health food stores. The best of Natren's products is a formula called Healthy Trinity, which consists of three types of friendly bacteria each suspended in an oil base (so they won't compete with one another and lose their potency). Although more expensive than any other formula, Healthy Trinity out-performs all others in our opinion and in the long run is no more expensive than any other good brand. Because it is super-strong, you need to take only one capsule a day. If you have problems finding it, call Natren at 800-992-3323.

Individualize your antifungal treatment by getting a Comprehensive Digestive Stool Analysis from Great Smokies Laboratories (800-522-4762). It will indicate which natural and pharmaceutical antifungals will work to control the particular form of candida you have. Without this information, you're shooting blindly in the dark. With it, you can get excellent results.

Some particularly helpful antifungals include:

Caprylic acid: A fatty acid found in coconut oil, this antifungal works in the intestinal tract. It is similar in effectiveness to nystatin, a pharmaceutical that can adversely effect liver function, but is very safe to use.

Citricidal and other citrus seed extracts: In addition to being effective as antifungals in the digestive tract, citrus seed extracts also kill off parasites like giardia and blastocystis hominis. If you take them an hour before or after meals you can avoid any upset stomach it might cause.

Flax oil and fish oils: These oils contain essential fatty acids, which boost the immune system. They are also antifungals.

Garlic and onions: Natural antibiotics and antifungals used for centuries. You can use deodorized garlic oil capsules if you want to avoid garlic breath.

Tanalbit is a non-prescription intestinal antiseptic used by many health care practitioners instead of nystatin and caprylic acid. It is made from natural tannins (resins found in tea) and zinc.

Drug therapy: If you use any medications, be sure your forms of candida will respond to the drug you're taking. And to avoid drug-resistant strains of candida from mutating, ask your physician to rotate your drugs frequently. If possible, include natural antifungals as well as pharmaceuticals.

When Candida Can't Be Controlled

If you've done everything possible to control an overgrowth of candida and still are unable to get well, there may be an underlying problem you haven't addressed: intestinal permeability, also known as leaky gut syndrome. When the fungal form of candida works its way across the intestinal mucosa it makes larger holes in the intestinal walls, allowing particles of food or bacteria to "leak" across this barrier.

Food allergies also enlarge the lining of the intestines, making it more vulnerable to harmful particles. Leaky gut syndrome will not get better by itself or with a simple change in diet and a few antifungals. It can be diagnosed by laboratory tests and treated by doctors familiar with it.

What to Do About Incontinence

We don't talk much about incontinence, but maybe we should. The statistics are nothing short of alarming:

● The majority of feminine hygiene pads sold, are used for urine leakage.

● Infant diapers and sanitary pads account for less than 25 percent of the profits for makers of such items; adult diapers and other absorbent products for adults provide over 75 percent.

● Experts estimate that incontinence affects more Americans than any other medical problem, condition, or disease. It is the leading cause of institutionalization of the elderly, second only to dementia.

● In 1995 alone, incontinence cost the U.S. economy $28 billion, nearly $4,000 per person.

The majority of incontinence sufferers are also female. And nearly 80 percent of in-home adult caregivers are women; with over half caring for someone (frequently a partner or parent) with incontinence. In short, you will probably be significantly affected by incontinence at some point in your life, either as a sufferer or a caregiver.

Now here's the clincher: It's also estimated that nearly 80 percent of all cases of incontinence are curable. Yet many cases go untreated because people simply don't know what to do. By the end of this article, however, you will know exactly what to do when you or a loved one is incontinent.

Pads and Diapers Aren't Always the Best Solution

One of the first things we need to understand about incontinence is that it can develop over the course of years and even decades.

For women, childbirth and hysterectomy are often first steps toward incontinence. Both have the effect of weakening the pelvic structures that support our urinary and bowel systems. Whether symptoms such as leaking are present or not, it is wise to follow-up each childbirth with a few weeks of Kegel exercises (which will be discussed later) to help recover pelvic muscle tone. (Kegels also speed healing of episiotomies.)

The incidence of incontinence among women who've had hysterectomies — 40 percent higher than average — is another little-known reason to avoid this surgery. It can contribute to incontinence in a number of ways. For starters, the uterus helps support the bladder in the abdominal cavity. In addition, if ovaries are removed, there is less estrogen to help maintain tissue health and muscle tone. Internal post-surgery adhesions (scarring) can also form, with hysterectomy as well as other abdominal surgeries, further altering the abdominal support structures.

Other Causes of Incontinence

Some other causes of incontinence are quite surprising. This too, often gets in the way of appropriate treatment.

For starters, constipation, interestingly enough, can cause urinary incontinence by putting enough pressure on the bladder to cause dysfunction. The solution here, of course, is to not be constipated. (See the section later in this book on laxative use and constipation solutions.)

Illness can cause temporary incontinence, too, by interfering with messages to the central nervous system from the bladder that it is full and needs to empty. Another complication of illness is dehydration, which can irritate the bladder and urethra. Both scenarios can result in incontinence. But when these primary illnesses and secondary bladder problems are resolved, so is the symptomatic incontinence.

In other cases, an actual urinary tract infection (UTI), can be the cause. UTIs can be related to kidney infection, poor personal hygiene, diaphragm use, and changes in the urinary tract that occur with aging. UTIs can also be sexually transmitted. In younger women, UTIs often have the symptoms of a burning sensation, frequent urge to urinate, fever, and even lower back pain. In older women, however, incontinence may be the only symptom of a UTI. Such cases can be confirmed with a urinalysis.

Simply drinking cranberry juice for up to a week is often enough to get rid of such an infection. Use unsweetened or fruit-sweetened cranberry juice. Otherwise, refined sugar may cause an infection to linger. The problem of recurring UTIs can often be halted by acidifying the urine with vitamin C supplements. More stubborn cases might require strengthening the immune system, or even a course of antibiotic treatment — in which case we also recommend taking the prescription drug Nystatin concurrently to prevent yeast overgrowth, and following up with a course of acidophilus to re-establish beneficial bacteria in your system. (For a long-standing problem, follow-up with Natren's Healthy Trinity probiotic supplement.)

Another common cause of incontinence in older women is vaginitis. Symptoms include painful urination, burning, itching, frequent urination, painful intercourse, and yeast infections. An over-the-counter remedy may be sufficient to clear up a one-time bout of vaginitis or even a yeast infection. If recurrence is a problem, however, this may indicate immune-system impairment and that you should build yours back up.

Incontinence is also a side effect of hundreds, if not thousands, of drugs, including diuretics, sleeping pills, sedatives, anti-depressants, painkillers, antihistamines, decongestants, narcotics, and even nasal sprays and alcohol. A good clue to whether a drug is causing incontinence is timing: Did the incontinence begin shortly after starting a new drug? If so, there are usually alternative medications or other remedies to use that won't cause incontinence. Remember, the more drugs a person takes, the greater the risk of side effects in general.

Other contributors to incontinence include dulled mental ability such as depression, confusion, and dementia. The common denominator here is that mental impairment can lead to less physical control, as communication between our brain and other parts of the body (i.e., the bladder) breaks down.

An environment that is no longer user-friendly can also be problematic, see function incontinence below.

Types of Chronic Urinary Incontinence and Treatments

There are five main types of chronic urinary incontinence:

Stress Incontinence. Caused by physical stress (such as weak pelvic floor muscles), compromised pelvic-region support (such as no uterus or a prolapsed — sagging or dropped — organ), lower back nerve injuries, and even constipation and excessive weight. This type of incontinence is usually limited to small amounts of leakage. Six out of seven sufferers are female. Kegel exercises can be especially effective. If prolapse is present, however, only pursue Kegels under the supervision of a doctor or other continence specialist.

Urge Incontinence. The bladder doesn't properly control the urine release reflex due to a number of causes, which may include instability of the detrusor muscle, bladder infection, muscle or tissue damage, tumors, kidney stones, diverticulitis, Parkinson's disease, MS, strokes, and many other illnesses, making it best to seek help from a doctor.

Overflow Incontinence. Indicates a blocked urethra or bladder that doesn't contract properly. Blockage can be caused by prolapsed (sagging or dropped) organs or neurological disease. This type of incontinence is best evaluated and treated by a doctor. If left untreated, it can lead to bladder infection and even serious kidney complications.

Functional Incontinence. This is caused by a person's inability or unwillingness to use a toilet. It is usually the result of physical or mental impairment and, in some cases, the primary cause of this impairment is drugs. Evaluating access factors and making appropriate changes can be helpful. This might include rearranging furniture to create more direct routes to the bathroom. Using canes, walkers, and other equipment to further improve a person's ability to get to the bathroom. Wearing clothing that can be easily removed for toileting. And finally, upgrading actual bathroom facilities for special needs, with such items as a raised toilet seat, bathroom grab bars, etc., which enhance ease of use. Many nursing homes diaper residents who are too much work to help with toileting.

Reflex Incontinence. This occurs when the brain doesn't receive the message that the bladder is full. Instead, the bladder contracts and voids itself, without the person ever getting an urge to urinate. It is usually caused by spinal-column nerve damage and is most effectively treated with toileting retraining and physical rehabilitation.

Mixed Incontinence. Most incontinent persons have two or more types of incontinence. Stress mixed with urge is most common in women; and urge mixed with overflow is most common in men.

Non-Surgical Solutions

Although many doctors offer incontinence treatment. It might be well worth the extra effort to track down a specialist. We recommend that you call the National Association for Continence at 1-800-BLADDER. This group can refer you to a continence specialist in your area. Look for a specialist who uses self-help and other non-invasive approaches first, including:

A healthy lifestyle. This provides the foundation for all good health. Poor habits, however, can lead to problems, including incontinence. Remember to eat a healthy diet — one that keep your bowel movements regular and includes plenty of water. Many incontinence sufferers initially cut back on fluid intake. This is a mistake that can be counterproductive by withholding fluids necessary for optimum performance of the urinary tract and other parts of the body.

Look for other simple solutions instead. Some foods and beverages, for example, can contribute to incontinence. These include alcoholic beverages, sodas, citrus juice and fruits, tomatoes, spicy foods, artificial sweeteners, and caffeine. If necessary, keep a food/incontinence diary to see if any foods or beverages make your incontinence worse. Eliminate anything that appears to worsen it. Caffeine (found in many beverages including sodas), chocolate, and some over-the-counter medications, can be especially irritating to an already compromised bladder. For caffeine withdrawal headaches, *nux vomica 30x* is a homeopathic remedy that works for many and is sold at most health food stores.

Retraining programs. These programs focus on identifying undesirable habits and correcting them. Continence specialists base retraining programs on individual needs and circumstances. At least 75 percent of women with stress and urge incontinence are able to reduce their incontinence by 50 percent with bladder retraining. It aims to restrict voiding to once every three or so hours by helping women wait out initial urges by sitting tight, contracting urine control muscles, then distracting themselves until the urge passes. Other helpful habits include: not voiding unless the urge to do so is present and not rushing to the bathroom, which can stimulate leakage.

Kegel exercises. They work like gangbusters for preventing and reversing incontinence — and you can do them just about anywhere and anytime. While watching TV, talking on the phone, even sitting in the car. Tightening the Kegel muscle group before coughing or doing other activities that would ordinarily stimulate involuntary leakage, can also reduce incontinence. Kegels are the first line of defense for anyone with mild to moderate stress incontinence and are also helpful in many cases of urge incontinence with improvement in 60 to 80 percent of cases. Remember, too, that a general exercise program can also help in the fight against incontinence by helping maintain good overall muscle tone.

To do a Kegel exercise correctly, simply contract the muscles you'd use to stop the flow of urine. Aim for 100 to 500 or more of these contractions daily, in three to five sessions spread throughout the body. As in weightlifting, contract, hold, and release slowly — and remember to relax your muscles completely between contractions. Results should be seen within a month, with continued improvement for three to six months.

Biofeedback therapy. This non-invasive treatment is used successfully by many continence experts. Look for someone who has experience using this technique.

The Next Step: Continence Devices

There are also hundreds of devices available to help keep us dry. It would be impossible to review them all. So let's just cover a few basic guidelines. In general, the simpler, the better. And steer clear, whenever possible, of products that are irritating. The Reliance insert, for example, is reported to have an extra high rate of irritation and infection. Because of discomfort, difficulty of use, and the frequency of infection, catheters are also best avoided. In short, it's best to consider as many devices as possible and pick the one that most safely and easily meets your needs. A continence expert can help you do this.

One class of devices of special interest to women are pelvic organ prolapse support devices. The most common complaint of these devices, such as pessaries, is improper fit. Keep trying. A proper-fitting support device can be well worth the effort, help you avoid surgery, and even help reverse a prolapse by making a successful Kegel exercise program possible. If you're a good candidate for a support device, a continence specialist may be able to help you find one to stop incontinence immediately. Although a device might sound unpleasant, the remaining options can be more so.

The Last Resort: Drugs and Surgery

The two most popular drugs prescribed for incontinence are imipramine (Tofranil) and oxybutinin (Ditropan). The first is a dual-action antidepressant. Both decrease bladder contractions by being anticholinergic. Both also have serious known side effects. Those for imipramine include postural hypotension and heart rhythm disturbances. Side effects with oxybutinin include dry mouth, blurred vision, constipation, increased eye pressure, heart irregularities, and delirium. Other incontinence drugs also have serious side effects, making them all best-avoided if possible.

There are also over 100 surgical procedures used to treat incontinence in women. These procedures, of course, are even more undesirable than drugs. Success rates vary. And even when a surgery is successful, it can result in other serious problems. In some patients, it can relieve stress incontinence, only to cause urge incontinence. All surgeries, of course, have the general risk of complications, and can result in internal adhesions (scarring) that further aggravate incontinence, or cause new or other problems. Furthermore, the older a patient is, the higher the likelihood that even minor surgery can be a major undertaking.

For all these reasons, it is critical to consult with more than one continence surgery specialist and find out as much as possible about any procedure you're considering, what specific results you can expect, and what risks you might be taking.

As you now know, there are many ways to stay dry. So many ways in fact, that finding which will work for you or a loved one often requires talking about the problem with a continence specialist. Take heart in knowing you're not alone.... That millions of others also suffer. And that the more we start talking about it, the closer we'll get to overcoming it.

Chapter 9

Pregnancy and Childbirth

Midwives vs. Obstetricians

Throughout much of Western Europe, midwives frequently handle all but the highest risk and most complicated pregnancies and deliveries, which are referred to obstetricians. Under normal circumstances obstetricians function as occasional consultants or backups, and are called in the event of unforeseen complications.

Statistics show that pregnancy outcomes with midwives are just as good if not better than pregnancy outcomes with obstetricians. This holds true for midwives who practice in the United States, as well. In late 1989, in fact, the *New England Journal of Medicine* published an article that reviewed midwife practices in this country. The review focused on birth centers — 73 percent of which were run solely by midwives. The result: Pregnancy outcomes were as good as those in hospitals, and C-section rates were dramatically lower.

The results of this review came as no surprise to the medical community. Just three years earlier, in late 1986, the Congressional Office of Technology Assessment recommended that Certified Nurse Midwife training programs be expanded.

So why aren't we hearing more about the outstanding maternity care provided by today's American midwives? Perhaps some of the answers can be found in the fact that obstetricians stand to lose a great deal of income if they begin sharing a significant portion of their market with midwives. American obstetricians are also exceptionally powerful. In fact, that's how they came to control the domestic maternity care market in the first place.

During colonial times in this country, maternity care, along with medical care in general, was dominated by midwives.

Typical midwife activities included treating sore throats and fevers, dispensing medication, attending labor and performing deliveries, and even "laying out" bodies for burial. Treatments most frequently made use of herbal and other natural ingredient remedies. These were most commonly based on established English tradition and were administered as teas, syrups, pills, vapors, poultices, plasters, baths, ointments, and salves.

What additional services doctors had to offer tended to be more dramatic — as might be expected in view of the higher status and fees they commanded even then. Most doctors possessed a few crude surgical instruments (stethoscopes and thermometers didn't even exist). These were used for procedures such as bloodletting and amputations. Doctors also set bones and pulled teeth.

The medications doctors prescribed were usually stronger, including such pharmacy items as calomel (a mercurial compound), laudanum (a liquid opiate), purple foxglove (digitalis), and quinine.

In addition, late 18th-century doctors were slowly making inroads into the realm of maternal care. Earlier surgeons had only attended births in dire emergencies (usually to dismember and extract an unsaveable infant). But by the late 18th century, many American doctors performed deliveries on a part-time basis in which they practiced "new scientific obstetrics."

Midwives Outperformed Early Obstetricians

Unfortunately, these early colonial obstetricians had a poorer record for delivery outcomes than their midwife counterparts. One of the most extensive records of childbirth during colonial times is contained in the personal diary of midwife Martha Ballard, who practiced in Maine during the late 1700s and early 1800s. She reported a maternal death rate of 0.5 percent, and a stillbirth rate of 1.8 percent. A male contemporary of hers, however, reported a higher stillbirth rate of 2.4 percent.

English statistics bear out the representativeness of these isolated incidences. Parish records indicate that English villages (which had few doctors available for delivery services) averaged maternal death rates ranging from one to 2.9 percent. But physician-run hospitals in London and Dublin reported maternal death rates ranging from 2.15 percent to over 22 percent!

Ballard noted in her diary a number of instances of physician shortcomings during deliveries. On one occasion, a doctor administered an opiate to a woman in labor. This caused her contractions to cease. Later she vomited, resumed contractions, and proceeded with an uneventful delivery. In two other entries, Ballard noted cases of doctors having difficulty dealing with breech births. In the first case, the infant was born dead with it's limbs badly mangled. In the second, Ballard was called in to take over and successfully delivered the baby.

Childbirth During Colonial Times

Historian Laurel Thatcher Ulrich, associate professor at the University of New Hampshire, recently analyzed Ballard's diary. In it, Ulrich discovered a rare and fascinating glimpse into everyday female life, and midwifery in particular, during this era.

The resulting book, *A Midwife's Tale*, has been highly acclaimed by historians and medical professionals alike. By the middle of her career, Martha Ballard performed two-thirds of the deliveries that took place in her immediate vicinity. Her descriptions of childbirth and the accompanying activities include three distinct stages:

First Stage Childbirth. Ballard describes the first stage as the "expectation" of labor. She was summoned at this stage and it lasted from several hours to several days and might not even include true labor. During this stage, Ballard reports patients staying on their feet and resting as necessary. In one entry she wrote that she knitted a stocking and helped the patient make a cake and a pie. Other entries describe Ballard sitting by bedsides throughout the night tending "ill" women, and sleeping when laboring women were "comfortable." Sometimes she even slept in the same bed.

Second Stage Childbirth. The second stage is described as featuring a new intensity of labor, at which time "the women" were called. Ballard required at least two assistants and in the large majority of cases, between two and four women were called. These women usually included nearby neighbors and relatives who sometimes lived farther away. They provided emotional and physical support such as lifting the laboring woman in and out of bed and dressing the infant.

After the delivery came a traditional celebration in which a meal was shared. And if it was late or the weather was bad, attending women frequently spent the night before returning to their homes.

Third Stage Childbirth. The third stage of birth, a lying-in period, began when the afternurse arrived and the midwife departed. Prior to a number of departures, Martha Ballard reports getting women up and changing their beds. For the next week or so, a woman who had just given birth was then tended by an afternurse and kept mostly to her room.

Although contemporary literature cautioned against it, rum was popular with women who were lying-in. One store manager in Maine wrote, "The women have been very fruitful this winter and had I not assisted many of them with tea, sugar, and rum in their lyings in, I do not know what would have become of them." During the course of lying in, a woman gradually became active in the care of her infant and household. The lying-in stage ended when she "returned to the kitchen."

Occasionally, Ballard was called back within a few days or weeks to treat postpartum complaints such as afterpains, hemorrhoids, hysterics, or delirium (perhaps postpartum depression), or sore breasts.

Rarely were a mother and child separated. In the event a mother was not able to nurse, neighbors filled in for her until she was again able. One of Ballard's entries reports neighbors taking turns nursing an infant after the mother died.

Compensation for Ballard's services was a flat fee of six shillings. It was paid in cash or in the form of goods. Ballard notes a generous payment of goods that consisted of two pounds of coffee, one yard of ribbon, and a cap border. A notably skimpy payment consisted of a bushel and a half of apples. Other payment items included piglets, candles, a "great" wheel, unwashed wool, codfish, teapots, thimbles, handkerchiefs, and snuff.

Length of labor did not affect compensation amounts. One delivery required eight river crossings and nine days spent on and off at the woman's home. For this, Ballard received a bonus — a present of a yard and a half of ribbon. Extra expenses, such as medicine, were added to the delivery fee.

The six shilling fee was higher than most women earned per day. For example, a full-time weaver earned four shillings a day at most. Ballard's husband earned six shillings for appraising an estate or a day spent "writing plans."

Obstetricians Manipulate Maternity-Care Market to Gain Control

Present-day attitudes toward childbirth appear to originate from the 1800s. During this time, male doctors gained control of childbirth among the upper and middle classes even though they didn't offer women higher survival rates.

Male-doctor dominated medical schools engaged in a variety of tactics to exclude women from admission because, according to Dorothy Wertz, author of *Man Midwifery*, "Doctors feared, not without reason, that if women were admitted to the profession, woman patients would prefer physicians of their own sex, especially for childbirth." To further confuse unsuspecting consumers, medical schools also established obstetrics as the first area of specialization in the medical field. Therefore, doctors who completed special obstetric requirements could make an official claim that they were more qualified than midwives to handle maternity care. Around this time, doctors also performed cruel experimental surgery on many women — developing maternity care "cures" that further manifested their self-endowed expertise and power.

Toward the end of the century, doctors continued expanding their maternity care market share by promoting their association with education and science — both of which were highly revered by the Victorians. But most working-class women could still not afford a doctor's delivery fees and continued to rely on midwives.

In response, doctors launched a virulent campaign against midwives, stereotyping them as ignorant, dirty, and irresponsible — in spite of the fact that many midwives continued to have better safety records than their assailants. Doctors also campaigned to promote the idea that childbirth was dangerous, so much so that "no precaution was excessive." This served as additional fodder to further alienate unsuspecting women from their midwives.

Legislation Suppresses Midwifery

In the wake of anti-midwife campaigns by doctors, an increasing amount of legislation was passed that further suppressed midwife practices. This, in turn, increasingly forced women out of their homes and into hospitals to give birth. By 1900, five percent of American women gave birth in hospitals; by 1935, 75 percent. Ironically, by 1930 the U.S. maternal mortality rate stood at one per 150 births or .66 percent. This represented enough of an increase over immediately preceding maternal mortality rates that many historians have attributed these extra deaths to the rise of modern-day obstetrics.

During the 1950s and 1960s, more efficient assembly line techniques developed during WWII were used to streamline hospital delivery services. Like autos moving through an assembly line, women were wheeled from one location to the next as their delivery progressed. The artificial breaking of waters, labor accelerating drugs, episiotomies, forceps, and C-sections helped expedite this system by minimizing delays in the birth process. By the late 1960s, 95 percent of American women gave birth in hospitals.

Midwives vs. Obstetricians Today

Today the maternal mortality rate is a mere one per 10,000 births or .01 percent. This is because the small minority of women who do experience delivery difficulty have the advantages of many gains that have taken place in obstetrical safety since the 1930s. It has *nothing* to do with the fact that the large majority of babies are delivered by obstetricians.

Huge fee discrepancies aside, the key distinguishing feature between obstetricians and midwives is philosophical.

Obstetricians view childbirth as dangerous (comparable to an illness) and tend to be interventionists. They receive training in medical schools, clinics, and hospitals where they rarely witness normal, spontaneous labor and birth. Instead, the labor scenarios they most commonly see take place in sophisticated delivery room settings in which women lie on an operating type table with their feet tightly secured in stirrups.

Women in labor are viewed and treated as surgical patients. Sometimes their pubic hair is still shaved as preparation for surgery and they are hooked up to fetal monitors and IV drug infusion equipment — including glucose to prevent dehydration (when a glass of juice would serve the same purpose).

Interventions might include breaking water, anesthetizing the patient, administering drugs to accelerate delivery, administering drugs to decelerate delivery, and cutting the womb or vagina to get the baby out. An obstetrician may later brag about a "tight" repair job. Too much tightness, however, can cause lifetime problems such as painful intercourse.

On the other hand, midwives traditionally approach childbirth as a perfectly normal and natural event and tend to be noninterventionists. After all, the large majority of deliveries do occur naturally and sponta-neously — with the body progressing to each new phase when it is ready.

Certified Nurse Midwives receive formal training in childbirth and are licensed by the state. *Lay Midwives* often have no formal training (although many have outstanding delivery outcome records) and it is illegal for them to practice in some states. Since midwife training varies, it is important to carefully evaluate one (as you should with any medical professional for that matter) before making a final selection.

During childbirth with a midwife, women are usually allowed to be as active as they feel they are able, and rest when they feel the need. Movement is not highly restricted and taking a walk is not uncommon. Instead of IV's, women drink water and juice to avoid dehydration. Actual delivery may take place with the woman in any of a number of positions including sitting or squatting.

These positions enable the laboring woman to work with gravity, reduce strain on the perineum, and (along with other midwife techniques) help avoid the "need" for an episiotomy. The *lithotomy* position, in which the woman lies on her back with feet in stirrups, is not as common. In general, it is the most ineffective and dangerous position for labor. The reason it is used in most hospitals is for the convenience of the obstetrician.

Fetal stress is also a less commonly encountered hazard since it is frequently brought on by invasive hospital routines and procedures that midwives do not practice. Finally, midwife delivered babies are frequently more alert at birth because they are not born under the influence of drugs that were administered to the mother.

In the event of an emergency, many midwives work in close proximity to obstetricians. Some midwives even work on the same premises.

To Choose a Midwife or Not

Today, the large majority of American women automatically turn to an obstetrician for prenatal care and delivery. This hardly qualifies as making a choice.

Yet there are many important individual choices that can be made to help ensure a better overall delivery outcome for yourself and your baby. These choices start with evaluating persons to whom you are considering entrusting your care, whether you consider midwives, obstetricians, or both. Since every woman is different, there is no single right or wrong choice. One will simply be best for you. And you are the best person to decide which maternity care provider best suits your needs.

Skip the Episiotomy

Abandoning the routine use of episiotomies, in which the vagina is cut to ease childbirth, has been recommended by a team of Canadian researchers. In a recent study, which included more than 1,000 births, they found that episiotomies may offer no medical benefits and definitely make recovery more difficult.

Childbirth Recovery Can Take Months

Traditionally, it had been thought that it only took six weeks to bounce back after childbirth. Now researchers are finding it can take several months and sometimes more, according to recently published study results from the *Archives of Family Medicine*. During the first month after delivery, 40 percent of the women in the study reported fatigue and breast soreness. One month after delivery, 10 to 20 percent of the women reported vaginal discomfort, hemorrhoids, poor appetite, constipation, increased perspiration, acne, hand numbness or tingling, dizziness, and hot flashes. Late developing problems which surfaced three to six months after delivery included pain during intercourse, respiratory infections, and hair loss — each of which was reported by 10 to 40 percent of the women.

Fertility Specialists Make Biggest Bucks

Fertility hormone specialists earn the highest salaries of all physicians, according to a survey by the William M. Mercer Company. These specialists enjoy an average salary of $259,750. That's almost twice as much as the average for all salaried doctors, which is $139,732. A recent issue of the *Townsend Letter for Doctors* suggested that during the last few decades, treating infertility has become a sizable "cash cow" for the medical establishment and that exploitation of patients seems to be ongoing.

High-Tech Job Hazards

Women who work in the fabrication areas of computer chip factories suffer a 40 percent higher miscarriage rate than other female semiconductor industry workers, according to a comprehensive new study by researchers from the University of California at Davis. The study took place over a four-year period and involved 15,000 workers at 14 different firms.

This study focuses new attention on potential workplace health hazards, especially in workplaces that use a variety of chemicals — many of which are so new that they have yet to be evaluated for workplace safety. One new chemical group called ethylene-based glycol ethers is used in computer chip factories and is the suspected culprit in the UC Davis study.

In addition to the higher miscarriage rate, the UC Davis study uncovered a higher rate of respiratory problems such as wheezing, more skin irritations, and more difficulty in conceiving for women. Critics point out that the study left many questions unanswered, such as the impact on birth defects and long-term chronic health problems.

Prior to the UC Davis study, animal studies from the early 1980s that scrutinized the relationship between glycol ethers and reproductive health came up with similar results, including lower rates of pregnancy in women and higher sterility rates in men, as well as an increased risk of miscarriage. The Davis re-searchers also suspected that propylene-based glycol ethers and other solvents might have played a role in their study in creating reproductive problems.

There are more than 35,000 computer chip fabrication workers in the U.S., of which about 70 percent are women. In addition, more than 630,000 U.S. workers in other industries such as professional cleaning services and printing (along with some workers in publishing, health services, business services and transportation) are also exposed to glycol ethers while on the job.

Gas Is No Laughing Matter for Dental Assistants

Female dental assistants exposed to high levels of nitrous oxide ("laughing gas" used in dental offices) were found to have significant fertility impairment in a study that has been published by the *New England Journal of Medicine*. Women who were exposed to the gas for five or more hours per week were only 41 percent as likely to conceive during a menstrual cycle as unexposed women. No fertility impairment was detected in women with lower exposure levels.

Swing Shift Miscarriage

Pregnant women who work a swing shift (those which start between three and four p.m.) are four times more likely to miscarry than women who work a day shift, according to a recently completed study by Canadian researchers. Women who work night shifts also had a higher miscarriage rate in the study.

Milk Drinking During Pregnancy Can Backfire

The most undiagnosed allergy in children is milk allergy, according to Doris J. Rapp, MD, a leading environmental medicine expert. Typically, milk allergies begin during pregnancy when a women consumes a lot of milk or other dairy products with the intention of boosting her chances of having a healthy baby.

Leg Cramps and Magnesium

Pregnant women are often plagued with leg cramps. A study reported in the *American Journal of Obstetrics and Gynecology* showed that when pregnant women were given 122 mg of magnesium lactate or citrate in the morning, and 244 mg of magnesium in the evening, their leg cramps disappeared.

This does not surprise us, since pregnant women are given high amounts of calcium to help the fetus form strong bones. However, we'd like to remind you that calcium causes muscles to cramp while magnesium causes muscles to relax. In addition, by increasing magnesium, many pregnant women find they have less constipation, as magnesium helps relax the colon.

Since pregnancy increases the absorption of calcium, we'd like to suggest that even if you're pregnant you do not overload on any one nutrient, including calcium. A diet high in whole grains, soy products, and dark-green leafy vegetables is also high in both calcium and magnesium.

If you're taking a prenatal supplement with 1000 to 1500 mg of calcium, you don't need a lot of high-calcium dairy products as well. Instead, increase your intake of magnesium-rich whole grains, beans, and a few nuts and seeds. (Note: Our favorite prenatal supplement is Optimox Prenatal. It contains 600 mg of calcium and 600 mg of magnesium.)

American Journal of Obstetrics and Gynecology, 1995;173:175-80

What often happens instead, however, is the growing fetus develops an over-sensitivity to cow's milk. Oftentimes, these babies kick excessively in utero. After birth, evidence of a milk allergy can arise among infants who are bottle-fed a milk-based formula, as well as nursing infants whose mothers continue to consume large quantities of dairy products. Symptoms include excessive frowning, perspiring, drooling, colic, and ear infections.

The solution is to limit intake of milk and other dairy products during pregnancy to the equivalent of one glass of milk a day or less, if any. There is no scientific evidence to support the idea that pregnant women need to consume milk to help the growing fetus develop strong bones. A good quality diet — without milk — can provide all the calcium a fetus needs for bone formation. Asian women are excellent proof of this. They consume little if any milk, yet their diets still include lots of calcium-rich foods including soy beans (foods such as tofu and miso), other beans, whole grains, and lots of vegetables.

As a result, Asian babies tend to be every bit as healthy as babies born in countries where lots of dairy foods are consumed, with one very important exception: There is a much lower incidence of colic and milk allergies among Asian babies. Asian women benefit, too, from consuming a good-quality diet that includes little if any milk, not only during pregnancy but throughout their adult lives. They enjoy lower rates of heart disease, arthritis, and osteoporosis — all of which milk and other dairy foods may contribute to.

After a baby is born, nursing mothers should continue avoiding dairy products. And in the event nursing is impossible, bottle-fed infants should be given soy-based formula. If milk products are reintroduced into the child's diet at a later date, watch out for allergy symptoms can occur such as hay fever, asthma, or behavior problems.

Assault in the Labor and Delivery Room

What you're about to read might sound farfetched. But if you'll bear with me and hear me out, you might be surprised to find yourself agreeing. Even if you're past your childbearing years, this is an important article for you to read. Although you aren't directly affected, the well-being of other women you know is being adversely affected. Perhaps that of a daughter, granddaughter, niece, or another younger woman you know.

Last week, I had an interesting chat with Teri Williams, my beloved doula (female labor companion). I mentioned I'd recently reviewed the new Mother-Friendly Childbirth Initiative and wondered what she thought about it. Like me, she thought it was great.

What I don't think is so great, though, is that the popular press has virtually ignored the much-needed birthing guidelines this exciting initiative sets forth. Why? Perhaps because it exposes the truth about the large majority of U.S. births: Women in labor, more often than not, are being unwittingly assaulted right in the labor and delivery room itself.

Consider what's going on in nearly every hospital across the country today:

* The overall C-section rate is approximately 25 percent.

* And the overall episiotomy rate is 80 percent, even higher for first-time births.

Now here are the dramatically different recommendations of the Initiative:

* A total cesarean rate of 10 percent or less in community hospitals, and 15 percent or less in tertiary care (high-risk) hospitals.

* And an episiotomy rate of 20 percent or less, with a goal of 5 percent or less.

* No routine use of electronic fetal monitors (EFMs).

You might be thinking such a radical departure from current procedures would endanger women and their newborns. Actually the opposite is true: They would benefit. Study after study shows that EFM use does not result in better birth outcomes (i.e. lower injury rates and higher survival rates). It does, however, result in higher C-section and episiotomy rates. And more C-sections and episiotomies result in overall worse, not better, birth outcomes.

In Norway, which has the highest maternal survival rates in the world, the C-section rate is around five percent and episiotomies are rare. In addition, most women give birth at home where EFMs are not used. Instead of a high-paid doctor who often shows up at the last minute to catch or cut out the baby, Norwegian women in labor have ongoing companionship and assistance from top-notch midwives, (who are also the primary prenatal care providers). Doctors, hospitals, and the big-gun medicine that come with them are reserved for high-risk pregnancies and deliveries.

Although all this may sound strange to many of you, the new Mother-Friendly Childbirth Initiative is, in fact, modeled after birthing practices in Norway and other developed nations that rank close to Norway's outstanding birth outcome rates.

How does the U.S. rank? Not to good. It has twice as many maternal deaths as Norway. Even many poorer countries are outperforming us, including Ireland, Spain, the Mediterranean island of Cyprus, and Israel.

When you take a good hard look at birthing in other countries, it's easy to see that there's absolutely, positively no defense for our current system of hospital-based, doctor-managed birthing. The facts speak for themselves. Most women giving birth in the U.S. are getting needlessly cut up, not to their benefit, but to their detriment. And if this type of rampant slashing was happening out on our streets or anywhere else, we'd call it assault.

Birthing is one of the greatest physical challenges most women will ever face. And we could have and deserve better birthing treatment. For a fraction of what we currently spend, we all could be given many more advantages for meeting the challenge with far greater success: The advantage of no routinely used EFM equipment, the advantage of mother-friendly doulas and midwives for routine deliveries, the advantage of giving birth at home without being labeled a kook, and the advantage of reserving high-paid doctors for high-risk births — when statistics show they do save lives.

These are some of the powerful birthing advantages that Norwegian and other more fortunate women enjoy, and which the Mother-Friendly Childbirth Initiative is promoting for us. Ultimately, these advantages can transform birthing into a much more positive experience, prevent countless obstetrical mistakes and injuries (including the large majority of C-sections and episiotomies), and save many more lives.

I'm afraid it might be decades, however, before the popular press in this country comes to its senses about birthing. So the American College of Nurse-Midwives, along with 25 other organizations serving women and children, sponsored the Mother-Friendly Childbirth Initiative. It's a blueprint for a shift from our current substandard system of high-cost maternity care, where fear of litigation and maximizing profits often drives decision-making, to a safer system of partnership and cooperation between the pregnant woman and her care givers.

This is not a legislative initiative, but more of a policy statement. To become a widespread reality, we must support the Initiative economically

— by choosing only birthing services providers who operate within the Initiative's guidelines.

Chapter 8

Health Hazards at Work, Home, and Travel

Is Work Making You Sick?

In 1990, the U. S. Bureau of Labor Statistics reported that 6.8 million employees were either injured or disabled while on the job. What's more, according to Ralph Nader, these "job casualties are statistically at least three times more serious than street crimes."

The severity of on-the-job injuries varies dramatically, from minor aches and pains to complete incapacitation. And in the wake of the increasing numbers of women in the job market, the rate of female job injuries has steadily risen as well.

One of the biggest on-the-job injuries varies dramatically, from minor aches and pains to complete incapacitation. And in the wake of the increasing numbers of women in the job market, the rate of female job injuries has steadily risen as well.

One of the biggest on-the-job injury culprits is the computer. According to federal government statistics, computers are linked to 40 percent of all workplace injuries. Many occupations that are dominated by women, such as secretary, data processor, telephone operator, and airline reservationist, require workers to spend nearly all their time in front of a computer, often performing repetitive tasks. A number of injuries can frequently result in such work environments. Here are some common work-related injuries and what you can do if you suffer from them:

● **Back Pain and Wrist Problems:** Spending long hours on end working at a computer station most frequently causes back pain and wrist problems — most often carpal tunnel syndrome (also common among factory workers). If you experience back pain, you'll feel it. In the case of carpal tunnel syndrome, symptoms can include numbness, tingling, and pain in the fingers or hand. This is the result of a nerve in the arm being compressed repeatedly as it passes through the wrist bones or carpals and a ligament under the skin. If you have any of these symptoms, do not ignore them. Take action right away since symptoms may become worse. Repetitive motion injuries such as carpel tunnel syndrome may even require surgery.

Oftentimes, back and wrist discomfort can be relieved simply by rearranging your work environment. For maximum comfort, adjust desks, tables, chairs, computer screens, telephones, and any other furniture and equipment in your immediate work area. Also, be sure you are exercising proper posture such as sitting straight up in your chair. A better quality chair that better supports the back might also be in order, such as the newer ergonomically designed ones. Periodic breaks can provide relief for overly stressed body parts — try standing on your feet and doing some stretching. Counteracting sedentariness during work with a regular exercise program can provide relief, too.

● **Eyestrain:** Working at a computer screen all day can also cause eyestrain, in which case you may experience blurred or double vision and/or headaches. Again, periodic breaks can provide relief. You may also find it helpful to adjust lighting in your immediate work area, as well as the contrast on your computer screen, or possibly switch to another brand of screen.

● **Radiation Exposure:** There's also the question of whether computer screens expose users to harmful radiation. Such injury has yet to be documented and many expects contend that computer screens are completely harmless. Still, other experts remain skeptical. To reduce the

Dental Assistants

Female dental assistants exposed to high levels of nitrous oxide ("laughing gas" used in dental offices) were found to have significant fertility impairment in a study that has been published by the *New England Journal of Medicine*. Women who were exposed to the gas for five or more hours per week were only 41 percent as likely to conceive during a menstrual cycle as unexposed women. No fertility impairment was detected in women with lower exposure levels.

possibility of risk, Louis Slesin, editor of *VDT News*, recommends keeping a computer at arm's length; keeping a computer turned off when it's not being used; and sitting directly in front of a computer — where the least amount of radiation is being emitted.

● **"Sick" Building Systems:** Finally, a phenomenon called "sick" building has been reported to exist in many larger modern office structures where the windows don't open. Instead of breathing fresh air, workers breathe stale, stagnant, polluted, and recirculated air day after day. Respiratory problems and other diseases can result. Initial symptoms may include a nagging headache and/or sore throat.

"Healing" a "sick" building is a big task. If an individual doesn't have a strong affinity for a job in a sick building, the easiest solution may be to find a new job. Otherwise, the situation can be addressed with company management and occupational safety groups, public and private. This, however, may take years of struggle before, if ever, the problem is corrected.

In the event that you are suffering work-related health problems, and are unable to correct them on your own, you may benefit by seeking help from a physician or other professional who specializes in treating occupational health problems.

Women Catch Occupational Hazards From Husbands

An analysis of more than a million deaths has discovered that women seem to share — at least in part — their husband's occupational hazards. For example, like their husbands, the wives of butchers had higher rates of multiple sclerosis (MS) because their husbands inadvertently brought home the cattle-borne brucella virus (thought to contribute to MS). Ben Flether, PhD, and psychology professor at the University of Hertfordshire, who conducted the analysis, suspects that "occupational stress is transmitted from one partner to the other when the husband brings his work home. In some cases, toxins are carried from workplace to home, too."

Homemakers at Greatest Risk of Job-Related Lung Cancer

Homemakers in Orange County were found to be at greatest risk of developing job-related lung cancer according to researchers reporting from the University of California at Irvine.

In addition to the possibility of second-hand smoke, researchers suggested that cleaning and cooking fumes could be partly responsible for the increased risk. Persons who worked in farming, factory, technical, and repair jobs also appeared to have a higher than average lung cancer risk, but to a lesser degree.

When Deep-Frying Causes Lung Cancer

Lung cancer from deep-fried foods? It seems a little far-fetched until you realize that when certain oils are heated to a boiling temperature, they release carcinogenic chemicals into the air. The more you breathe them, the more you may be increasing your risk for lung cancer.

This unusual association was discovered when researchers noticed that Chinese women have some of the highest amounts of lung cancer in the world. The cooking oils tested in a study published in the *Journal of the National Cancer Institute*, were unrefined Chinese rapeseed oil (canola oil is a from a variety of rapeseed) and peanut oil.

To reduce your exposure from carcinogenic compounds released when heating cooking oils, have good ventilation, and lower the heat when you cook. Since we hope you're not deep-frying (re-heated oils are carcinogenic and most people re-use large quantities of oil used for deep-frying), you can use peanut oil if you're concerned, for any stir-fried dishes.

Carpet Alert

Some synthetic carpets contain as many as 120 chemicals that can produce an alarming number of adverse health reactions in chemically sensitive individuals. Reactions can include difficulty concentrating; headaches; nausea; thirst; and burning of the eyes, nose, and sinuses. Even some natural fiber carpets may be chemically treated and, in turn, produce adverse health effects. This is because toxic chemicals found in carpets, such as ethylbenzene, formaldehyde, methacrylic acid, toluene, amines, and styrene, can be released through vapors that are then inhaled into the body.

What to do?

Wood flooring with natural fiber area rugs (that are not chemically treated) are generally considered to be the safest choice for your health. If this isn't an option, chemically treated carpeting can be treated with AFM Carpet Guard, a silicone finish that forms an insoluble water and odor resistant barrier, and can be mail-ordered from Allergy Relief Shop at 800-626-2810 or American Environmental Health Foundation at 800-428-2343.

What Nobody's Told You Yet About Tainted Meat

Everybody blamed everybody else in the recent tainted meat scare in the Pacific Northwest.

The fast-food chain which served the bacteria-laden burgers blamed the supermarket chain from which it purchased the meat.

The supermarket chain retorted that if the hamburgers had been properly cooked, the bacteria would have been destroyed.

Others said that the USDA was responsible for not finding the contamination in the first place.

Government authorities countered back, saying that while the USDA may be able to do more to insure the safety of our meat supply, meat, by its very nature, will never be completely sterile.

And as the accusations flew back and forth, over 400 persons became ill and several children died. The cause: eating hamburgers that contained high quantities of a particular strain of E. coli bacteria, a bacteria found in the feces of animals and humans.

While we may certainly need better quality control and meat inspection from government agencies, and while it is the responsibility of restaurants to cook meat products well enough to destroy most harmful bacteria, we are still not completely powerless against E. coli bacteria meat contamination. There is something we can do to protect ourselves from getting sick when we are exposed to this harmful bacteria, as well as others.

Pregnant Women, Elderly Women, and Young Children at Highest Risk

E. coli, Camplylobacter, Salmonella, and Listeria are some of the harmful bacteria living in dairy products, seafood, poultry, eggs, and red meat. And it's pregnant women and young children who are among the people at highest risk of getting sick from these bacteria, along with the elderly and immune-impaired.

To give you an idea of the magnitude of this problem, Salmonella, found most commonly in eggs, causes from two to four million people to become ill, and 2,000 to die, annually throughout the United States. By comparison, the recent problem with E. coli is small. Such food-borne illnesses will always continue to some degree.

A little talked about avenue of defense against food-borne illnesses does exist, however, and it is right inside our bodies. People who get sick from harmful bacteria often have fewer beneficial microorganisms in their intestines. And it's these beneficial microorganisms that keep the harmful bacteria (or pathogens) under control. Therefore, it is possible to better protect yourself, your children, and other family members against harmful bacteria by taking simple steps to increase helpful microorganisms. During pregnancy, these steps can actually begin with you before your child is born.

By Adulthood, a Healthy Person has Several Pounds of Helpful Bacteria

Microorganisms are everywhere — on the foods we eat, on everything around us, in the water we drink, and in the air we breathe. We can't avoid them, and there is no need to do so. They are not only all around us, they also live inside our bodies. In fact, your intestinal tract contains from 400 to 500 different species of microorganisms. Some of them are helpful, others harmful.

How do we get these microorganisms into our intestines in the first place? We're not born with them. In fact, newborn babies have no microbes in their intestinal tracts. Instead, they pick up beneficial bacteria from their mothers as they travel through the birth canal and by drinking breast milk.

Until a baby is weaned, 99 percent of its intestinal flora is comprised of a type of bacteria called Bifidobacteria, which is an entire group of microorganisms that helps strengthen the child's immunity. If the child is born vaginally and breast fed, it can get a lot of Bifidobacteria, especially if the mother has high levels of Bifidobacteria. That's because the actual quantity of bifido found in breast milk is affected by the amount found in a mother's intestinal tract.

Unfortunately, we are seeing more of a decline in this beneficial bacteria than ever before, even in babies who have been breast fed. Researchers believe this is due to the effects of environmental pollution. Because bifido helps nutrients in the intestinal tract become absorbed, babies who are not gaining weight, or premature babies, may need additional amounts.

Babies also pick up some helpful microorganisms through skin contact with their mothers. Throughout a baby's life, therefore, opportunities exist for the repopulation or diminishing of these bacteria, both the beneficial and harmful ones. Washing infants excessively, especially with antimicrobial soaps, washes off some beneficial bacteria, so keep your baby clean, but don't try to sterilize it's skin. Some of baby's good bacteria can protect it against infantile diarrhea and infections.

After a child is weaned, another strain of microorganism, acidophilus, enters the intestines from food, the environment, and additional contact with human skin. Eventually, balance is achieved, and colonies of Lactobacillus remain more prevalent in the small intestines throughout our life, while Bifidobacteria predominates in the large intestines. The average adult with healthy colonies of these bacteria is carrying around several pounds of them in his or her intestinal tract.

E. Coli and Other Sources of Food-Borne Illnesses

Although there are a number of harmful bacteria that cause illness, the one most in the news today is E. coli, a bacteria found in feces which finds its way onto the flesh of beef and poultry. When meat is inspected, it is examined visually, not placed under a microscope. But bacteria are too small to see, and the speed with which carcasses are inspected at slaughterhouses is too fast for inspectors to find and eliminate all cases of fecal contamination.

Cooking meat until it is well-done can eliminate these bacteria, although it may not destroy its toxic by-products which can produce diarrhea. Still, there will always be people who either do not cook meat sufficiently, or who prefer it cooked less well.

In addition, food-borne illnesses may not only be coming from high levels of harmful bacteria on and in our food. An article in the *Annals of Internal Medicine* reported that the reason harmful bacteria, like E. coli, may be appearing in greater numbers in our bodies could be because they are becoming more resistant to antibiotics like penicillin.

Antibiotics have been used for over 40 years in factory-farmed animals like beef and dairy cattle to reduce pathogenic bacteria. But these harmful bacteria don't just cooperate and die, they mutate into other strains which may require stronger antibiotics. Over time, many harmful bacteria become better able to withstand the drugs designed to kill them. Therefore, the number of harmful bacteria remain unaffected, or worse yet, can increase.

In addition, when a person eats this meat, the antibiotic residue doesn't just disappear, it also gets into the intestines.

Now we are looking at a vicious cycle: highly resistant harmful bacteria, and stronger antibiotics given to animals raised for food.

As the antibiotics in meats get into a person's body, they strip away the helpful bacteria on the intestines. This leaves empty spaces where harmful bacteria, or pathogens, can attach.

A child is especially vulnerable to this phenomenon. Since your child's intestine is young and small, it may not have strong colonies of helpful microorganisms. And over time, the antibiotics in milk and meat products can actually upset a child's delicate intestinal bacterial balance.

What's the outcome? It has been well-documented in medical research that poor balance of intestinal bacteria increases susceptibility to illness, food-borne illnesses as well as others.

Fortunately, there is a solution. The balance of beneficial bacteria can be restored. In turn, this renewed balance will increase resistance to illness. Lactobacillus acidophilus is a beneficial bacteria that is particularly effective against E. coli bacteria, which caused the recent tainted meat scare. (An especially effective strain of acidophilus is called strain DDS-1.)

How to Restore the Balance of Beneficial Bacteria

To increase beneficial bacteria, start by feeding the beneficial bacteria that is already present. This will enable them to flourish, keeping the pathogens that cause food-borne illnesses in check.

Eat lots of fresh produce. Oligosaccharides, sugars found in vegetables and fruits, help beneficial Bifidobacteria grow. These bacteria aid in forming healthy stools and improve the breakdown and utilization of fats. When you eat refined sugar from cookies, cakes, candies, and ice cream, you're feeding more pathogens and less of the good bacteria.

Also include fermented milk products in your diet, like yogurt and kefir. While most people believe all yogurt is high in Lactobacillus acidophilus, it actually is higher in Lactobacillus bulgaricus — a bacteria that helps bifido and acidophilus thrive.

If you suspect you need to further boost the helpful bacteria in yourself or your children, acidophilus and Bifidobacteria supplements are

Safer Water

Nearly 75 percent of all drinking water in this country is chlorinated to kill bacteria. Unfortunately, chlorine by-products in water are carcinogenic. A group of 28,000 postmenopausal women in Iowa were evaluated for exposure to chlorine and a connection to getting cancer. The more chlorine they were exposed to, the greater their risk was for getting colon and other cancers.

Interestingly, the greatest exposure is not in the water we drink, but the water we bathe in. For that reason, if you get chlorinated city water or if you chlorinate your well water, we suggest you may want to purchase an inexpensive shower de-chlorinator. This small attachment lasts for about a year and removes chlorine from shower water. It's a small price to pay to lower your risk for cancer. Plus it can get rid of itchy winter skin fast. To order one of these filters, call Subscriber Service at 800-728-2288.

Morris, Kelly, "Water, water, everywhere — but is it safe to drink?" *Lancet*, August 23, 1997.

available. Those which contain the highest potencies are found in the refrigerated section of health food stores. Here are situations in which you might want to use them.

Bifidobacteria: All babies and nursing mothers need Bifidobacterium infantis, one of the predominant bacteria found in babies' intestines. It may be added after any exposure to antibiotics, and used with babies who are formula-fed. Bifido produces lactase, the enzyme needed to digest milk sugar. Since 80 percent of the world's population lacks sufficient lactase to digest milk, adding this bacteria at an early age can help your child's digestion.

Acidophilus: Children who show signs of deficiency of helpful bacteria, like thrush or colic, can take acidophilus as soon as they're eating solid foods. Consider using acidophilus after vaccinations, too. While powdered acidophilus is strongest, liquid acidophilus is less expensive and can be helpful after some stomach aches.

Bifidobacteria and Acidophilus: You can increase your absorption of nutrients and protect yourself from getting infections by taking Bifidobacteria and acidophilus regularly. You can use acidophilus after a course of antibiotics to retard the growth of Candida albicans, a yeast that causes vaginitis. Remember, acidophilus lives mostly in the small intestines and Bifidobacteria lives in the large intestines.

Lactobacillus bulgaricus: This bacteria, which is found in yogurt, helps acidify the colon, creating a poor environment for harmful bacteria. It also feeds acidophilus and Bifidobacteria.

Some brands of beneficial bacteria contain the medium in which they were grown, called supernatants. These brands retain their potency longest, since the supernatant contains food for the living bacteria. Tablets or capsules which do not need to be refrigerated are usually lower in potency.

Different bacteria require different living conditions. Like some cats and dogs, they don't coexist well together. Therefore, buy them separately, not mixed together in the same jar. This will also allow you to use the amount of each you want, depending on your needs.

Where Good Bacteria "Park"

To better understand why we need plenty of helpful Lactobacillus and Bifidobacteria, think of your intestinal tract as being a long parking lot with trillions of individual slots along its walls. These slots are attachment, or parking, sites. When the attachment sites are filled up with good bacteria, there's no place for the harmful pathogens to attach. All they can do is move on by, looking for somewhere else to park.

When you take strong drugs, like broad spectrum antibiotics or chemotherapy, these medications wipe off some helpful bacteria and leave attachment sites for pathogens to park and grow.

The result can be more putrefaction, or infections like diverticulitis, in the lower intestines. The balance of bacteria in your intestines can be upset by a number of conditions including digestive problems, immune disorders, and even extreme stress.

Food Sources of Beneficial Bacteria

Yogurt can be purchased at the market or made at home. The best quality yogurts have the highest amount of beneficial bacteria. If you buy ready-made yogurt, any added sweeteners, artificial or natural (including fruit), will tend to lower helpful bacteria content.

It's simple and inexpensive to make your own yogurt. You don't need a yogurt maker. Just pick up some milk, whichever type you prefer, plus some yogurt starter from your health food store (Natren Yoghurt Starter, or Yogourmet, are two of the best). Next, follow the easy directions for heating, cooling, stirring, and pouring. Then wrap a towel around your jar of yogurt mixture, place it in an empty cooler, and close the lid. In about eight hours, you'll have a cultured yogurt that's high in beneficial bacteria.

Sweet acidophilus milk contains some acidophilus, but not very much. It may help keep your beneficial microorganisms fed more than correct a deficiency. Use it to feed the bacteria in your intestines.

Any fermented food contains bacteria that will feed your beneficial bacteria, including sauerkraut, tofu, miso soup, pickles, and olives. Some are high in sodium, so use in small quantities, and only if your health permits the extra sodium.

During Pregnancy

If you're pregnant, it may be wise for you to increase your beneficial bacteria. It can help keep your baby well and support its immune system (an overgrowth of pathogens can be responsible for infant diarrhea, diaper rash, thrush, and many infections). It can also help you avoid urinary tract infections, vaginitis, and constipation.

Planes, Trains, and Health Hazards

My family had a big scare not too long ago when my grandparents returned from a three-day whirlwind trip to New York City. They went to attend my cousin's wedding and had a great time. But shortly after their return flight landed back in San Jose, my grandmother landed in the hospital with a severely inflamed leg.

She's recovered and back home now. Still, her experience is a good reminder to us all of the need to take extra good care of ourselves when we travel — especially on long airplane rides. For people prone to blood clots (my grandmother, for example, has a maternal family history of fatal clotting disorders), long plane flights can be life-threatening.

"On long flights, particularly transoceanic flights, it is important that people prone to blood clots keep their blood moving by taking a few simple steps," says Dr. Wayne J. Riley, director of the Travel Medicine Service at Baylor College of Medicine in Houston. The same goes for long rides in cars, buses, or trains.

Reducing Your Risk of Blood Clots

To avoid discomfort and potential complications during these times, Riley recommends walking the length of the plane, bus, or train at least once an hour. If you're in a car, stop hourly, get out and walk around for a while. He also suggests:

● Flexing your ankles up and down when sitting. Blood tends to collect in the lower extremities and this simple exercise will encourage its movement.

● Avoid really tight clothing. It can restrict the free movement of blood throughout the body.

● Avoid sleeping for long periods.

● Drink lots of water. Good hydration is important for blood volume and circulation.

● Take one adult-size aspirin before departure. This helps prevent the formation of blood clots.

● Wear thigh-high support stockings or panty hose, and avoid any hose that cuts off at the knee.

To this list I would add:

● Don't eat high-fat meals or snacks (which can make blood sluggish and more prone to clotting) on the days you're in transit.

● In addition, eat very little, if any, sugar for several days before traveling. Sugar may adversely affect insulin levels and increase blood stickiness (and clotting potential).

These tips will make for a more comfortable ride, even if you have no history of blood clots.

If You Have Varicose Veins or Foot Fungus

One sign that you may be unknowingly at risk of blood clots is varicose veins — even if they don't bother you. Mine really acted up the last time I flew between California and the east coast. Taking aspirin before my flights as suggested above, then on an as-needed basis (as well as following some of the other tips), helped me keep vein inflammation to a minimum.

This is much more important than many of us realize. Excessive vein inflammation can develop into phlebitis, a painful and serious complication that often requires medical attention. And varicose vein complications result in approximately 100,000 deaths annually. Many of these deaths are the result of clots forming in inflamed and/or inflammation-damaged veins. So if you have varicose veins, play it safe, and follow the above tips for long plane flights and other forms of travel.

The cause of my grandmother's leg inflammation turned out to be a staph infection, and her doctor suspects a crack in the sole of her foot and foot fungus were contributors. Today, we hear a lot about the unsightliness of foot fungus, but not much about the health risks. They're very real. A cut or crack is especially prone to infection when fungus is present, and the infection can spread in the foot and up the leg. This is most common in diabetics, but it can happen to others, too. You are especially vulnerable to this when your immune system is under extra stress, such as the extra stress that comes with physically demanding travel. The solution? Traveling or not, always give your feet hygiene priority. Keep them clean, fungus-free, and well-manicured.

Does This Mean Some People Shouldn't Travel?

Does all this mean that you should cancel your travel plans? Probably not, although you should certainly check with your doctor if you have concerns. Vacation travel, though, provides its own type of healing benefits. The emotional healing, nourishment, and rejuvenation that come with getting away from our daily surroundings and routines. For most people, these health benefits outweigh the travel risks. Just be sensible and make the extra effort to deal healthfully with potential travel-spoilers, including long plane, train, bus, and car rides.

Chapter 9

Depression, Fatigue, and Low Energy

Are You Depressed?

What's the best thing to take for depression? Prozac? Other anti-depressants? How about making a few dietary changes first. You may avoid unnecessary medications. A number of depressed people were evaluated for sugar and caffeine — substances that can make you feel energetic and feel good when you first consume them, but actually cause a let-down afterwards. When they eliminated sugar and caffeine, many found their depression was reduced. At the end of three months with no caffeine or sugar, the people whose depression had lessened were still less depressed.

Clinically, many health practitioners have seen a reduction or absence of depression when their patients have stopped drinking coffee and tea and avoided sugar (and honey). Try this for two weeks. If diet can help your depression, you'll know.

St. John's Wort: Why All the Fuss?

It's hot. It's the latest remedy for depression. You can find it anywhere from health food stores to mainstream drug stores. But is it safe for you to take if you're depressed? Maybe. It depends on many factors from why you're depressed to how depressed you are.

St. John's wort has never been an appropriate remedy for severe depression. Nor do we believe it should be used over a long period of time, especially since there are no long-term studies that would give us information about side effects with long-term use. Still, St. John's wort seems to be a safer answer for many people than current medications.

Remember that no food, vitamin, mineral, or herb works in the same way for everyone. Everything we ingest can cause some side effects, and our bodies vary tremendously in the quantity that is beneficial or harmful. So as good as it may be, St. John's wort is not for everyone. But then, neither is Prozac, one of several popular antidepressant medications that can have numerous side effects. A number of large, double-blind studies have shown that St. John's wort can be as effective as an antidepressant with very few side effects.

What Is It and What Makes It Work?

St. John's wort is an herb called *Hypericum perforatum*, a shrub with bright yellow flowers that grows in Northern California and Southern Oregon. It's also cultivated throughout the world, where it has been used for centuries. In Germany, for example, millions of people take St. John's wort every year.

This plant contains a number of chemicals that appear to help regulate your body, including hypericin, flavonoids, xanthones, phloro-glucinol derivatives, essential oils, and carotenoids. Some of these ingredients are antiviral (against the herpes and hepatitis C viruses, Epstein-Barr virus, and influenza types A and B), some antibacterial (ointments can help heal burns more quickly), and others antifungal. St. John's wort has been used for numerous conditions in addition to depression.

It is thought that one action of St. John's wort is that it may inhibit your brain's uptake of serotonin in a similar way to Prozac, Paxil, and Zoloft, thus alleviating depression. The roots of the plant contain an anti-fungal agent, which has been shown to reduce Candida albicans.

Michael T. Murray, ND, has also found St. John's wort to be helpful for people with fibromyalgia — non-specific muscle pain — because he believes the central cause for this condition is low serotonin levels, which amplify the sensations of pain. The herb is one of a number of nutrients he uses for fibromyalgia. The others are magnesium and 5-HTP (5-hydroxytryptophan, a precursor to serotonin available only through compounding pharmacists — to find one, call the International Academy of Compounding Pharmacists, 800-927-4227).

When to Consider Taking St. John's Wort

Researchers agree about when to use St. John's wort for depression. It is most appropriately used for mild to moderate depression, not when your depression is severe. But Dr. Michael Murray cautions against using St. John's wort for a long time as a crutch. We agree with him. Diet, hormone levels, lifestyle, and attitude need to be evaluated and the appropriate changes need to be made. St. John's wort may be an excellent tool to use — but not instead of addressing any underlying problems.

Dr. Murray finds that only 25 percent of his depressed patients need to take the herb for more than six months. For people who may have a genetic tendency toward depression, long-term use may be appropriate. But not for most people.

What About Side Effects?

St. John's wort has fewer side effects than any antidepressant medication, but it has a few. The most common are gastrointestinal irritation, allergic reactions, fatigue, and restlessness. No toxicity has been reported in Germany, where more than three million prescriptions a year are given. However, if you suspect any reaction, stop taking the herb for three to five days and see if the symptom goes away.

What Should I Do About Continuing My Antidepressant?

First, talk with your doctor. Some people do best with a combination of medications and this herb, but they risk a phenomena called the "serotonin syndrome," a series of side effects including confusion, fever, shivering, sweating, diarrhea, and muscle spasms. If you continue taking any medications, be closely monitored by a health care practitioner who can recognize if you're getting yourself in trouble.

Dr. Michael Murray is both a naturopath and writer on herbs. He begins giving his patients St. John's wort extract while they're still taking their antidepressants. Then he reduces their antidepressants for two weeks, stopping them completely if all is going well.

Before You Begin ...

Don't fool around with your body and be your own doctor. If you're depressed, you need to do more than pop a few pills or take a tincture a few times a day. Your body needs specific nutrients. Either find a health practitioner to work with (doctor, naturopath, nutritionist) or run, don't walk, to your local health food store or book store and get a copy of *St. John's Wort: Nature's Blues Buster*, by Hyla Cass, MD.

I have personally known Dr. Cass for a dozen years. A psychiatrist who has used nutrition, herbs, natural hormone therapy, and lifestyle changes with her patients for decades, she is extremely knowledgeable about how and when to use St. John's wort, and what else you need to do. Her book, published by Avery Publishing (1998) is one of the best ones available.

What Doctors Don't Tell
Women About Depression

You may be depressed every month before your menses, have lived with depression all your life, or have occasional long periods of depression. If you ask your doctor what you can do for it, you may be handed a prescription for Prozac or another antidepressant.

But as Dr. Peter R. Breggin explains in his book, *Toxic Psychiatry*, (St. Martin's Press, 1991), drugs commonly prescribed by doctors for anxiety and depression have numerous negative side effects. For example, known Prozac side effects include nausea, chills, fever and diarrhea, insomnia, bizarre dreams and even hallucinations, tremors and convulsions, migraines, arthritis, and irregular heartbeat. In addition, prescription drugs often don't address the origin of depression.

What doctors don't tell you about depression is what they don't know. And much of what they don't know about numerous conditions is nutritional information. There have been many scientific studies on the nutritional aspects of depression, but most doctors confine their practice to working with pharmaceuticals. You can often change your biochemistry by eating differently and by taking supplements to increase low levels of vitamins, minerals, and other nutrients.

Begin by looking at when you're depressed and why. During a long, dark winter, depression may be due to lack of sunshine (commonly referred to as Seasonal Affective Disorder or SAD). Enough time in the sun (or use of special therapeutic lights) will wash this type of depression away. You may be having difficulties at work, a relationship may be ending, or you could be moving. These may be expected causes for a depression that will leave as you come to terms with these changes. But if you can't find a seasonal or emotional reason for depression, look to when you're experiencing the depression and what you're putting into your body.

Depression and PMS

We have learned the most about premenstrual depression from a research gynecologist and endocrinologist, Dr. Guy E. Abraham, who has been conducting and publishing studies on nutrient deficiencies and PMS for more than 20 years. His studies show that you can correct premenstrual depression, anxiety, and mood swings with a diet high in magnesium and vitamin B_6, and lower in calcium. He suggests twice as much magnesium as calcium.

In 1993, a study on depression was published that showed a connection between the hypothalamus (in the brain), pituitary gland, and thyroid. All have an influence on the amount of magnesium we have in our bloodstream and brain. The doctors who conducted this study observed that magnesium seems to help regulate our moods. In fact, the study showed that the most depressed people had the lowest levels of magnesium.

A diet to reduce and eliminate PMS-related depression is high in whole grains and beans (which contain B_6 and magnesium), and low in dairy products (which are high in calcium). Nuts and seeds are also high in magnesium, and many women have eliminated them in an effort to keep their weight down. Small amounts added to your cereal or salads usually do more good than harm.

If you are taking a multivitamin with minerals, be sure it has plenty of vitamin B_6 (Dr. Abraham advocates up to 300 mg daily) and more magnesium than calcium. Since magnesium helps calcium get into your bones, lowering your calcium intake should not put you at greater risk for bone loss but, and there are a number of studies supporting this idea, give you significantly better insurance against osteoporosis.

What you're eating may be contributing to your depression, and if you're depressed you may not be eating foods high in the nutrients you need, like B$_6$ and magnesium. If you are drinking more than 700 mg of caffeine a day (four to five cups of coffee or cola), or taking medications that contain a lot of caffeine, you may be contributing to your depression. Limit caffeinated beverages to one cup a day.

Large amounts of refined sugar also has been shown to contribute to depression. If you are drinking sugar-sweetened colas throughout the day, there is little doubt you would benefit from eliminating both the caffeine and sugar. Look at your diet and stop all caffeine and refined sugar for two weeks. Your depression should be noticeably lower. Alcohol and cigarettes have also been linked to depression. For two weeks, stop all alcohol and reduce your smoking as much as you can.

Nutrient Deficiencies and Depression

Numerous studies show lower levels of vitamins and minerals in depressed people. They include some of the B vitamins like folic acid (found in dark green leafy vegetables), riboflavin, thiamine, B$_{12}$, and B$_6$. A diet high in whole grains and beans will contain these nutrients. In addition, you may want to take a multivitamin with 50 mg or more of vitamin B complex. Whenever possible, take this in a divided dose — half with breakfast and half with lunch — for better absorption. Always take them with food to eliminate stomach discomfort.

Along with magnesium, vitamin B$_6$ is one of the most important nutrients for depression, since it is needed to help various amino acids work.

Depression and Amino Acids

Your brain contains chemicals called neurotransmitters that send various messages from one cell to another. Two particular neurotransmitters have been found to be low in people with depression: serotonin and norepinephrine. When you take large quantities of specific amino acids, you can stimulate the production of these brain chemicals. Many anti-depressant medications do this, but often with toxic side effects. Amino acid therapy can be a more natural and safer solution.

Serotonin is produced with the help of 1-tryptophan, an amino acid used for more than 20 years without side effects. Several years ago, one contaminated batch of this nutrient purchased from a single Japanese manufacturer caused serious health problems and resulted in a few deaths. The FDA then took 1-tryptophan off the market despite protestations from doctors, patients, and amino acid distributors that it was safe. Now, in a concessionary move, 1-tryptophan has been made a prescription item much more expensive than ever — but available.

Tryptophan is the least abundant amino acid you can find in food; large quantities of food must be eaten to affect a chemical change. Tryptophan is relatively high in turkey and soy. Since high dietary soy intake is also associated with a lower incidence of breast cancer (as well as

---

Women and Depression

A study out of McGill University in Canada, conducted by Dr. Mirko Diksic, shows that more serotonin, the "feel good" chemical, is made in the brains of men than in women.

An important amino acid, tryptophan, is used by the brain to manufacture serotonin. It's possible, according to Dr. Diksic, that women may be more depressed than men if their brains can't make enough serotonin, especially during stressful times when serotonin is needed.

One answer is to take tryptophan, now a prescription drug and quite expensive. Another is to take an over-the-counter form of tryptophan called 5-hydroxytryptophan (5-HTP), also expensive ($36.95 for a one-month supply from Vitamin Research Products, 800-877-2447). But a lower-cost method would be to make sure you have enough vitamin B_6 and magnesium (approx. 500 to 1,000 mg/day) in your diet or supplements. Without these important nutrients, tryptophan (found in poultry and beans) can't be used.

Dr. Diksic speaks about the effects of stress in the depletion of tryptophan. But vitamin B_6 and magnesium are also used in greater quantities when we're under stress. We've found that increased amounts of B_6 and magnesium reduce premenstrual depression, and we're suggesting these two nutrients may be even more vital than buying expensive tryptophan if you tend to get depressed frequently.

Then, if these nutrients don't do the trick, you may want to consult with your doctor about taking tryptophan. First things first.

Diksik, Dr. Mirko. *National Academy of Sciences*, 1997, 94:5308-5313.

many other serious health threats), you may want to add soybeans to soups, tofu to stir-fried vegetables, and add veggie burgers made from soy (we think the Boca Burgers taste the best) to your diet.

L-phenylalanine and l-tyrosine are amino acids available through health food stores that increase the production of norepinephrine. Amino-acid treatments can be a bit complicated, so you may want to coordinate yours with a physician or health care provider familiar with this approach. (To find one, you can call the American College for the Advancement of Medicine at 1-800-532-3688.)

If you'd like to go ahead on your own, consider the following protocol based on conversations with several doctors: l-tyrosine, from 500 to 3,500 mg in the morning as soon as you awake, and the same amount mid-afternoon without food. If you feel this program is not working as well for you as you'd like, substitute the afternoon dosage of l-tyrosine for 1,000 to 3,000 mg of l-phenylalanine or d-l-phenylalanine in the afternoon. Take this amino acid with food.

All amino acids require adequate vitamin B_6 and magnesium to be utilized. You can be sure you're taking enough if your multi-vitamin is one of dozens of women's PMS formulas with extra B_6 and magnesium. Additional information on how to use these supplements may be found in *The Way Up From Down*, a book on amino-acid therapy and depression, by Priscilla Slagle, MD (St. Martin's Press, 1992) or from a physician familiar with this approach.

Exercise All Your Options

Depression is stagnant energy that sits and weighs you down. Inactivity is known to contribute to depression, while exercise stimulates brain chemicals that lift your mood. It doesn't seem to matter whether or not you do aerobic or non-aerobic exercise. Anything will do. Begin with a 10-minute walk every day and gradually increase the time. While it may be difficult to get yourself moving, just changing your diet and taking a walk may make it unnecessary for you to take prescription drugs for depression — or to be depressed.

Treating Depression Helps Women Abstain From Alcohol Abuse

Depressed female alcoholics who were treated for depression were more likely to remain abstinent than those whose depression went untreated, according to a study that appeared in the Journal of the American Medical Association. "The relationship between women, alcohol, and depression is a complicated one, where physiological, social, and psychological issues all come into play," explained Barbara Mason, PhD, associate professor of psychiatry at the University of Miami School of Medicine and lead authors of the study. Her study looked at 71 patients with primary alcohol dependence, with 28 of these exhibiting secondary major depression.

Patients were abstinent from alcohol for one week before being randomly assigned to six months of outpatient treatment with either desipramine (an anti-depressant drug) or identical placebo capsules. Physicians have traditionally believed that depression will clear once an alcohol abuser abstains from drinking.

But Dr. Mason's study suggests that treating diagnosable depression in recently abstinent alcoholics may make their relapse more likely. It found that those treated with desipramine remained abstinent significantly longer than those taking the placebo. It also found a significantly greater depression response in those receiving desipramine (82 percent) than those receiving the placebo (22 percent). Desipramine belongs to a class of drugs called tricyclic antidepressants.

Although the actual mechanism of action is unknown, the leading theory suggests that these drugs restore normal levels of certain chemicals in the central nervous system, called neurotransmitters, by preventing their re-uptake once they have been secreted. Desipramine is selective for one neurotransmitter in particular, norepinephrine, which is altered during alcohol withdrawal.

Fatigue

To Look and Feel Your Best, Spring Clean Your Body

Springtime is when life begins to renew itself once more. Plants that have been dormant in winter begin to sprout. We think of spring cleaning our homes, perhaps as an unconscious way of complementing the changes occurring in nature. However, we often forget that we are part of nature, and spring is the perfect time to clean our bodies as well.

Janet was a college student who came to see me complaining of fatigue. Her family has a history of breast cancer, so I was especially concerned when she told me she had time to eat only fast foods and frozen dinners. Many of these foods are heavily processed (luncheon meat sandwiches) and high in fat (French fries and cheese). She ate few vegetables and drank enough coffee and soft drinks for a small family. All of this explained why she was fatigued, but her diet was doing something much worse. It was turning her body into a toxic-waste dump and increasing her risk for breast cancer.

I told Janet she needed to do some spring cleaning. She looked puzzled until I explained that the body needs to be cleaned and maintained just like our homes. Janet's face lightened, and she agreed to eat more

Chronic Fatigue and Vitamin B$_{12}$

Many women suffer from a debilitating cluster of symptoms called Chronic Fatigue. This is not an easily identifiable disease, but rather a syndrome that seems to originate from a past virus or viruses. While the condition is complex, the tonic effect of vitamin B$_{12}$ injections has been seen in various studies.

People were given from 3,000 to 5,000 mcg of vitamin B$_{12}$ every two to three days. After a number of weeks, from 50 percent to 80 percent of them noticed increased energy and a feeling of well-being. Continuation of the injections was necessary for patients to continue feeling well. Although vitamin B$_{12}$ does not address the cause of Chronic Fatigue, if it can help someone function better or feel better while they're pursuing a cause-and-cure approach, we think it may be a good idea.

Br J Nutr 1973;30:277-283.

salads, less fried foods, and reduce her coffee intake for two weeks. She drank flavored mineral water instead of sodas and made fast nutritional meals for herself like fat-free refried beans and corn tortillas piled high with salsa and sprouts.

Janet soon realized that the fatigue was gone and life was enjoyable once again. Her increased energy convinced her to continue eating better, and she understood the long-term benefits of spring cleaning.

People Hibernate, Too

Winter is when plants and animals store food and conserve energy and when we tend to overeat and eat foods with more fats and sugars, which keep our bodies warm. In spring, the weather is warmer and we don't need so many dense or fatty foods. We stop to think about how we look and feel. What can we do about the extra pounds we'd like to shed? We can change our diet and spring clean ourselves from the inside out. In the process, not only will we feel better and have more energy, but like a freshly cleaned house, we'll look better, too! Because no matter how well-cared for your skin might be, what's inside will still be reflected on the outside.

A Bit of Chinese Wisdom

Chinese medicine has talked about the concept of spring cleaning for centuries. The Chinese think in terms of eating foods that are in season because seasonal foods contain the nutrients our bodies need at those times. Root vegetables, grown in winter, contain starches that are burned as fuel to keep us warm. Spring and summer fruits and vegetables cool us when the weather is mild or hot. Lemons are a refrigerant, keeping us cool in summer when we drink lemonade.

The Chinese also associate various elements with the seasons: fire, earth, metal, water, and wood. Wood is the element that is associated with all living things: plants, animals, and people, and the season in which wood predominates is the spring. Each season has not only its own element, but specific body organs and glands. Spring is liver time, and the liver has an amazing ability to regenerate itself. It also is the organ that stores toxins the body doesn't know how to excrete. So it's important to give our livers additional support through detoxification, and there is no better time to do this than in the spring.

Your liver is a workhorse. Every day it performs more than 300 separate functions including filtering toxins in your blood and sending them out your body through natural, solid, and liquid waste pathways. Whatever your body can't get rid of, it stores in your liver and in fat cells. Once a year, it's a good habit to take any dietary burdens you can off the liver and to help remove stored toxins.

Avoid New Toxins and Flush Out the Rest

An important step in spring cleaning your body is to stop putting toxins into it. This means eliminating foods with added chemicals, additives, and preservatives like hot dogs, luncheon meats, diet sodas, processed cheese, and ice cream. Diet foods are often packed with unnecessary chemicals that increase the liver's burden. Start reading labels!

In addition, reduce coffee consumption, for even when it's organic it contains over 100 unwanted chemicals your liver has to eliminate. Commercial decaffeinated coffee is worse, often containing additional chemical residues from the decaffeinating process.

Also eliminate alcohol for a few weeks while you're detoxifying. It takes three full days for your liver to eliminate the ethanol in one drink.

Finally, buy organic produce, free from insecticides and pesticides, when you can. Not only is organic produce free of chemical residues that add unnecessary burdens to the immune system — studies have shown that organic foods have up to two-and-a-half times the minerals of non-organic food. To further increase organic-produce consumption for yourself as well as your family, consider growing your own produce. Or begin sprouting garbanzo beans, mung beans, and lentils to add extra nutritional punch to your salads.

It's in the Water

When you spring clean your body, you're helping it remove stored toxins which can lead to fatigue or illness. Start sipping more clean water (purified or distilled) throughout the day to allow your body to release toxins naturally. Try to drink half a glass an hour, or whenever your mouth is dry, rather than a glass or two at once. Even if you aren't thirsty, sip water every half hour for a few days.

As you increase the amount of water you drink, you'll notice your mouth feels dry more often. That's because when you don't drink enough water, your body gets used to being dehydrated and shuts off the thirst sensation. Drinking more water awakens the body to its dehydrated condition. Water is your best first detoxifier.

Increase your fresh fruits and vegetables to add more fiber to your diet. This helps move toxins out of your intestines where they can sit and ferment, causing a buildup of harmful bacteria and toxic gasses associated with colon cancer, inflammatory bowel disease, and other illnesses. They also contain high amounts of vitamin A and other nutrients important to liver function.

Many people use various herbs or fasts to detoxify. They can be effective but can cause headaches and fatigue. You can give your body a good spring cleaning without any side effects — except more energy — just by eating more vegetables, especially green salads and sprouts, high in cleansing chlorophyll and vitamin A, and drinking more water.

It's Time to Improve Your Health by Gardening

If you've yet to become a gardener, we strongly urge you to do so. Here's why: Gardening is great exercise. It utilizes a wide variety of different movements including stretching, aerobics, and weight lifting. Gardening also gets you out into the fresh air and sunshine. These are important nutrients for good health. If you're extra sun-sensitive or will be out for more than 15 or 30 minutes, cover up well with a wide-brimmed hat, long-sleeved shirt, and sunscreen as needed.

What will you grow? Flowers can be fun and rewarding. Or maybe you've been wanting to add to or revise part of your landscaping. Around here, we aim for easy-care, low maintenance flowers and landscaping, and concentrate our greater efforts on cultivating fresh, organic herbs and produce.

If you're a beginner or want to learn more about gardening, take a class, or read up on it. You might try the *Herb Quarterly*. It is beautifully illustrated and is brimming with fascinating articles, savory and healthy recipes, and much more. You can get a sample issue for half-price by sending your name, address, and $3 to: The Herb Quarterly, P.O. Box 689, San Anselmo, CA 94979-0689.

Don't have space for gardening? You'd be surprised at what you can grow in pots and other large containers. If you have only a window, look for a sprout kit at your health food store, and grow your own sprouts.

Finally, gardening is great for the lifting your spirits. Digging, planting, watering, and other garden activities all provide quiet times for reflection in the great outdoors. This is especially important for those of us who spend lots of time indoors and with machines. One outstanding Chinese doctor we know recommends gardening for this very reason. It helps create better balance in our lives, and in turn, better health.

Spring Planting Tips for Better Health

Whether you've never grown a single bean or are a seasoned gardener always on the lookout for a new tip, here are a number of quick and easy ways to have your own fresh-grown, organic produce.

Plant fruit and nut trees. Once a fruit or nut tree is established, it can provide 10, 15, maybe even 20 years of great-tasting, home-grown, organic produce — with minimal maintenance. Fair-sized bare-root trees are now in stock at most nurseries for $10 to $20 a tree.

Start a vegetable garden. A vegetable garden can be simple or elaborate. Beginners should think about the produce they eat the most (or would like to eat more of). Then ask your local nursery person how easy these items are to grow in your area, and try a few easy ones and maybe a difficult one your first year. Tomatoes, peppers, basil, parsley, beans, peas, and squash are usually easy to grow, and various combinations of them produce a wide variety of tasty dishes.

Go for the greens. Those luscious, exotic salad mixes that cost a lot in the store are a lot easier to grow then you might imagine. Simply prepare soil in a "salad" plot, large pot, or window box, mix up several varieties of lettuces (no iceberg), sprinkle them over the soil, then sprinkle another quarter inch of soil over the seeds, keep moist, and your salad will start growing.

Think edible. Many crop-producing plants and trees can be just as attractive as decorative ones. Cherry and pomegranate trees have especially beautiful blossoms; citrus and avocado trees are evergreens and can be used for screening or a continuous show of green leaves in warmer climates; hardy strawberries quickly spread and work double duty as ground cover; asparagus and artichoke plants feature beautiful ferns. Grapes are easy-to-train vines and uniquely suited to arbors.

The beauty of perennials: less work. Any plant that is not an annual will live for years and sometimes decades, and that means less work for the grower. Non-annuals include trees, grapes, berries (such as raspberries, blueberries, and strawberries), asparagus, artichokes, and rhubarb.

Sprouting. Sprouts, such as bean sprouts, are rich in enzymes, vitamins, and minerals, making them a true power food to add to salads. The easiest way to get started is to purchase a sprout kit at your local health food store. No space? No problem! You can grow sprouts in a jar on your kitchen counter.

With a little foresight and planning ahead, you can enjoy a variety of homegrown, organic fruits and vegetables with minimal effort. What's more, gardening is great exercise, and you can share any extra produce with others — another great way to lift the spirits and help you feel great.

Question and Answer

Q. I've been tired and sick for more than a year and have been taking vitamins and echinacea, but I'm not getting any better. Blood tests show I have a virus called Cytomegalo-virus (CMV). What do you suggest I do next? Who, other than a medical doctor, might be able to help me? I've tried medical doctors and they haven't had answers that have worked.

A. Drs. Michael Rosenbaum and Murray Susser have indicated in their book, *Solving the Puzzle of Chronic Fatigue Syndrome* (Life Sciences Press), that CMV is one of a number of viruses that has been associated with chronic fatigue. They are both MDs, so their book offers a more thorough program than you, as a lay person, can devise.

In addition, we have found documentation linking high concentrations of calcium to Epstein-Barr virus and CMV. David L. Watts, PhD, speaks about studies that showed when calcium was blocked from entering lymphatic cells, Epstein-Barr virus was inhibited. If you are eating a lot of dairy, or taking high amounts of calcium supplements, you might want to lower your calcium intake for a month to see how this affects you.

Finally, we suggest you contact ACAM (the American College of Advancement in Medicine at 800-532-3688) for doctors in your area who use a number of approaches in addition to conventional medicine. When you have been sick for so long, you may want a medical doctor who uses complementary medicine. Many of them use herbs, homeopathy, and nutritional supplements.

Low Energy

High-Energy Eating

Some people function best on a high-protein diet, such as the one featured in *Enter The Zone*, a popular new diet book by Barry Sears, PhD. For many others, however, a high complex-carbohydrate diet is the best one for feeling satisfied after meals and providing a steady stream of maximum energy. Here's why....

Simple carbohydrates, found in refined starches, sugars, and fruit, burn quickly. They may give you a quick energy boost, but then your energy level may also crash just as quickly if not backed up by another slower burning energy source such as protein or complex carbohydrates. When a crash occurs, your thinking becomes fuzzy, your muscles lose their strength, and you feel generally fatigued.

Slow-burning, complex carbohydrates also improve your body's ability to burn fats. Eat more complex carbohydrates and you just may lose weight, as a result of burning extra fat, without even trying!

In addition, complex carbohydrates fill you up and cause you to feel satisfied longer. Brown rice, millet, oatmeal, lentil soup, and beans of all kinds, are filling foods. Because they digest over a longer period of time than white flour products and sugars, your stomach is not giving you a signal that it's empty as quickly, and energy from these foods is released for hours, not just minutes. You'll have more energy and you won't crash afterward.

Pasta for Breakfast?

Which food burns slower and leaves you feeling more satisfied: pasta or white bread? A recent study compared how quickly each of these wheat products affects blood sugar levels and satiety (fullness). In this study, pasta and bread, both made from white flour, were shown to have very different burn rates. Pasta burned slowly and gradually declined to a level called baseline. Bread burned rapidly, but also dropped quickly below the baseline. People who ate pasta for breakfast, rather than bread, were less tired after lunch.

Is Wheat Best for You?

Let's say you switch to eating more whole grains and the grain you're eating is predominantly is wheat: cereals, crackers, pasta, bread, cookies, wheat tortillas. If you find you're more tired than you were before you ate so many carbohydrates, stop all wheat for two weeks. Watch your energy during that time and at the end of two weeks, eat a little wheat. If you have any negative reactions — such as fatigue, headache, etc. — you may need to avoid wheat for a few months.

Emphasize eating other grains like millet and brown rice. Make cornbread without wheat, have corn tortillas and baked corn chips. Eat oatmeal or wheat-free granola for breakfast. Try some rice noodles for dinner and ad barley to soups. Some people have wheat sensitivities, others just find that wheat products burn too quickly to give them lasting energy.

How Much Protein?
Let Your Energy Be Your Guide

How much protein do you need to consume for maximum energy? The answer depends on who you ask. Different experts will give you different answers. *In Becoming Vegetarian,* author Vesanto Melina, RD, *et al,* recommends around 49 grams of dietary protein daily for a 135-pound person. We agree with this general recommendation, but also consider it an approximation — different people have different dietary needs. How much protein you actually need to consume may be more or less than Melina's suggestion of 49 grams. In our opinion, it's best to let your energy be your guide.

If you've been experiencing fatigue for no apparent reason, such as lack of sleep or a health condition, you might try increasing your protein intake for one month. Do this by decreasing your intake of fast-burning foods, such as refined flour and sugar. Instead of these foods, consume a little more animal protein and/or beans, peas, and tofu. For some, a protein powder might be an easy solution. At the end of one month, if your energy level has increased, you will know a lack of protein was playing a role in your lack of energy.

In fact, these concerns are so widespread that you can even find wheat-free bread at most health food stores.

Rice vs. Wheat for Energy

All grains burn at about the same rate, right? Not according to a Cornell University study published in the American Journal of Clinical Nutrition. They followed over 3,000 women in China, some on a wheat-based diet, some on a rice-based diet. The study looked closely at blood test markers that are associated with diabetes, obesity, high blood pressure and coronary heart disease. The results were surprising.

Women who ate a lot of wheat had high triglycerides, indicating they were storing sugars in their fat cells and not burning them up as energy. Those who ate a rice-based diet appeared to burn up the sugars, rather than store them. Rice contains a higher amount of amylose, a particular kind of starch that slows down the absorption of glucose. In plain language, this means that you'll get longer-lasting energy from eating foods made with rice than wheat.

Choose Slow-Burning Starches

In addition to rice, legumes and most vegetables turn into energy slowly and steadily, while potatoes, carrots, and sweet corn burn quickly.

Pass on These Energy Bars

Yohimbe Strength and Energy Formula bar by Mega Pro. Yohimbe is an herb that induces erections in men, and the advertising on this energy bar talks about a "rock hard physique." When asked about how much yohimbe was in the bar, and how it could be metabolized without citric acid (little did the sales rep know we were knowledgeable in the use of yohimbe), we were told there wasn't enough in it to do anything, so the lack of citric acid wasn't important.

This Yohimbe bar also contains Damiana (said to be an aphrodisiac) and Guarana (which contains a chemical almost identical to caffeine). The Guarana might give some energy, but the rest is placebo. The same company makes an Energy Max bar. Since there are much better products out there for your money, pass these two up!

If you're having a baked potato for a meal, include some brown rice or beans to slow down how quickly the meal turns to sugar. Add lentils, split peas and all kinds of beans to what you've been eating.

If beans give you gas, this is not an insurmountable problem. Take two Beano enzyme tablets with your first mouthful. Beano helps digest beans, grains and vegetables and it really works! You'll find Beano in pharmacies, supermarkets and some health food stores. Often, after you've eaten small quantities of beans over a period of time, your body will produce the enzymes needed to digest them and you may not need to take extra enzymes.

Canned beans are fine to use if you don't have the time to cook dried beans. They can be rinsed free of sugar and any preservatives and added to instant soups or salads. If you're cooking beans, throw away the water they've been soaking in, then cook them slowly over a low flame in fresh water. They're less likely to cause flatulence when cooked in this manner. An herb used in Mexican cooking, epasote, also removes the gaseous quality of beans.

Tired After Lunch?

If you get tired after you eat lunch, as opposed to late afternoon fatigue, you may be eating too much fat and not enough carbohydrates. In two human studies, people who ate more fats and less carbohydrates were less alert than those who ate more carbohydrates and less fats. They also had a more difficult time concentrating on tasks that required sustained attention and were less cheerful.

People on a high fat diet experienced a drop in alertness two-and-a-half hours after eating, when the foods they ate had left their stomach. Researchers believe this is due to a chemical reaction which occurs after fats are absorbed. For now, you may want to substitute your hamburger and French fries or ham and cheese sandwich with potato chips for some leftover rice or pasta with veggies, or a carton of instant bean soup — and watch your afternoon energy increase.

Wells AS, Read NW, Craig A, "Influences of dietary and intraduodenal lipid on alertness, mood and sustained concentration," *British Journal of Nutrition* 74, 115-123 (1995).

High-Energy Meal Ideas

Breakfast: Don't skip this meal! Your body needs fuel in the morning. Contrary to popular diets, fruit and fruit juice is not sufficient for most people. It's high in fruit sugars and gets digested too quickly to give you lasting energy. You may want to begin with a little fruit or diluted juice, but follow it with a whole-grain cereal. Cream of brown rice and oatmeal are two good hot cereals. Fat-free granola, Nature's Path Millet Rice flakes, or New Morning Oatios are good-tasting cold cereals that will keep your energy up. Van's International makes both organic whole wheat frozen waffles and some that are wheat-free. Look for them in health food stores and top them with a little fruit, or fruit jam.

Lunch: If wheat doesn't make you sleepy, you could have a sandwich and salad. Otherwise, look for soups like lentil, split pea, black bean — either canned, dried or homemade. Add a grain to it (throw in a little leftover brown rice or have rye crackers or rice cakes) to give you a complete protein for longer-lasting energy. Remember, mixing grains and legumes makes a complete protein, which also provides slow-burning energy.

Dinner: Keep your portion of animal protein low. About the equivalent of a half a chicken breast is sufficient when you're eating plenty of grains and beans. Make sure you add brown rice, millet, rice noodles or pasta to your protein and vegetables. Or skip the animal protein for a high-energy vegetarian meal like stir-fried vegetables over brown rice, leftover vegetables with rice and beans in a corn or whole wheat tortilla, or a veggie burger like Boca Burgers with oven-baked potato slices and cole slaw.

Snacks: Baked corn chips with or without bean dip, popcorn, whole grain crackers, fruit-juice sweetened muffins or cookies like Nana's (made with organic grains, raisins and maple syrup). Avoid snack foods made with evaporated cane juice or unrefined sugar like Sucanat. The minerals they contain may not be sufficient to keep your energy from spiking and dipping.

Give this kind of a program a few weeks, and see how your energy improves. Animal protein can take several hours from the time you eat it until it becomes energy. Complex carbohydrates turn to energy in a fraction of that time. Sustain your energy throughout the day with good quality whole foods rather than sugar and caffeine. You'll love the difference good foods make in your energy level! And if you prepare meals for other family members, too, they'll appreciate the difference as well.

Chapter 10

Diet, Digestion, and Weight Loss

No Time to Eat Well? No Problem!

This chapter goes right along with the preceding one because the better you eat, the better you'll feel. You probably already know what foods you should be eating — low in fat, high in fiber, plenty of vegetables, and a little good-quality protein — but do you find the time to prepare meals that fit this picture?

What follows is a dietary plan that will give you the most energy and help you be your proper weight. At the same time, it's probably the best protection against illness for both you and your family.

Many women know which foods are healthier than others but not how to put them together into an acceptable meal everyone in the family will eat. Besides, cooking healthy meals that taste good takes time, doesn't it? Not necessarily.

Over the years, I've found a simple formula that has helped hundreds of my patients eat the way they want and need to. It's based on one of my favorite eating out experiences as a child when I was taken to a Chinese restaurant and could choose one item from column A and one from column B. The excitement of creating my own taste sensations is one I've always remembered.

The formula I've given to my patients begins with the first question: which ethnic foods do you like to eat and what sauces or condiments give foods that flavor? Begin with tomato sauce if you like Italian. For Chinese-flavored foods, you want soy sauce with perhaps a little grated fresh ginger (it's easy to keep a small piece of ginger root in your vegetable bin). Curry turns a meal into an Indian one, and curry powder can be mixed with a can of lentil soup, then pureed together for a curried lentil sauce to pour over vegetables. For Mexican-style meals, think of salsa and corn tortillas.

Think of any other ethnic food you like— perhaps from the country where your grandparents are from — and the flavors that could turn a starch, vegetable, and protein into a meal that has a taste you enjoy. Your list of sauces and condiments, then, might look something like this:

tomato sauce with garlic
soy sauce with ginger or oyster sauce
curried lentil sauce
salsa

Next, begin a column of starches — those low-fat, filling foods that add bulk to our meals. This column might include any or all of the following:

brown rice
pasta (any kind)
potatoes
corn or whole wheat tortillas
couscous (cracked wheat) or millet

Your next column is for vegetables. We all have our favorites and not-so-favorites. But add some of these for quick, easy meals:

mixed Chinese vegetables (frozen or prepacked)
green beans
broccoli
mixed vegetables (fresh or frozen)

Then there's the protein column. Protein may or may not include animal protein. When it does, you can keep this protein to a small amount. Here are some ideas for protein: beans (black beans for chili, fat-free refried beans for Mexican food, pureed garbanzo beans for hummus, white beans to add to pasta sauce, pureed lentils with curry powder)

chicken, turkey, fish, meat
eggs
tofu (soy bean curd)

Now you're ready to mix and match. Let me give you a few ideas and you can see how easy this is.

Italian: Toss steamed broccoli or asparagus with tomato sauce and pasta. Serve with salad (add garbanzo beans or white beans for protein) and garlic bread (use a little olive oil instead of butter). If you like, put a little ground turkey or chicken in the sauce.

Indian: Combine mixed sautéed vegetables with diced potatoes, winter squash or yams, or eggplant (whichever you prefer) and a good helping of frozen peas. Add small chunks of chicken if you want and pour over rice or millet. Add curried lentil sauce. Serve with mango chutney. If you like Indian food, but your children don't, serve their vegetables with tomato or soy sauce for a flavor they may prefer.

Chinese: Combine mixed sautéed Chinese vegetables (or add bean sprouts to frozen mixed veggies) with a little diced tofu, which adds

---

Broccoli Sprouts — The New Wonder Food

Three-day old broccoli sprouts, started from seed, have been found to have 30 to 50 times as many isothiocyanates as those found in mature broccoli.

Isothiocyanates are chemicals that stimulate detoxifying enzymes found in our bodies that are believed to significantly lower the risk of cancer. Sulforaphane is one isothiocyanate that appears to be a potent detoxifier.

Broccoli, cauliflower, brussels sprouts, kale, cabbage, Chinese cabbage, and bok choi are just some of the cruciferous vegetables that contain significant enough amounts of isothiocyanates to be considered cancer-fighters. Two pounds of them eaten each week appear to reduce the risk for colon cancer, according to scientific studies. By contrast, an ounce or two of the sprouts would do the same thing.

We expect numerous products to come on the market containing powdered broccoli and sulforaphane. Because all foods contain more than one or two helpful ingredients, and the interaction of all nutrients appears to give greater benefits than any one isolated chemical, we suggest you get your isothiocyanates in one of two ways. Either eat more cruciferous vegetables or add broccoli sprouts to your diet.

If you're sprouting them yourself, you'll want to buy organic seed. This is not so simple, if you want more than a small packet. But if you really want organic broccoli seed, call Pat at Harmony Farm Supply and Nursery (707-823-9125). He'll make every effort to find it for you. Minimum order: 1 pound. Price: unknown, as it can fluctuate widely depending on its availability. But if it can be found, chances are, Pat can find it for you!

Angier, Natalie. "Researchers find a concentrated anticancer substance in broccoli sprouts," *NY Times*, September 16, 1997.

texture but not much taste. If you want to buy just a small amount, Mori-Nu brand comes in small boxes and does not have to be refrigerated until after it's opened. Keep some in your pantry. Add a little soy sauce and fresh grated ginger if you like and serve over rice (white or brown) with oyster-flavored sauce (ready-made sauces are available in many markets, and some are vegetarian).

Mexican: Corn or whole wheat tortillas with fat-free refried beans (either pinto or black), a little leftover rice, shredded chicken if you like, and topped with salsa and romaine lettuce. Serve with a salad or put out various raw vegetables that can be added to these tostadas (tomatoes, cucumbers, sprouts, chopped carrots, avocado).

Mediterranean: If you like this taste, try pureeing a can or two of garbanzo beans and adding fresh garlic (1 or 2 cloves) and lemon juice. Now you have fat-free hummus. The hummus sold in stores has a lot of olive oil and sesame seed paste (tahini), so it's fairly high in fat.

Next, make some couscous (cracked wheat) or millet (cooks like rice, but takes less time) and add lemon juice and a bunch of finely chopped parsley. Finely chop two or three tomatoes and add. Now you have tabouli.

Serve with a salad that has a lot of cucumbers, tomatoes, and onions with a dressing of olive oil and lemon juice. Add some whole wheat pita bread and you have a Middle-Eastern meal.

Easy to Be Prepared

These meals do not have to take a lot of preparation. Some foods can be made ahead of time, others can be bought frozen, like vegetables and boneless chicken breasts. Some, like beans, can be canned.

Rice, millet, couscous, and even pasta may be made in large quantities some evening after dinner when you are going to be home. After they've been cooked and cooled down a bit, put them in plastic containers or zip lock bags and store in the freezer. When you come home tired and rushed, simply take out a bag or two of your starch and heat it in the microwave. Sauté a package or two of frozen vegetables in a wok with a little olive oil, add your seasoning and present your family — or yourself — with a delicious, healthy, low-fat meal.

Healthy meals do not need to be boring or take a lot of time when you have a few easy formulas to follow.

A New Definition of Food Quality

Whole grain or refined? High fat, low fat or no fat? Organic or non-organic? When there are so many factors to look at, how can we possibly make the best food choices? Is it better to eat a non-organic bread made with refined flour or an organic white bread? Do we pick up a bag of organic corn chips fried in safflower oil or are non-organic baked chips better? If you're confused, you're not alone. This is enough to tax even the most careful shopper.

What does it cost to eat better quality foods? The answer comes in

All Complex Carbos Are Not Alike

Now that we're becoming familiar with the difference between complex carbohydrates (starchy vegetables and beans, for instance) and simple sugars (white sugar and honey), there's new information that will either confuse us further — or give us more energy. We've been told that complex carbos turn into sugar more slowly than simple sugars, and for that reason provide more constant energy over a longer period of time. By switching from a high-sugar meal to a high-starch meal, we'll be more energetic and healthier. But all complex carbos are not alike.

Some starchy foods raise our blood sugar and insulin levels higher than sugar. And the longer it takes for foods to turn into sugar, the more sustained our energy. Fats slow down the absorption of simple sugars, so an ice cream cone containing fats doesn't cause a sugar rush and sudden energy drop. But a baked potato could! It all depends on the glycemic index, which tells us how fast certain foods turn into sugar. If you're eating a diet high in complex carbohydrates that turn to sugar quickly, you may be having periods of low energy. Even if the foods are healthy foods.

Potatoes, sweet corn, and grains (even whole grains like brown rice) are higher on the glycemic index than beans. Keep plenty of garbanzos, black beans, kidney beans, navy beans, etc. in your diet. Sweet potatoes are lower on the glycemic index than white-fleshed potatoes, so eat more of them for better energy. If you're eating grains, corn, or potatoes, add a little fat to them to slow down their conversion into sugar. Just a half teaspoon of olive oil or butter will give you more sustained energy.

Ref: Blaak, EE, Saris, WHM, "Health aspects of various digestible carbohydrates," *Nutrition Research* 15, 1547-1573 (1995).

the form of another question: what does it cost you when you're sick? Even if you have an HMO with no deductible, illness costs you the most precious commodity of all: time and quality of life. Some of the most devastating illnesses have been associated with our diets: breast cancer, colon cancer, and autoimmune diseases. You can't put a price on your health.

That said, we grocery shoppers spend a little over $80 a week, on average, to feed a family of three or four. Purchasing the best quality foods possible doesn't have to cost much more. It can even cost less. That's because the least processed foods have the highest nutritional value — foods like brown rice, millet, corn tortillas, beans and vegetables. These foods tend to be the least expensive, even when they're organic. Many of these foods can also be made in large quantities and frozen for future meals, to allow you extra convenience as well as more variety in your diet. Even rice and millet can be cooked ahead, put into zip-locked baggies, frozen, then thawed, without losing taste, texture or nutrients.

My priorities for quality foods are based on the effect certain foods and chemicals have on women's health. Some of these, like pesticides, affect the health of children and men, as well. The same estrogenic effects of the organochlorines found in pesticides that contribute to breast cancer increase men's risk of prostate cancer. So I'd like to share some of my shopping insights with you to make your choices easier. There are two important areas to consider in the foods we eat: harmful substances and helpful substances.

Perhaps the most harmful to women are foods that have been heavily sprayed with pesticides, herbicides, fungicides and insecticides. They contain organochlorines—chemicals that mimic the effects of estrogen. The best information we have to date about the risks for breast cancer is the length of time a woman has been exposed to estrogen. If you increase your estrogen exposure by eating a lot of non-organic fruits and vegetables you could be increasing your risk for a disease that has increased since chemicals on plants have been used commercially.

A report in the June 1997 issue of *Nutrition Action Newsletter* showed that strawberries, cherries, apples, and grapes were among the foods containing the highest amounts of pesticide residues, according to a Washington D.C. consumer group called the Environmental Working Group. The head of an organic foods company told us that artichokes were among the most heavily sprayed of vegetables. Some of the least toxic kinds of produce appear to be broccoli, cabbage, cauliflower, onions and sweet potatoes.

A study out of Mount Sinai Medical Center in New York discovered that women who had high levels of a derivative of DDT (called DDE) developed breast cancer four times more than women with low levels of this poison. For your health, and for the health of any children and other family members you're feeding, we strongly suggest you buy, raise, and eat organic produce whenever possible.

Question: In view of the fact that strawberries are the most heavily sprayed crop of all, is it better to eat a) sprayed strawberries for nutritional value? b) no sprayed strawberries because of pesticides?

(My answer is "b," no sprayed strawberries.)

● Whenever possible, buy organic. In the past, we've bought the largest, most beautiful apples, the most perfect-looking tomatoes, lettuce without a sign of insect damage. Now we are realizing the cost to our health that eating perfect-looking foods brings. Pesticides, insecticides and herbicides are contributing to health problems, and nothing neutralizes the chemical residues that get inside the food. A 1995 study from the US Agriculture Department showed 10,329 pesticides on and in 7,328 fruits and vegetables. The apples were washed and cored; bananas peeled, and other produce was tested after it was washed and prepared for cooking.

It's also important to realize that many pesticides and herbicides that are too toxic to be used legally in this country are manufactured here, shipped to other countries, then sprayed on produce which is shipped back to us for our consumption. This is called The Circle of Poison. These poisons are killing the people who apply them and causing birth defects in their babies. The smaller quantities we consume are probably also contributing to many of our illnesses.

Best solution: Shop at farm markets at peak growing seasons and buy local organic produce. Ask your supermarkets to carry more organics and buy them so the stores will find organic produce profitable. Supermarkets can often buy in larger quantities than health food stores, bringing the cost down. Grow some of your own produce. A 2'x3' planter box will hold 6 lettuce plants, 4 potato plants, one tomato plant, 3-4 spinach or chard plants, 3 pepper plants, or 2 squash or cucumber plants. You can put one on your patio if you don't have gardening space.

● Wash all non-organic produce with detergent. You can wash some of the harmful chemicals off with detergent or sprays designed to clean produce. One brand, Healthy Harvest — 203-245-2033 — prints a chart on their package showing how effective their product is in reducing pesticides from the surface of produce.

● Eliminate or reduce fried foods. All foods that are fried commercially are fried in reheated oil. When oil is reheated it becomes rancid and is then carcinogenic. It's safer to eat foods that have not been fried, like baked egg rolls, baked French fried potatoes, and baked chips. How, then, do you choose which chips to buy: baked and not organic vs. organic and fried? Consider your entire diet. If you eat mostly organic produce, a bag of non-organic baked chips may be fine. Corn is low on the pesticide list. If you're not so careful with the amount of organic foods in your diet, the organic chips would be better. But limit the amounts in either case. Best solution: Take some organic corn tortillas and bake them in your oven. Break up into smaller pieces and enjoy baked organic corn chips!

● Keep fat content low. I disagree with the fat-free diets that are popular. They don't provide essential fatty acids necessary for a woman's reproductive system (before or after menopause) and for all of our immune systems. Essential fatty acids are essential for good health and essential to eat because our bodies don't make them. Have a variety of helpful fats: monounsaturated like olive oil and canola oil; polyunsaturated like safflower oil; and essential fatty acids like flax seeds or oil and fish oils. Note: if a product says "Lite" it means it has 50 percent or less fat content. Lite cream cheese can be 50 percent fat. Choose the fat-free over lite. You'll get enough fat in your diet from other sources, like salad dressing, eggs, a little avocado, soy products (may contain as much as 50 percent fat!).

● Read labels. Labels show the ingredients of a product in descending order by weight. Often, these ingredients are separated to make it look like there is less of something—like sugar—than there is. Sugars can include obvious sweeteners like brown sugar, corn syrup and honey, as well as many sweeteners ending in "ose" like fructose, maltose, dextrose. The combination of all sweeteners indicates the proportion of sugars in the food.

Look at the amount of fats and sodium in the product. Compare similar products and look for one that's lowest in sodium and fats. Look for disguised sugars. "Very low sodium" is 35 milligrams or less; "low sodium" means 140 milligrams or less per serving. "Light sodium" or "lightly salted" is 50 percent or less added sodium.

Packages marked "low fat" must be 3 grams or less for a food, and 30 percent or less fat calories for a meal. A product marked "lite" can contain as much as 50 percent fat. Ideally, no matter how much fat is in any one food, you want to keep your fat intake to between 20 percent and 25 percent of your daily calories. To calculate this, look at the number of grams of fat in a food, multiply by 9 (each gram of fat contains 9 calories) and divide into the total calories.

Finally, if you see a lot of chemical names on an ingredient list, you're probably looking at a lot of additives and preservatives — more potentially harmful chemicals to avoid when possible.

● Eat the least-processed food possible. It's difficult to control the amount of sugars, fats, sodium, additives, and preservatives when you eat out frequently or eat a lot of packaged foods. You can, by spending a little extra time initially, and finding some processed foods low enough in these ingredients to mix with fat-free, salt-free, sugar-free produce. A frozen pizza (with cheese or soy cheese) can be topped with vegetables sautéed in a little broth or water, thereby reducing the total fat and salt ratio of the meal.

● Get more information: Some books you may want to read on the subject of good quality foods include: Living Foods for Optimum Health, Brian R. Clement, Prima Publishing, 1996. Long Life Now, Lee Hitchcox, D.C., Celestial Arts, 1996.

Fat-Free, Sugar-Free, Nutrient-Free

Whether or not you take nutritional supplements (which we'll discuss later), you're reading this book because you're concerned about your health and are doing, or wanting to do, something to improve it. At the same time, you're hearing the messages from large corporations that manufacture highly refined foods, and from the advertising companies they hire, that their products are good, safe, and even necessary in your diet.

There's big money to be made if the public can only be convinced that these nutritionally devitalized foods are fine for us to eat every day. Billions of dollars flow through our economy to support the premise that highly processed foods not only can, but should, be eaten in large quantities. Newspapers, magazines, television, and billboards proclaim the superiority of one nutritionally deficient food over another. Advertising agencies charge vast sums of money to convince you that fat-blockers, fat-free foods, and sugar-free foods with artificial sweeteners are safe. If this is true, why are so many of us tired and sick? Why are our disease rates (such as breast cancer and heart disease) higher than those in many other countries where highly processed foods are not nearly as prevalent?

The truth is, we are living in a world that grows more polluted each day, and these pollutants cause our bodies to need more nutrients, not less. To de-smog your body from the inside out, you need more antioxidants — chemicals that destroy the free radicals caused by smog and rancid fats. Antioxidants — vitamins A, C and E, to name a few — are found in fresh fruits and vegetables. Canned fruits and vegetables have less of them. Whereas highly processed foods have many vitamins and minerals processed right out of them.

Our lives are more stressful than ever, not easier. We are assaulted daily by the stresses of making a living; banging our heads against the glass ceiling that limits our advancement in the corporate world; balancing work with family; finding time to do the shopping, cooking, and cleaning; finding time for relationships; finding time to sit down and read a book or take a walk in the country. No wonder we want to bury ourselves in a big bowl of fat-free, sugar-free frozen yogurt at the end of a hectic day and

Problems With Sorbitol and Isomalt

We keep looking for a safe sweetener that won't add extra pounds and tastes good. In a recent study, two low-calorie sweeteners, isomalt and sorbitol, were added to standard-sized chocolate bars and given to a number of subjects. It was found that the chocolate with sorbitol wasn't digested well in the small intestines and resulted in fermentation in the colon. Chocolate with isomalt was better digested.

The fermentation produced by the sorbitol lasted a full six hours. All fermentation leads to changes in intestinal bacteria feeding the pathogenic (bad) bacteria that cause disease. Fermentation also reduces the colonies of good bacteria that keep your immune system strong and protect you from vaginal candida. So if you are going to eat a little sugar-free chocolate occasionally, reach for something sweetened with isomalt and not sorbitol.

Br J Nutr 71, 1994:731-737.

inhale its sweet taste. No wonder we buy fat-free cakes and cookies, and pop low-fat meals in the microwave for a quick dinner. What's so wrong about this?

What's wrong is we're looking at only one aspect of the frozen yogurt — low-fat — and ignoring the consequences of consuming artificial sweeteners and the excessive calcium contained in dairy products, which is unable to be absorbed into our bones. Unabsorbed calcium finds its way into our joints, where it becomes arthritis, and into our arteries, where it becomes atherosclerosis, increasing out risk for heart disease.

Fat-Free and Sugar-Free Often Mean Nutrient-Free

In many cases the foods you're being told are fine to eat are not just tasty and low in fat, they're low in vitamins and minerals as well. Fat-free,

---

Sugar or Aspartame?
Both Contribute to Weight Gain

Aspartame may contain fewer calories than sugar, but women who drink soft drinks sweetened with aspartame tend to consume more calories, according to a study published in the *International Journal of Obesity Related Metabolism Disorders*. The first day the women in this study were given aspartame-sweetened sodas, they ate fewer calories. But the second day their caloric intake was significantly higher. It didn't matter whether or not the women knew which type of sweetener was in their drinks. They still ate a higher calorie diet even though neither drink caused an increase in their appetites. If you're using aspartame as a substitute for sugar for weight control, you may be fooling yourself. Try drinking flavored mineral water for just two weeks and get rid of your aspartame-sweetened foods and drink. If necessary, add a little apple juice or black cherry juice to the mineral water. See what happens to your caloric intake and your weight.

Lavin, J.H., et al. "The effect of sucrose- and aspartame-sweetened drinks on energy intake, hunger and food choice of female, moderately restrained eaters," *Int J Obes Relat Metab Disord*, 1997;21:37-42.

sugar-free cakes and cookies are also free from the magnesium found in whole grains. It's this same magnesium that helps calcium travel to the bones and protect us against osteoporosis, the same magnesium that allows our heart and other muscles to remain healthy and supple. White flour has been stripped of most of its vitamins and minerals. When it's enriched, a few are put back, but not magnesium. In fact, not even half of all of the vitamins and minerals that were removed.

The issue is not the amount of fat or sugar that has been left out, but whether or not the food you're considering contains sufficient vitamins and minerals to support you and contribute to your health. Only whole foods will give you the balance you need, and it is this balance of nutrients that can give you the edge to stay healthy. For example, sugar is not a dietary culprit until it is extracted from its original source, such as sugar cane, or beets. But once sugar is removed from these foods it ceases to be a whole food and can wreak havoc with our bodies.

Most of the fat-free crackers you find in supermarkets are made from refined flour and are low in vitamins and minerals. You can find fat-free whole grain cookies, muffins, and crackers in health food stores and in the health food section of many supermarkets. These products are usually sweetened with fruit juice, a much safer alternative than artificial sweeteners which have been linked to numerous health problems from headaches and dizziness to a few reported incidents of death. Eye problems and sugar-cravings have been associated with the use of aspartame, a common artificial sweetener found in desserts and sodas.

Fat-Free or Sugar-Free and Nutrient-Dense

When you're looking for fat-free or sugar-free foods, first look to see if the food originally contained plenty of nutrients. If only the fat has been removed, as in the case of fat-free, baked corn chips, you may have found a food that's worth eating. By baking corn chips you simply omit frying them in re-heated, rancid oils. Baked chips, then, are healthier than regular fried chips. If you dip them into a fat-free bean dip — made from healthy black or pinto beans — you have a fat-free snack that's high in nutrients. Or if you dip pieces of raw carrots, jicama, and broccoli into them as well, you up your ante of vitamins. Air-popped popcorn is fat-free, but is still a whole grain food.

But fat-free cereals are often made from refined grains, low in nutrients, with some vitamins and minerals added back to make the product sell. Fat-free frozen entrees that often contain devitalized white rice and list numerous chemical additives and artificial flavorings are going to give you less vitamins and minerals to carry you through the day. And the fat-free or sugar-free desserts you may be eating every night as a treat are often packed with artificial ingredients but not much in the way of nutrients.

Why You Crave Fats and Sugars

Many women crave high-fat foods because they have a need for essential fatty acids, specific fats that support the immune system and contribute to a healthy reproductive system (before and after menopause). These fats are found in highest quantities in flax seed and raw walnuts. Try grinding one to three tablespoons of flax seed in a seed or coffee grinder and adding it to your breakfast cereal or a glass of juice. Or add two or three walnuts to your cereal or salad. It may reduce your fat cravings. If you need more essential fatty acids, you may actually lose weight after you begin adding them to your diet.

Some people crave fats or sugar as a learned response. When fatty or sweet foods were given as a reward or just part of a normal everyday diet for years, our taste buds become accustomed to them. By reducing fats or sugars for a few weeks, often the craving goes away. But reduce fats and sugars in a diet high in whole grains, beans, and vegetables — high in nutrients. Then, if you have a favorite food that is high in fats, you're better off eating a little of it once in a while, and stick to a diet of low-fat natural foods for your daily regime. No low-fat, fat-free, or sugar-free fake food can take the place of the real thing.

When It's Chocolate — Why Organic?

At a recent health products trade show, we decided to get samples of various kinds of organic chocolates and have a panel of people taste test them for you. After all, not everyone is going to stop eating chocolate forever just because it's high in fats and sugar. So my goal with this report is to steer you toward the best-tasting, best-quality chocolate available, plus encourage you to limit your intake to small amounts. I might add that in researching this article, even I was surprised at the size of the hornet's nests I discovered inside all the pretty candy wrappers.

The organic chocolate bars that have begun to appear on the market are not just another gimmick to sell a higher-priced candy to people interested in unadulterated foods. Organic means sustainable agriculture, women's economic and health rights, the wasting of natural resources, and your personal health as well. And yes, it also involves taste.

Why Not Vanilla or Raspberry?

What is it about chocolate that draws us to its flavor more than any other? Well, women are the largest consumers of chocolate, and we think some of the reason for this is that it is high in magnesium, a mineral often found to be deficient in women. Your craving for chocolate may just be your body's way of asking for magnesium-rich foods. If so, nuts, seeds, and beans are better sources for increasing your dietary stores. You'd have to eat too much chocolate, complete with sugars and fats, to get enough magnesium. It's better to eat only a little chocolate occasionally as a treat.

Can Chocolate Help Reduce LDL Cholesterol?

Yes, according to a study in the *Lancet* (vol 348, 1996), but not by eating your favorite candy bars or ice cream. Chocolate is naturally rich in polyphenols, chemicals that can lower the harmful, sticky LDL cholesterol levels that contribute to atherosclerosis. And there are as many LDL-lowering polyphenols in half a large chocolate bar as there are in a glass of wine. But here's the problem: the chocolate, or cocoa, must be de-fatted. Otherwise, the fatty acids in chocolate will negate the polyphenols.

Fortunately for your cholesterol, if not for your taste buds, onions and apples contain high amounts of polyphenols. As, of course, do the grapes from which wine is made. So if you see something in the news telling you that chocolate lowers cholesterol, be aware that this is only when the cocoa has been defatted and the product is fat-free. Don't let the media's enthusiasm for getting your attention result in a misunderstanding that could cost you your health.

Kondo, K. "Inhibition of LDL oxidation by cocoa," *Lancet*, 348, 1514 (1996); *Int'l Clin Nutr Rev*, July 1997.

We need more magnesium when we're under stress and just before we menstruate — two times we tend to reach for a chocolate bar or chocolate ice cream. Unfortunately, the ice cream (or frozen yogurt) often perpetuates our chocolate craving, because it's not just our body's need for more magnesium that causes the craving, but an imbalance between calcium and magnesium: too much calcium and not enough magnesium. This means that if you're eating a lot of dairy products the high amount of calcium they contain can help create your chocolate craving.

Chocolate is also high in copper, especially dark chocolate. In fact, people who eat a lot of dark chocolate can increase their dietary copper intake more quickly than by using any other food. Copper appears to be an anti-tumor, anti-carcinogenic, anti-inflammatory substance (remember those copper bracelets used for arthritis?). But better sources of copper, without the fats and sugars that can promote these conditions, include potatoes, chicken, whole grains, and beans.

In the Beginning There Were Cocoa Trees

Chocolate, in the form of cocoa trees, originated more than 2,000 years ago along the eastern slopes of the Andes in Central America. The trees produce cocoa beans, which were revered by the natives and used as a fertility symbol, as well as a symbol of prosperity. Cortez took the beans back to Spain with him, where he proclaimed the beverage they produced to be both a delicious medicinal drink and an aphrodisiac. From Spain, chocolate traveled to France with a Spanish princess who married Louis XIV in the 1600s.

Seventeenth century nobility drank hot chocolate in chocolate houses throughout London and continued the myth of chocolate as an aphrodisiac and healing drink. But the surge in chocolate consumption came in the late 1800's when a Dutch inventor, Van Houten, made a press that extracted cocoa butter out of the beans. The cocoa powder that was left could be mixed with sugar, more cocoa powder, and the cocoa butter to make a richer, smoother drink or to be formed into bars. While the Amerindians of the Andes were among the first people to eat chocolate, the Dutch turned the beans into a confection, which was then made in England and now here in the U.S.

Once expensive, chocolate is now cheap to make and is at the top of an $8 billion confectionery market with Hershey and Mars making half the products consumed each year. One of the reasons it's inexpensive is because the people who grow cocoa beans are underpaid. At the same time, they're being poisoned.

Pesticides — The Circle of Poison

Some pesticides which can be used only on a restricted basis in this country are being manufactured in this country, exported to other countries, and shipped back to us in cocoa beans. Lindane is the pesticide found most often in cocoa beans. The Environmental Protection Agency (EPA) has classified lindane as probably being carcinogenic. Some researchers believe it is more toxic to humans than to the laboratory animals used in studies.

Cocoa beans come from the Ivory Coast, Ghana, Malaysia, and Brazil. The beans we import mostly come from Brazil and Malaysia. Brazil is the second largest producer of cocoa in the world, and most of it is grown on large plantations, which have taken over small farmlands and dispossessed the people who once lived and farmed there. Women are paid half the salary of men, although they each do the same amount of work. When they plant small cocoa trees, they're paid $1 for every hundred they plant, or one penny per tree!

Women also spray the trees with pesticides, but because these

Chocolate Taste-Test Results

Here's how the organic chocolates we tasted rated with our happy testers:

#1 Green & Black's — the unanimous favorite. Their organic dark chocolate rated highest with everyone, with their milk chocolate coming in a close second. If you or your favorite store can't find it, call American Natural Snacks at 904-825-2057. Casey van Rysdam or John McNichols will tell you where to find it. Worth hunting down!

#2 Rapunzel Natural — made in Switzerland and found in many health food stores. The winner, until people tasted Green & Black's.

#3 Newman's Own Organics — We love this company's generosity in donating all profits to charity, but their chocolate tasted a little thin compared with the others. Many tasters commented that it tasted like Hershey's, not like a gourmet bar. If you like Hershey's, you'll love Newman's Own. Found easily in many health food and other stores.

chemicals are so toxic and frequently cause birth defects, they must often show proof of sterilization before they're allowed to do this work. Not only are they giving up their own health, they're giving up the possibility of having families.

In Malaysia, conditions are no better. Eighty percent of the people who spray cocoa trees are women who put pesticides and herbicides like paraquat in pumps they carry on their backs. They often mix these by hand and blow out any blockages in the sprayers. The workers rarely wear any protective clothing other than occasionally rubber gloves (although U.S. safety regulations suggest protective clothing, respirators, goggles, and gloves), so the deadly chemicals drip over them as they work.

These women know what they're working with. Drinking pesticides is the most popular way of committing suicide in this country. And paraquat, an herbicide used to kill weeds around cocoa trees, is responsible for more deaths than any other weed killer. But when you're poor, you'll do anything ... and they do. Why aren't these chemicals banned? Because their use produces more cocoa beans. Although the Malaysian Health Minister has asked plantation owners to improve the health conditions of their workers, the Minister of Agriculture is not willing to ban chemicals that are cheap and effective.

Manufacturing Chocolate

The chocolate you eat today comes from cocoa beans. The chocolate you eat a few years from now may be created in a laboratory. At the very least, cocoa trees will have been genetically altered through biotechnological research to produce larger yields and more uniform beans. This research is currently being carried on at Pennsylvania State University, funded by the cocoa industry and candy manufacturers. It includes making the plants resistant to pests. Sounds good, doesn't it? But when plants are identically resistant to anything, once a pest finds a way to attack it — by mutating as pests do — it will be able to attack all cocoa trees. Then more pesticides will be needed. If you don't want to eat genetically altered foods, consider chocolate. Today it may be grown naturally. Tomorrow it may be another genetically engineered product.

Organic Chocolate — The Safe Alternative

A very small percentage of today's chocolate is organic. It's expensive to produce, but the product does not contain the toxic chemicals found in ordinary chocolate. And the land on which it grows is not poisoned, either. One British chocolate company we spoke with, Green & Black's, gets cocoa grown in Togo and Belize. When Hershey's helped fund a program to plant hundreds of acres of cocoa trees in Belize, paying $1.75 a pound for the beans and suddenly dropping the price to 55 cents a pound, this company stepped in and helped reform the cocoa growers into an organic collective that could again make a living from a product that was not poisoning them. Green & Black's is not the only company that supports environmental health and the economic health of cocoa growers. All manufacturers of organic chocolates do the same. So when we buy organic chocolates we not only eliminate some toxic chemicals from our diet, we support sustainable agriculture and economic and personal health in other cultures.

Organic Chocolate — The Tasty Alternative

Have you noticed that some chocolate products don't taste very chocolatey? It's because of the amount of dry cocoa beans in it. And the smoothness is due to the amount of cocoa butter (fat). We found the organic chocolates we tasted to have a fuller flavor than many non-organic brands — especially the less expensive ones.

The higher the amount of dry cocoa powder, the stronger the chocolate taste. This is why bittersweet chocolate tends to have a stronger taste than milk chocolate. And it's the reason some brands are more chocolatey than others.

We found that Green & Black's 70 percent solids bittersweet chocolate was the most flavorful, smooth bar we tried. Green & Black's is made with more cocoa solids than cocoa butter. The solids have the flavor. Other brands contain a greater percentage of cocoa butter for a smooth, rich taste. But they are not as flavorful and are higher in fat. If you like bittersweet chocolate, you might find you eat less of Green & Black's than other brands. By the way, having more cocoa solids means the product is higher in magnesium and copper, as well. They both come from beans — even cocoa beans!

Nutrition in a Can

They're fast. They're tasty. They're filled with vitamins and minerals. And you can buy them by the case almost anywhere. So what's wrong with drinking Ensure, Resource, Boost, SlimFast, and other similar canned meal replacement drinks? It's better to drink one and get plenty of vitamins than to skip a meal, isn't it?

We don't think so.

Meal replacement drinks were designed to get calories into hospital patients who could not eat solid food, or people in convalescent homes who were unable to eat properly. They consist of lots of sugars, water, and protein with inexpensive vitamins and minerals added. The problem with inexpensive nutrients is that they're poorly absorbed. Take Ensure, for example. It may say it contains 25 percent or more of the Recommended Daily Allowances of a vitamin or mineral, but the amount found in a can of Ensure isn't the amount that gets into your body.

Ensure contains such minerals as potassium chloride, calcium phosphate, and thiamine chloride, for example. The chloride, phosphate, and hydrochloride forms of nutrients are not as well absorbed as the citrate, malate, fumarate, aspartate, or gluconate forms. This is because our body contains citrate, malate, fumarate, aspartate, and gluconate, and it recognizes and uses larger amounts of the minerals, which are bound to these chemicals.

So don't compare vitamins and minerals in mass market drinks like Ensure with those in health food company drinks like Recovery, Naturally Complete, Vigoraid, and Balanced. They may look the same, but they don't perform as well. Technically, they may have the same amount of a nutrient, but the amount your body can use varies tremendously.

Is Cancer in the Mix?

This is the difference between a good quality product and a cheap one. But it's not what alarms us. We are very upset that many of the mass market drinks, including strawberry and orange cream flavored Ensure, contain food dyes like red dye number 3, which is a known carcinogen that has been shown to promote the growth of breast cancer cells! More than that, this food coloring, like many pesticides, is estrogenic. For women who want to guard against breast cancer, repeatedly ingesting drinks with red dye number 3 is totally counterproductive.

While you might argue that there's not much of any dye in a single can of Ensure, we suggest you take a look at the majority of people using it. Sick people. Infirm people. People with cancer, AIDS and other weakened immune systems, children who don't eat much variety of food and need more calories, and even women recovering from breast cancer. In our opinion, these people can't afford to be eating any amount of dangerous products. They need all the help they can get. They need the best quality nutrients in a product that's easy for their bodies to absorb.

Food dyes are in everything from candies to hot dogs, lunch meats, and snack foods. And just because a particular dye hasn't been found to cause breast cancer or other problems doesn't necessarily mean it's safe. It could mean it hasn't been thoroughly tested. Our suggestion: read labels carefully and pass up those products with dyes and other artificial ingredients.

These original supplemental drinks (Ensure, Resource, Boost, and other mass market drinks) served their purpose. They brought our attention to the needs of busy and sick consumers who need a fast way to get calories and vitamins. Now their popularity has driven a number of health food companies to come out with products made with healthy ingredients and nutrients the body can more easily absorb. So stop buying chemicals-in-a-can. There are healthier choices.

The best of the best, in our opinion, are products called Recovery Power Foods, made by the same people who founded Earth's Best Baby Foods more than a decade ago. Their products include the ready-made drinks, packets you can mix with water, drink mixes, and supplemental nutrition bars. All of them come with information on fruit, starch, and fat protein exchanges for diabetics and people on other restrictive diets, including those who simply want to lose weight.

They have a ready-to-drink liquid supplement in 8 oz boxes. Each serving contains 270 calories, 10 grams of protein, and six grams of fat. But not just any fats. Recovery drinks have a variety of essential fatty acids (to boost the immune system) and medium chain triglycerides (fats that are easily digested). Made from rice and whey protein, these beverages are low in lactose and contain no soy — a protein some people have difficulty digesting, especially when they're elderly or sick. The sweetener, fructose, has no corn protein in it, so if you're sensitive to corn, you can still use these products. The vitamins and minerals are expensive, high-quality nutrients chosen for their ability to be well digested and absorbed. This is a very sophisticated line of products that work. If you can't find them in your health food store, call the company, Great Circles, at 800-872-0611.

Westbrae Natural has a new product called West Soy VigorAid made from organic soybeans. The company has added 50 mg of isoflavones, nutrients found in soybeans that protect against breast and prostate cancer, boosting the nutritional value of their beverages. These drinks also contain essential fatty acids to help the immune system, and are lactose free. From 240 to 260 calories per serving, with 50 calories from fat, three 8 oz boxes (choose vanilla or chocolate) sell for about $3.99. You should be able to find them in health food stores around the country. If you have any problems, call Westbrae Natural at 800-776-1276.

Pacific Foods' answer to Ensure is called Naturally Complete, 8 oz and 32 oz boxes of a drink made from whole grains and soybeans with added vitamins and minerals. An 8 oz box will give you either 170 or 200 calories (chocolate has 30 calories more than vanilla), and sells for around $2.99 for a set of three. The larger box costs from $3.49-$3.99.

Balanced, which comes in 11 oz cans, is made by American Natural Snacks from organic soybeans and contains no lactose. It's higher in calories than the two above (230 with 25 calories from fat), but a little lower in nutrients. But remember, these are still better absorbed than the nutrients in mass market drinks. Their quality far surpasses Ensure. For more information, call them at 800-238-3947.

Whether you're using these drinks as a meal replacement for a weight loss program, a way to boost your nutrients with a healthy snack, or looking for a drink to help a sick person, the elderly, or the very young get high-quality nutrients, you are no longer limited to using Ensure. Leave dangerous food dyes and poorly absorbed nutrients behind.

Finally, if you think a meal replacement drink can truly take the place of a nutrient-dense meal made up of whole foods — it can't. A better name for these beverages might be meal supplement drink. When circumstances permit, it's always better to return to eating whole-food meals, rather than continue using these drinks.

Olestra: Fat Free and Dangerous

No sooner had we published the above section "Fat-Free, Sugar-Free, Nutrient-Free" in a recent issue of *Women's Health Letter*, than we were assailed by information from Proctor & Gamble heavily promoting their new fat substitute made from sugar and fatty acids: olestra. P&G calls olestra Olean, knowing how much we want to be lean. Olestra, or Olean, sounds like a miracle. It passes through the digestive tract without being digested or absorbed, which means you can eat cookies or potato chips made with Olean and not gain weight, get intestinal gas, or raise your cholesterol.

Sound too good to be true? It is. Even the FDA thinks it may not be a totally safe product. Although it approved the use of olestra, it did so with qualifications. For now, olestra may only be used in snack foods. Perhaps they believe snack foods aren't eaten in large quantities. We think this is being shortsighted. Some people eat little else! Why would olestra not be safe to use in more foods? Consider this:

Olestra frequently causes cramping and diarrhea. Studies showed that just one ounce of chips made with olestra caused diarrhea in fully half the people being tested! That's a high price to pay for a few crunchy chips. But diarrhea wasn't the only negative side effect. Some people had intestinal cramping. Others had rectal leakage and soiled their underwear. Sound gross? Read on...

While the best studies are those with people, not laboratory animals, olestra was found to cause changes in liver cells in some mice. Although none of the mice actually got cancer (who knows what might happen over a long period of time?), you might not want to be a guinea pig until long-term human safety studies are conducted. With all the fat-free potato chips (even Lays has jumped on the fat-free bandwagon) and baked corn chips, with all the fat-free desserts available in supermarkets, health food stores and bakeries, why would you even be tempted to experiment with Olean? Fat tastes better, you say? Perhaps, but olestra presents still more risks than those we've mentioned.

Remember: olestra passes through your digestive tract intact, without being digested and without being absorbed. So do any fats which are eaten at the same time. And your body needs some fats. Essential fatty acids (EFAs), found in nuts and seeds (walnuts, flax seeds, etc.) and oils (especially safflower), help support your immune system. Dr. Uzi Reiss, a prominent Beverly Hills gynecologist, has said that EFAs may be the most important nutrient for a woman's reproductive system both when she is pre- and postmenopausal.

We've all heard of the importance of vitamins A and E, and beta carotene — antioxidants which have been shown to protect against heart disease and some forms of cancer. Vitamin D is another fat-soluble substance that helps keep your bones strong and dense. Vitamin K, another fat-soluble vitamin, helps your blood clot. Olestra was shown in studies — one actually conducted by P&G — to lower the body's levels of these vitamins.

P&G will be adding some — but not all — of these fat-soluble vitamins into Olean, their olestra product. But if olestra passes through the body without being absorbed, adding them will only help the P&G Olean advertising campaign. It won't do you any good.

Ed Bauman, PhD, director of the Nutrition Training Program at IET (Institute for Educational Therapy) in Cotati, California, believes in eating real foods, not food substitutes like this one. And he's particularly concerned about people on medications who eat foods with olestra. We spoke with a pharmacist in Santa Monica, California, who is also concerned. While medications are not fat-soluble, many of them carry warnings that you should not take them with or near oil-soluble vitamins or foods that contain them. If your medications should be taken an hour before or two hours after meals, it might not be safe for you to eat a handful of chips or cookies made with olestra and then take your medication. This means carefully planning when you can eat foods made with olestra around your medication schedule — or risking that your medications may not work.

Fatty acids are found in more natural remedies, like anti-fungals used to control an overgrowth of Candida albicans yeast. The caprylic acid found in many of these products is a naturally occurring fat found in coconuts. Lauric acid, another fatty acid, breaks up Epstein-Barr virus cells, causing them to die. Many people with chronic fatigue have the Epstein-Barr virus as part of their illness — and women have a much higher rate of chronic fatigue than men.

We understand that some foods made with Olean may taste better to you than those that are fat-free. But there are many fat-free healthy snack foods already on the market that taste just fine. And eating them won't prevent you from absorbing the nutrients you need from the other foods you eat. Or cause unnecessary side effects like cramping, diarrhea and rectal leakage. We think fake foods may have serious long-term effects on your health. Invariably, when something like Olean sounds too good to be true, it turns out it is.

Avoid Holiday Weight Gain
With Thermogenics

Most women know they're going to gain weight every year between Thanksgiving and New Year's and go on a diet on January first — or second. That's the time the media is set to blitz you with New Year's resolutions and ideas for taking off the pounds you've just put on. We think this is backward reasoning. Sure, you can dive into holiday foods now and start to lose weight next year, or you can try something new today that will result in little or no weight gain.

We think there's more to this weight issue than simply pushing yourself away from the foods you typically eat at holiday time. Holidays bring with them an assortment of memories, both positive and negative. And these memories are often associated with particular foods and beverages. To recapture some of the feelings you want, you're likely to eat and drink more fatty and sweet foods than usual. That is, unless you can find a way to have a smaller appetite and burn up more calories than usual.

We think there's value in considering another approach — using thermogenic agents today to avoid your usual holiday weight gain tomorrow.

What Are Thermogenic Agents?

Thermogenesis is a process by which your body burns fat to produce heat. When you can increase thermogenesis, you burn fats more quickly. Some thermogenic agents — both herbs and drugs — increase your metabolism and decrease your appetite as well. This gives you three ways to avoid weight gain. Pharmaceutical companies are now looking into another type of weight loss pill called beta-3 agonists, which increase thermogenesis. And, of course, there are always amphetamines — the usual diet pills that women have been getting hooked on for years. But more natural products exist today at a fraction of the cost of drugs, and they're less toxic, milder, and have fewer side effects than pharmaceuticals.

The Best Natural Diet Pill

One herb, ephedra, also known as Ma Huang, may be a key ingredient in the most effective natural diet pill around. It has been used in China for more than 5,000 years and is safe when taken in small quantities for most people. Its active ingredient, ephedrine, is used by pharmaceutical companies in many asthma medications.

What's wrong in using just plain ephedra or ephedrine to decrease your appetite and increase thermogenesis? It has some limitations for weight loss use, like a feedback system that turns off its fat-burning qualities, causing it to stop working after a while. By adding another ingredient to it, like caffeine or white willow bark (similar to aspirin), you can turn off this feedback mechanism and keep the active ingredient, ephedrine, working.

You can find ephedra, which contains ephedrine, in health food stores, either by itself or combined with caffeine (EC) at a much lower cost than medications containing ephedrine. All ephedra products should say on their labels that the ephedrine is standardized, meaning you are guaranteed a particular amount in each tablet or capsule. If it's not, it may be too weak — and not work — or too strong and give you unnecessary side effects. Studies show that just 10 mg/day of ephedrine burns more calories than 20-40 mg. Don't take more than you need!

The herb, ephedra, contains various quantities of ephedrine. Only standardized formulas contain the same amount in each tablet or capsule. If you're not sure how much ephedrine is in a particular formula, call or write the manufacturer and ask them. With one company we called, just two capsules contain 11 mg of standardized ephedrine.

What's So Good About EC?

Larry S. Hobbs, author of *The New Diet Pills* (Pragmatic Press, 1995), calls the combination of ephedrine and caffeine "the ideal diet pill." Why? Because it decreases your appetite, accounting for 75 percent of your weight loss, and increases thermogenesis for the remaining 25 percent of weight loss. If you keep taking EC over a period of months, thermogenesis increases. The more overweight you are, the slower your metabolism is likely to be. EC increases your metabolism. Meanwhile, you enter the holiday eating fray with less of an appetite. So go ahead, indulge a little and have tastes of whatever you like. Just eat less. It's easy when you don't have an urge to eat more.

Larry Hobbs has thoroughly researched EC and other ephedrine combinations. He found that women who take EC lost 100 percent more body fat and 72 percent less muscle than women who took a placebo. He also provides a list of suppliers for these and other thermogenic agents, which are eye-openers. For example, TwinLab supplement company makes an EC combination called Metabolift that can cost as little as $1/day if you buy the large-sized bottle, or you can buy their Ripped Fuel Thermogenic Protein Drink, which will set you back nearly $10/day! Look for other brands in your health food stores.

A less-expensive route would be to purchase plain ephedrine. BDI Pharmaceuticals makes Mini Thins, which contain 25 mg of ephedrine. Break up Mini Thins to get the right dosage and it will cost you between 6 and 14 cents a day. Add to that three or four cups of healthy, yet inexpensive, green tea (40-60 mg of caffeine per cup) and you have a very affordable formula that works just as well.

But ... It's Not for Everyone

The research we've read indicates that ephedra plus caffeine (EC) is safe for many people, but not everyone. It is a stimulant, and many people prefer to not use stimulants or can't use them. We never recommend stimulants when anyone is under unusual stress. This just gives your body another stress to deal with.

The most common side effects from EC include nervousness, insomnia, hand tremors, and heart palpitations — symptoms that seem to decrease over time. EC could initially increase your blood pressure or cause constipation, but these symptoms usually disappear with use. And if you have a thyroid problem, it's not recommended to use it. To reduce your chance for any side effects, begin with a lower dose and gradually increase it over a few weeks. If it keeps you awake at night, take it earlier in the day. And if you still have problems, it's not for you. Try something else.

We has always advocated eating properly over using any pills, even ones considered to be ideal and natural. At the same time, we're aware of the painful struggle thousands of women have every year around holiday eating. If you've tried eating smaller meals, avoiding fats and refined sugars, limiting your alcohol intake, and it hasn't worked, we're suggesting there are other options.

Trying non-stimulating herbal formulas is another possibility, but when you need the strongest, safest method to fight the biggest yearly battle, EC seems to give the biggest and fastest results.

Irritable Bowel Syndrome

If you're one of the many people who reaches for an antacid whenever you get stomach pains or bloat after a meal, we've got news for you. You may not have simple indigestion or need an antacid at all, even if an antacid makes you feel better temporarily. You could be one of the 15 percent of Americans who suffers from irritable bowel syndrome (IBS). Other IBS symptoms include diarrhea and/or constipation. And while IBS is rarely life-threatening, it's uncomfortable and can drain your energy.

The problem with taking an antacid or other medication that offers symptomatic relief is that you never get to the source of your problem and eliminate it. You just find a Band-Aid approach and cover up the discomfort. The only time to take an antacid is if a medical doctor has determined that your body is making too much acid. Taking any unnecessary medications can lead to other problems. They all have side effects, including antacids.

Stomach acids like hydrochloric acid are important to your digestion. They help you break down the foods you eat into small enough particles to be absorbed. Antacids neutralize them, making it difficult for you to thoroughly digest your food. So you begin by missing out on some of the vitamins, minerals, proteins, and fats your body needs that are in the foods you eat. But that's not all. Partially digested foods often ferment in the intestines causing more gas. They also upset the balance of friendly bacteria needed for a healthy immune system and to guard against vaginitis, candida, and pathogenic bacteria like streptococcus and E. coli. They can also contribute to colon problems.

Find Out What You've Got

Frequently, stress and food sensitivities cause irritable bowel syndrome, which puts it more in your control than your doctor's. Other more serious colon problems like colitis and Crohn's disease are forms of chronic relapsing inflammatory bowel disease, and may require medication as well as lifestyle changes. These more serious illnesses may be genetic or could be caused by an auto immune problem. Don't confuse them with IBS, which can respond well to stress management and dietary changes.

Begin by having an examination from your doctor and rule out the more serious problems like colon cancer, colitis, and Crohn's disease. Then, if you are told you have IBS, prepare to change your life before reaching for a medication that may only control symptoms. Ask your doctor or other health care practitioner to monitor you as you make some lifestyle changes.

Diet and Stress — Common Causes of IBS

Have you been under stress for three months or longer? Studies show that digestive disturbances occurring after prolonged stressful periods of our lives are usually symptoms of IBS.

Not a lot of stress in your life? Then it's time to look to your diet and begin to make some changes. IBS can be caused by food allergies or food sensitivities, by causing an irritation to the intestinal lining. Try avoiding a food or foods completely for two to four weeks, and then reintroducing them into your diet. This will let you know whether or not a particular substance is causing your digestive complaints without having to get expensive tests.

It may be that IBS isn't caused by stress, but its symptoms are more likely to be present when you're under stress. This is because stress often leads to poor digestion. When you're anxious, your body doesn't make enough digestive enzymes and acids to break down the foods you eat, leaving partially digested foods to ferment and cause IBS symptoms. Any technique or tool that breaks your stress cycle can calm down your intestines and help you feel better.

Dietary Irritants — and Solutions

Food allergies always cause a negative reaction; food sensitivities cause problems periodically — when you eat too much of a certain food, when you're under stress, or when your body's out of whack (like an imbalance of friendly bacteria in the intestines, or a suppressed immune system, for instance). Any food can contribute to IBS, but some are more commonly associated with it than others.

The foods most commonly associated with IBS are: wheat, corn, dairy, coffee, tea, and citrus. If you crave any of these, look out. Craving a certain food is often a symptom of a problem.

Many people have sensitivities to more than one of these foods. If you eat wheat, corn, or dairy daily, stop eating one or all of them — 100 percent — for two full weeks. Read all labels carefully and ask questions when you're eating out.

Some prepared foods, like veggieburgers, for instance, have wheat or flour (made from wheat) in them. Cornstarch, corn oil, and high fructose corn syrup are ingredients you need to avoid when you're eliminating corn. And to completely avoid dairy products, shop for foods marked "vegan" in health food stores. Vegans are vegetarians who don't eat eggs or dairy.

The more processed the foods you eat, the more likely you are to find some of these ingredients lurking in them, so simplify your diet for a few weeks. Rice is rarely a problem for people with IBS. Use it as your primary starch. You can find rice crackers, rice cereals, rice bread and even rice noodles (these can be found wherever Asian foods are sold).

Instead of dairy, use rice milk or soy milk in your cereal, beverages, and cooking. A number of delicious frozen desserts that resemble ice cream include: Sweet Nothings (their non-dairy fudge bars are remarkable!), Rice Dream, It's Soy Delicious, and Ice Bean. Avoid those with a lot of sugar like Tofutti. Sugar can upset the intestinal flora and cause diarrhea.

Keep your refined sugar intake very, very low. Use fruit-juice sweetened foods instead. Beware of the unrefined cane sugar found in a lot of "health foods" these days. We have not seen enough studies to convince ourselves that it doesn't cause at least some of the bowel problems associated with refined sugar like gas and diarrhea.

At the end of two weeks, have a small amount of the food you've been avoiding: a piece of bread, a little milk or cheese, some baked corn chips. If your symptoms reappear, you need to avoid the offending food longer.

Helpful Supplements

Three supplements are key in reestablishing balance to your intestines: fiber, probiotics and peppermint oil. If you're constipated, increase your fiber by eating more whole grains and vegetables. Because adding more fiber increases your need for water, drink water throughout the day. Half a glass an hour, whenever possible, is ideal, and better than drinking two or three glasses at a time, which can cause bloating.

Probiotics are friendly bacteria, like Lactobacillus acidophilus and bifido bacteria. Adding these to your diet daily for two or three months is important for keeping large enough colonies of "good" bacteria present, which fight disease-causing bacteria. One sign you don't have enough probiotics is vaginitis and systemic Candida, caused by an overgrowth of pathogenic Candida bacteria. In a moment, we will focus on the causes and answers to this common health problem.

Peppermint oil has been found to relax the smooth muscles in the intestines and prevent the cramping some people get with irritable bowel syndrome. It works by blocking the intestines' ability to utilize calcium. Calcium causes muscles to cramp; magnesium and peppermint oil cause muscles to relax. The first step you take might be to remove large sources of calcium from your diet (dairy products) and supplements. Next, if you are constipated, consider taking a little extra magnesium. It causes looser stools and helps muscles relax. If you have loose stools or diarrhea, try Enzymatic Therapy, or another brand of peppermint oil found in many health food stores.

A Final Comment

We support your desire to take more responsibility for your health and to use more natural methods of achieving it whenever possible. But we caution you to first get a diagnosis from a health care practitioner to rule out any serious problem and help you decide what options are open to you. Next, look for the simplest step to take first. In the case of IBS, perhaps you can begin by simply chewing your food better and eating when you're relaxed. This has a great effect on your body's ability to digest.

Keep a food diary and see if certain foods seem to trigger your symptoms. Most importantly, don't oversimplify and automatically reach for an over-the-counter or prescription medication that alleviates symptoms without addressing the cause of your problem. Irritable bowel is not indigestion, and antacids are not its solution. But it may be just as easy to eliminate or control.

Bran Can Irritate Irritable Bowel Syndrome

Over the past few years, nearly everyone has hopped on the bran wagon. A high-fiber diet — particularly one containing bran — has been touted as a way to prevent everything from colon cancer to digestive disorders.

But while there is no doubt that bran is a healthy addition to the American diet, it may not be the wonder food it's been cracked up to be.

According to a study recently published in the *Lancet*, bran may actually exacerbate irritable bowel syndrome — a condition it is often used to treat.

Irritable bowel syndrome is a functional disorder of the intestines characterized by bouts of constipation, diarrhea, abdominal pain, gas, and bloating. While the cause of the disorder is unknown, experts have speculated that it is caused, in part, by fiber depletion, so they have advocated a high-fiber diet — particularly bran — as a treatment method.

Two British physicians who suspected that bran appeared to make the situation worse conducted interviews with 100 syndrome sufferers who had tried bran. Fifty-five percent of those interviewed reported that bran made their symptoms worse; only 10 percent said that bran improved their symptoms. The remaining 35 percent said their symptoms remained the same. And the symptoms most likely to worsen were bowel disturbance, swelling, and pain.

According to the authors, these responses indicate that the treatment most commonly recommended for irritable bowel syndrome can actually make the condition worse. This "despite the strong placebo effect that might be expected from something so widely advocated as being beneficial by lay publications and the medical profession."

This is not to paint bran as an enemy, however. On the contrary, an editorial that accompanied the Lancet study indicates that while there is little proof that bran is successful as a treatment for irritable bowel syndrome as a whole, it can be quite effective in treating one of its symptoms — constipation.

"If the constipation component of IBS is targeted, a beneficial effect can be expected," the editor wrote, adding that bran softens stools, prevents straining, increases the weight of stools, and speeds up intestinal transit. And, he added, it is both safe and cheap. "Nevertheless, bran is no panacea for IBS and some patients either refuse it or cannot tolerate it."

So what should you do? The study authors suggest that consumers should be advised to judge for themselves whether bran is useful for them. If it is not, they may wish to consider reducing their intake. If it is, they should continue to use it. "The importance of an adequate intake of fiber in the diet in both health and disease cannot be disputed," they wrote. "However, as with other dietary constituents, it should not come as a surprise if excessive supplements may in some instances be detrimental."

The Hidden Dangers of MSG

If you simply can't get well and have tried just about everything, we may have important news for you. You may be reacting to the MSG (monosodium-glutamate) occurring in many manufactured foods during their processing. MSG-reactivity is more than the Chinese restaurant syndrome, a condition that leaves you with a headache or burning feeling after eating Chinese food. And it affects 30 percent of people in this country. That's right. A full third of our population may be reacting to MSG in processed foods.

MSG Reactions

Whether foods with MSG cause these symptoms or aggravate an underlying problem is not known for certain. But here are a number of symptoms that people with MSG-sensitivity have reported after eating foods containing the manufactured form of free glutamic acid, which is a man-made form of MSG. This information comes from Truth in Labeling Campaign (P.O. Box 2532, Darien, IL 60561; phone 312-642-9333).

The symptoms include: swelling, muscle stiffness and achiness, joint pain, rapid or irregular heartbeat, sudden drop in blood pressure, angina, depression, dizziness, disorientation, anxiety, sleepiness, migraines, nausea, diarrhea, stomach cramps, irritable bowel, bloating, shortness of breath, chest tightness and/or pain, runny nose, sneezing, rash, flushing, extremely dry mouth, blurred vision, and difficulty focusing.

Now, before you point a finger at MSG as being a causative factor for everything that is or could ever be wrong with you, remember that these are symptoms that occur in people only after they eat foods containing processed glutamic acid. While it's true you may be eating foods with this chemical every day, the amount of MSG ingested may be responsible for any symptoms. You may not react to a small amount of MSG, but only to a larger quantity. This amount can vary from person to person You may want to look at the foods and ingredients you eat that contain MSG and see if your symptoms — or those of any member of your family —can be associated with their ingestion.

MSG Reactions From Processed Foods

Why processed foods? To answer this, we first need to look at just what MSG is. It is a form of free glutamic acid — a naturally occurring chemical found in protein — that is found in many processed foods. Naturally occurring glutamic acid is different from the glutamic acid found in processed protein foods. This difference is significant. People sensitive to MSG have adverse reactions to the glutamic acid in processed foods, but not to the glutamic acid found in unprocessed proteins. And what's more, these reactions may be immediate or occur up to two days after you've eaten foods with MSG.

All Glutamic Acid Is NOT Alike

Unfortunately for us, the consumers, the FDA does not differentiate between these two forms of glutamic acid. In fact, they say the two are functionally and chemically identical. But that's not true. Bear with me while I explain why. This simple lesson in biochemistry can keep you from getting sick!

Natural glutamic acid found in unprocessed proteins is L-glutamic acid. The manufactured glutamic acid is a combination of L-glutamic acid, D-glutamic acid, and pryoglutamic acid. Does this look to you like two chemically identical products? Of course not. But the FDA, which is highly influenced by special interests, plus over-worked and understaffed, can't afford to address the reality of MSG, so it appears that they're sweeping it under a rug so no one will see it. Meanwhile, millions of us are getting sick without knowing why!

Processed Foods Containing MSG

MSG is always found in calcium caseinate, sodium caseinate, gelatin, texturized protein, hydrolyzed protein, yeast extract, yeast food, and yeast nutrient.

MSG is often, but not always, found in the following: malt extract, barley malt, bouillon, carrageenan, maltodextrin, whey protein, whey protein isolate or concentrate, pectin, enzymes, natural flavorings, seasonings, soy sauce, soy protein, soy protein isolate or concentrate, anything fermented. It can even be found in the milk solids added to low-fat milk products!

Even some soaps, shampoos, hair conditioners, and cosmetics that are hydrolyzed or contain amino acids may cause sensitive people to have an MSG-reaction. Fillers and binders used in prescription and over-the-counter drugs, as well as nutritional supplements, may contain MSG.

Why "No MSG" on Labels Means Nothing

Right now, there are no regulations that say MSG must be labeled if

Eat Fish — Decrease Rheumatoid Arthritis

If you have a history of rheumatoid arthritis (RA) in your family, you may have heard that fish oil capsules can reduce some of its inflammatory symptoms. RA is a chronic inflammatory disease with unknown causes.

Now a new study suggests that eating more broiled or baked fish can reduce the risk of getting RA. The study, published in *Epidemiology*, concluded that eating more than one serving of fish (excluding tuna) a week produced a significant reduction in risk for getting RA.

Other nutritional factors discussed in this study include: A high protein intake reduced the risk for RA., and a diet high in calories increased its risk.

Remember, high protein doesn't just mean animal protein. Soy products (soybeans and tofu) contain a chemical, genestein, shown to reduce the risk for breast cancer. And all legumes lower cholesterol, increase fiber, and balance blood sugar levels throughout the day.

Shapiro, J.A., et al. "Diet and rheumatoid arthritis in women: a possible protective effect of fish consumption," *Epidemiology* 7, 256-263 (1996).

it is in a product. Some manufacturers put "No MSG" or "No MSG Added" on their labels even when their products contain ingredients like hydrolyzed protein or yeast. They can get away with it because the FDA is no longer coming after the manufacturers. Remember, this agency is really overworked and understaffed. Unfortunately, we can't rely on them alone for the safety of our foods — especially when the consequences are not life-threatening. The FDA is busy hunting down sources of deadly bacterium in foods which may kill several hundred people a year, rather than scrutinizing the thousands of products that could be making millions of people sick, but not sick enough to die.

Any product that has a little bit of protein in it and has been exposed to heat, enzymes, or hydrochloric acid during manufacturing, can contain MSG. The amounts may not be significant, but they could add up. Remember, people who are sensitive to MSG often react in a dose-dependent way: the more they ingest, the worse they feel.

MSG Is Everywhere — What Can I Do?

We're not trying to frighten or overwhelm you, but the sad truth is that products containing MSG are, indeed, everywhere — from the foods we eat to the shampoo we use and the vitamins we take. Not all, of course, but MSG is in some of them. We just want to alert you to a substance that is so common it just may be the reason you can't get well.

If you'd like to see whether or not an MSG-sensitivity is responsible for any of your health problems, begin by using the least-processed foods, supplements and cosmetics you can find. If necessary, write to the manufacturer of your favorite natural products asking them to show you documentation that the finished product they're selling you does not contain MSG. That is the only way you can know for sure that the product is MSG-free. (Hint: Many large companies have 800 numbers. Call 800 information — 800-555-1212 — to see if you can locate the company you want information from.)

Get back to basics with the foods you're eating. Stop eating any processed foods for two weeks. If you've been using protein powders and tofu, switch to eating lentils, split peas, and beans. Instead of buying instant or canned soups, make them from scratch. Cooking beans isn't time-consuming if you use an electric crock pot.

A diet based on whole grains and beans, a little animal protein if you like, plenty of fresh vegetables, and a little fresh fruit is not so difficult.

Especially if it can help you identify or eliminate a potential problem like MSG-sensitivity. We know that MSG is almost everywhere. But we're also aware of how many people suffer from the many symptoms that could be due to the exposure to too many products containing this chemical that is formed during the manufacturing process.

Chapter 11

Skin Problems

Are You a Victim of Environmental Aging?

by Howard Murad, MD*

Did you know that the condition of your skin is a reflection of lifestyle and environment?

Studies have shown that the cumulative effects of exposure to sun, stress, smoking, drinking, and even harsh home and office environments can have a dramatic impact on your body's largest organ — your skin. It is these day-to-day influences that result in what I refer to as "environmental aging."

Environmental aging can add years to the appearance of the skin — and its effects can take years off the average lifetime. But what is most frustrating to me as a dermatologist is that environmental aging can and should be prevented. In fact, after more than 20 years of observing the lifestyles and habits of my patients, I firmly believe that environmental aging is unnecessary aging.

Proper skin care is a lifestyle decision, and many of my patients don't realize the long-term effects of sun exposure, prolonged bouts with stress, consistent exposure to alcohol and even occasional smoking. My goal is to provide each of my patients with the information necessary to make informed decisions about the ultimate health and condition of the skin. Here are a few of the most common environmental factors that are sure to add years to anyone's appearance.

---

* *Dr. Howard Murad is an Assistant Clinical Professor of Dermatology at UCLA, a dermatologist, researcher, and pioneer in the development of innovative product ingredient systems. He is the Founder and Director of the Los Angeles-based Murad Skin Research Laboratories.*

Sun Sense ... We all know that the sun is the skin's most formidable enemy. But it never hurts to be reminded that the number of reported skin cancer cases is growing every day.

The first rule of thumb for the "environmentally conscious" is that it is never too early to learn about sun sense. Eighty percent of all sun damage occurs among teenagers ... and that damage is cumulative. The sunburn they acquire today may appear in the form of wrinkles 10 to 15 years down the road. For more mature skin, these golden rays present an even greater danger. Too much sun can also weaken the immune system, making mature skin a prime candidate for skin cancer and other diseases. Sun over-exposure can also contribute to superficial bruising (ecchymoses) by weakening the tiny blood vessels in the upper skin layers, allowing them to rupture easily.

Up in Smoke ... Smoking and drinking alcohol are not only unhealthful for the body, but they are extremely damaging to the skin. The mechanics of smoking can enhance the fine lines and wrinkles around the lips and eyes and the toxins in the smoke-bred free radicals (uncontrolled atoms that have been unequivocally linked to premature aging). You might also be surprised to know that wound healing is dramatically altered when

The Tell-Tale Signs of Environmental Aging

- Do you have rough, dry areas on skin that is often exposed to sun?
- Do you have growths or moles (which may be pre-cancerous)?
- Do you have dry, brittle nails?
- Pinch the skin on your hand. Does it take more than a second to bounce back?
- Can you see fine lines (pre-wrinkles) around your eyes?
- Does your neck or chest look crepey?
- Do you have rough, dry skin on your elbows, knees, and feet?
- Do you bruise or bleed easily?
- Is the skin on your legs rough and parched?
- Have you gained or lost more than 20 pounds in a short period of time?

If you answered yes to any of these questions, you are probably a victim of environmental aging.

you smoke; studies have shown that it takes nearly twice as long for a wound to heal on a smoker versus a nonsmoker.

Drinking alcohol dehydrates the skin and pollutes the body. As the body's largest organ, the skin has the important function of detoxifying the body of internal impurities. The consumption of alcohol can greatly overtax the entire system, thus leaving skin dull and dry.

It's in the Air ... The quality of the air in your home, office, and the city in which you live can have a great impact on the overall health of your skin. For example, dry heat, when combined with a harsh, cold environment, can parch the skin and later translate into fine lines and wrinkles. Traveling may also lead to aging. Did you know that one transcontinental flight produces as much unhealthful radiation as one chest X-ray?

Smog is another air quality problem that wreaks havoc on the skin. The residue from smog sits like a filmy, grimy layer on the surface of the skin and some of the toxins are actually absorbed into the skin. What isn't absorbed can clog the pores, give a dull, gray cast and cause oiliness, breakouts and dryness. Smog also produces free radicals in the body which can be doubly harmful for the skin.

Up All Night ... Starving the body of sleep can put undo stress on one's external organs as well as the internal ones. Wrinkles and fine lines under the eyes can finally start to show after extended periods of inadequate sleep. Another interesting fact: A lifetime of sleeping on one side of the body can cause long, crease-like wrinkles down that side of the face. Visible signs of these habits may not appear until 10 to 15 years later, but they will eventually surface.

The Hazards of Home ... The home environment, a place where the majority of people spend at least eight hours per day, can also cause environmental aging. Years of exposing skin to chemical cleaners, deodorizers, and disinfectants can be extremely dehydrating to the skin. And the pesticides and insecticides used in lawn and garden care can be irritating and, in some cases, dangerous. Any substance that is harmful to one's body is also harmful to one's skin. Radon (a type of radiation found in older homes) is one example of this. Many common household products can also cause unusual skin reactions and have intense aging effects.

Other environmental agers include poor eating habits, working conditions (such as exposure to chemicals), and unhealthful beauty products.

Combating Environmental Aging

The good news is that almost all types of environmental aging can be prevented by first identifying the causes, finding ways to steer clear of those causes, and then protecting yourself through continuing education and proper treatments.

Smoking and habitual drinking can have far more devastating effects on your health than wrinkles. Smoking is the number one preventable cause of death; it is also a preventable cause of environmental aging. Even smoking less than half a pack a day drastically alters the aging process with each and every puff.

Drinking can also take its toll on the skin. Occasional or social drinking won't cause undo harm, but it should be done in moderation and preferably include drinking lots of water before, during, and after alcohol consumption.

Smog, unlike the sun, is unavoidable for many people. People who reside or work in a metropolitan area are exposed to smog every day. To combat the effects, regular cleansing and use of an alcohol-free toner as an instant skin refresher during the day can help.

Harsh heat or cold can also contribute to environmental aging. It's important to always keep a protective layer between the skin and those elements. I suggest using a moisturizing body lotion that fits your skin type and apply it after showering and before bedtime. During colder seasons, you may try using a thick, rich cream, but for warmer weather, use a light lotion that won't trap sweat or bacteria. Key ingredients for a lotion include glycolic acid (a naturally occurring substance derived from the sugar cane plant), vitamin E, and one of the newest topical ingredients, vitamin C.

Relief from dry weather may also be found in the use of a humidifier for the home or office, especially during the winter months.

To protect the skin from environmental agers in the home, one should always wear rubber gloves when washing dishes or using abrasive cleaners and detergents. Garden gloves and protective clothing should be worn when using pesticides and insecticides and when working in the garden. Of course, potentially harmful chemicals should never come in contact with skin. To protect skin and nails, one should never peel acidic fruits with bear hands. A better method is to use a peeler or cut the fruit with a knife.

Everyone knows that stress ages a person before his or her time. People who work in high-pressure environments may pay the price in wrinkled, unhealthy skin. Again, plenty of rest and good eating habits can help. A poor diet can lead to nutritional deficiencies that wreak havoc on the skin, nails, and hair. People who are prone to breakout and other chronic skin problems may want to ask their dermatologist, doctor, or nutritionist about dietary guidelines.

Work conditions may also contribute to the aging process. Pilots are notorious for having fine lines and creases around their eyes due to dehydrating pressure systems and glare from the sun (which causes them to squint). People who work at a computer all day may also experience eye strain. If you have glasses, wear them in order to avoid the wrinkles that can develop over time from squinting.

Proper nutrition is also a preventative measure in the fight against environmental aging. Look at your eating habits and make sure your diet is not comprised of all processed foods. Vitamin deficiencies can also contribute to environmental aging and can cause noticeable changes in skin, nails, and hair. Topically, vitamins such as A, C, and E are known antioxidants and have proven beneficial in minimizing the damaging effects of free radicals.

Sunscreens: Solar Perplexes

When summer's heat approaches and outdoor activities increase, store checkout displays fill up with sunscreens. There are oils and lotions; scenteds and unscenteds; brands promoted by bikini-clad models and brands touted for their moisturizers — the choices are endless. But for consumers wishing to avoid sunburn and overexposure to cancer-causing ultraviolet rays, one factor — the sun-protection factor (SPF) — is crucial. Medical professionals routinely advise consumers to use a sunscreen with an SPF of 15 or more. These sunscreens have already been proven to prevent sunburn and swelling. Now researchers have proof that these sunscreens may prevent some forms of skin cancer. Unfortunately, a potentially deadly skin cancer, melanoma, is not one of them.

Researchers found that regular use of sunscreens prevents the development of solar keratoses — skin lesions caused by the sun that greatly increase the risk of, or can lead to, skin cancer. Researchers monitored 431 people with solar keratoses. Half were given sunscreen to apply daily to their heads, necks, forearms, and hands, while the other half were given a cream without sunscreen. At the end of seven months, the number of lesions decreased by an average of one-half per person in the sunscreen group and increased by an average of one per person in the non-sunscreen group. Members of the sunscreen group were 40 percent less likely to develop new lesions and about one and a half times more likely to have their lesions disappear.

The researchers, who reported their findings in the *New England Journal of Medicine*, discovered that both the number of new lesions and the probability of remission were affected by the amount of sunscreen used — better results correlated with the use of more sunscreen. They concluded that health officials should continue to recommend the use of sunscreen to reduce the risk of skin cancer.

That was also the conclusion of the commentary that accompanied a January 1994 study. The authors of the commentary stated that regular use of sunscreen with an SPF of 15 during the first 18 years of life can cut the lifetime incidence of non-melanoma skin cancer by 78 percent.

The bad news was the finding of the study itself: Sunscreen may not provide protection against melanoma, the most serious form of skin cancer. The study, which appeared in the *Journal of the National Cancer Institute*, found that mice exposed to ultraviolet rays developed melanoma tumors despite being treated with sunscreen. While this does not negate sunscreen's benefits, the researchers suggest that sunscreen use could actually accelerate the onset of melanoma by enabling people to endure longer sun exposure, and ultimately more exposure to ultraviolet rays.

So where does this leave you? You can now rest assured that using a sunscreen with an adequate SPF will provide protection against premature aging caused by sun exposure, sunburn, and some forms of skin cancer, but you must remember that this protection may not always be adequate. Try to avoid prolonged exposure to the sun, particularly between 10 a.m. and 2 p.m., when its rays are most intense. When you must be in the sun for an extended period of time (long enough to get a sunburn), apply a sunscreen with an SPF of 15 or higher and wear clothing that is tightly woven, not sheer. Protect your face and eyes with a wide-brimmed hat and sunglasses.

What's most protective against skin cancer is a sunscreen that includes antioxidants, like vitamins C, E, and beta-carotene. One antioxidant sunscreen is Oxy Screen, which contains all three. It is distributed by Ecological Formulas in Concord, California.

Eczema: Itchy Winter Skin

"Oh, the weather outside is frightful" goes the song. Such words may be especially true for the estimated 15 million Americans who have eczema. For these people, their dry, inflamed skin may worsen dramatically when the temperature drops, indoor heat goes on, and the air inside and out becomes arid.

Eczema, in fact, is a generic term used by patients and many physicians to describe various types of dermatitis. However, most commonly it is used to describe one particular skin condition, atopic dermatitis (AD), a disease that causes itchy, inflamed skin. Atopic dermatitis typically affects the "flexures of the skin" — insides of the elbows and the backs of the knees — as well as the face and the hands, but in severe cases, it can cover most of the body. The skin looks red, cracked, feels itchy, and there are often marks from scratching. In more severe cases, the cracks allow for the development of infection, which leads to yellow crusts or little pinpoint pus-containing bumps.

The Facts About Eczema

About 10 percent of Americans have eczema during infancy and childhood, and in about 40 percent of these cases the disease resolves by adulthood. But that means about 60 percent of the remaining cases — or about 15 million Americans — experience eczema throughout their lives. The tendency to develop eczema is part of what is known as an atopic "triad," which is genetic and includes asthma, hay fever, and atopic dermatitis. If one parent has AD, asthma, or hay fever, the chances are about 50 percent that their child will have one or more of the three diseases. If both parents are atopic, chances are even greater that the child will be, too, according to the Eczema Association for Science and Education.

"The atopic triad really refers to people in whom there's a tendency for inflammatory and immune cells to overreact," says Jon Hanifin, MD, professor of dermatology at the Oregon Health Sciences University in

Portland. "In some people, the cells are most prevalent in the lungs, and they get asthma; in others, they are found mostly in the mucosal surfaces and the people get hay fever. In patients with eczema, the cells are most prevalent in the skin. Of course, some people can have problems in two or all three of these areas."

It is not surprising, then, that many of the same allergens that increase one's risks for asthma and hay fever are suspected of triggering some eczema outbreaks. These allergens include animal dander, dust mites, pollen, and certain foods.

Dry, Dry, Dry

In winter, however, the most common trigger factor for eczema is severely dry skin, a condition that can set off a vicious spiral of circumstances. The dry skin cracks, making it more prone to infection. It may also feel itchy, and the resulting scratching and rubbing can cause the skin to thicken; once it has thickened, it is less able to absorb medications and moisturizers and so becomes more difficult to treat. Although in most people eczema is localized to specific small areas of skin, in severe cases the dermatitis can become so widespread that it covers large portions of the body. "These cases are terribly disabling, and occasionally even require hospitalization," says Dr. Hanifin. "The skin is so cracked and weeping that it begins to lose heat, and the heart begins to pump overtime in an effort to regulate the body temperature. These patients lose so much heat that they become chilled and sick. So a problem that was once limited to the skin can become a systemic disease, and even be life-threatening."

The best approach to eczema (and to all skin conditions) is prevention. In winter, prevention is focused on one simple goal: avoiding excessively dry skin.

The Best Prevention Program
Starts With Nutrition

Your skin is your largest organ of elimination and its condition tells you something about the foods you eat and the nutrients (vitamins, minerals, and fats) that make their way into its cells.

Omega-3 and Omega-6 Fatty Acids: The fats you eat that go into your skin keep it moist from the inside out. In an effort to keep thin and follow a healthful, low-fat diet, many women eat too little or the wrong kinds of fats. Omega-3 and omega-6 fatty acids are two kinds of fats that have been found to help improve eczema. Cold-water fish, like salmon, tuna and halibut, are high in omega-3 fatty acids. These good fats are also sold in health food stores under the name of "MaxEPA." Before you begin taking the capsules you might want to increase your intake of cold-water fish as part of your nutritional program for eczema. Doses of MaxEPA capsules that have been found helpful in eczema, according to published scientific studies, range from three to nine grams a day, taken in divided doses.

Omega-6 fatty acids can be found in evening primrose oil. Since you're not going to find evening primroses in your grocery store, this fat is only available in capsules. However, there is an excellent and inexpensive form of both omega-3 and omega-6 fatty acids in the form of flax seed. Flax seed capsules and flax oil can be found in most health food stores. So can the less expensive flax seeds. You can take a few tablespoons of these hard, shiny seeds and grind them in your coffee or seed grinder, then add them to your breakfast cereal, sprinkle over a salad, or use to garnish a bowl of soup. The oil deteriorates rapidly in light, so use the freshly ground flax meal within 15 minutes. Don't grind up a week's supply all at once.

Vitamin A: High doses of vitamin A have been found helpful in some cases of eczema. But don't rush out and buy a lot of vitamin A. It can be toxic to children and pregnant women. It's best to have a high vitamin A intake supervised by your health care practitioner. Of course, it's never harmful to increase your intake of vitamin A (or it's co-factor, beta carotene) by eating more fish, fresh vegetables and fruits.

Vitamin C, on the other hand, can safely be taken in high quantities. Its most common side effect, if taken in excess, is loose stools. So you can self-monitor your vitamin C intake. A study published in 1989 suggests that vitamin C may help eczema by boosting the immune system. If this is how and why it works, make sure you're not on a junk food diet or consuming large quantities of medications (even over-the-counter ones), alcohol, or foods high in sugar. They can suppress your immune system. Vitamin C is high in broccoli, bell peppers and potatoes, as well as citrus fruits.

Selenium with Vitamin E, and Zinc, have been found to be helpful in cases of eczema. Interestingly, these minerals both support the immune system. In addition to finding them in whole grains and fresh produce, they are included in many vitamin/mineral supplements. A study reported in *Dr. Wright's Book of Nutritional Therapy* (Rodale Press, 1979) showed improvement in 39 out of 40 cases of eczema in people who took 50 mg. of chelated zinc three times a day. Because there is controversy over the safety of high amounts of zinc, it would be best to take this amount under the direction of a health care provider who understands mineral supplementation.

Food Sensitivities have been implicated in many cases of eczema, and an elimination diet seems to be the best way to clear up the skin. Sensitivities to egg and dairy are among the most common, but you could be sensitive to anything you eat frequently — even if allergy testing does not indicate a problem. To identify a sensitivity, select one or two foods you eat regularly, beginning with dairy and eggs. Eliminate them 100 percent for two weeks. Then introduce them one at a time over a two-day period. If your skin began to clear up when you eliminated them and you have skin eruptions or other symptoms after re-introducing them, avoid these foods temporarily. Test at three-month intervals to see if and when you can tolerate those foods.

Multiple food sensitivities are often associated with a lack of hydrochloric acid (HCI), an acid produced by the stomach which assists in the digestion of proteins and influences the production of other digestive enzymes. While we do not suggest you self-administer HCI, your doctor can evaluate you for HCI insufficiency (achlorhydria). Since antacids stop the production of HCI, anyone with eczema should seriously consider not taking antacids. If you think your digestion warrants HCI supplementation, talk first to your health care provider about the amount to take and when to take it.

Other Prevention Tips

Routine use of mild moisturizers helps fight dry skin from the outside. Environmentally friendly, fragrance-free, and hypo-allergenic formulas tend to be the mildest and, therefore, least likely to irritate the skin. Creams and ointments are best, says Dr. Hanifin, as lotions may not be emollient enough, and in some cases may contain solvents that increase moisture evaporation from the skin. The cream or ointment should be applied immediately after bathing or any other time skin becomes wet. "I give patients my three-minute rule," says Dr. Hanifin. "Apply the moisturizer to the skin within three minutes of bathing or showering.

Waiting any longer could cause too much moisture loss from the skin due to evaporation." For people whose hands are frequently wet during the day — a common cause of hand dermatitis — Dr. Hanifin recommends keeping hand cream right beside the sink and applying it automatically after every wash.

Other ways to prevent dry skin include the use of lukewarm — not hot — water to wash the skin, and minimizing the use of harsh soaps, detergents, and other harsh substances (on yourself as well as clothes) that can irritate and strip the skin of natural oils. Excessive rubbing or scrubbing of skin also should be avoided. Running laundry through a second rinse cycle can help remove detergents more thoroughly. Also try skipping fabric softeners which are chemical-laden and can also irritate sensitive skin.

Chlorine in shower and bath water can also dry out the skin. An easy way to remove most of it from your shower water is to install a Hydro Spray showerhead (call 800-728-2288 for more information).

Some people like to use humidifiers in the home or office to increase the ambient humidity, making skin less likely to dry out. "I don't think this works very well," says Dr. Hanifin. "The minute you leave the humidified room and go into another room, skin begins to dry out again."

There are other important ways to prevent a flare-up of eczema, particularly in winter. First of all, avoid irritating fabrics such as wool. Instead, keep warm with layers of non-irritating fabrics such as cottons and soft synthetics. If you are participating in any vigorous physical activity, peel off these layers as your body begins to heat up to prevent excessive heating and sweating, which can lead to a prickly heat type of itching. Extremely vigorous exercise is not recommended during a flare-up of eczema; it's best to wait until the skin clears again. At night, keep your thermostat set fairly low, and don't overdo night clothes or bedding. "Night sweats" caused by too many warm layers can also lead to prickly heat types of rashes.

The New Wrinkle-Fighter: Renova

by Alison Lapinski, RPh*

Fine lines, wrinkles, rough and dry skin. In our eternal search for a way to help keep our skin smooth and wrinkle-free, a potential solution has appeared on the horizon in the form of a new prescription cream called Renova.

This cream contains the active ingredient tretinoin, which is the same compound contained in the popular acne drug Retin-A. The principal difference between the two is that Retin-A is formulated as a drying agent to treat acne lesions, while Renova's formulation is to be an emollient to moisturize rough, dry skin.

For several years, women have used Retin-A for the non-FDA approved use of reducing fine lines and wrinkles. Individuals using it for acne observed that the fine lines and wrinkles on their faces were also disappearing. It is not known how this occurs, but it is thought that tretinoin acts on the growth and differentiation of epithelial cells in the skin. This somehow "plumps" up skin lines and smooths them out.

When this discovery became public, people raced to their physicians to obtain prescriptions for Retin-A.

But be warned, many insurance companies have refused to pay for these prescriptions, since they feel they are not being used for the FDA approved use of treating acne.

These findings with Retin-A have spurred more studies on the active ingredient tretinoin, and the formulation of Renova, only this time in an emollient base for rough, dry skin. These studies were conducted with individuals using Renova along with a comprehensive skin-care program for 24 weeks.

These studies have shown that 30 percent of the people using Renova for fine wrinkles and spotty discoloration had moderate improvement, 35 percent of the individuals had minimal improvement, and 35 percent had no improvement. Of those individuals using Renova for rough skin, 16 percent had moderate improvement, 35 percent minimal improvement, and 49 percent had no improvement. Most improvements were noted during the first 24 weeks of therapy. After the initial 24 weeks of therapy,

---

* *Alison Lapinski is a pharmacist in Joliet, Illinois, and a consumer advocate for safer pharmaceutical choices.*

when the use of Renova and the comprehensive skin-care program were discontinued, most of the beneficial effects were gone.

The reality is that Renova comes with no guarantees. Renova's manufacturer clearly states that Renova doesn't eliminate wrinkles, nor does it repair sun-damaged skin. Additionally, they state that it may help treat fine wrinkles, spotty discoloration, and rough skin, but doesn't cure these conditions. In fact, they recommend the preventative measures of using a sunscreen with an SPF of 15 or higher, wearing protective clothing such as a hat or sunglasses, avoiding direct sun exposure, and using moisturizing creams. Who's to say that these aren't bringing about the reported improvements?

If you feel that this is not enough for you, and you wish to try Renova, it is imperative you follow a few important instructions:

1. After thoroughly washing your face and letting it dry for 20 to 30 minutes, apply a small amount of cream to your face, carefully avoiding the eyes, ears, nostrils, and mouth. The best time for this application is before bedtime.

2. Stay out of the sun, because Renova increases your sensitivity to sunlight. Avoid sun lamps.

3. Do not use Renova if you are taking any of the following prescription medications; tetracycline, thiazide diuretics (i.e., Dyazide, Maxzide, Hydrochlorothiazide), phenothiazines (i.e., Mellaril, Thorazine), sulfa drugs (i.e., Bactrim, Septra), and fluroquinolones, (i.e., Noroxin, Cipro). When any of these are combined with Renova, there is the possibility of developing a phototoxicity or increased sensitivity to sunlight.

4. Avoid using skin cleansers, hair removers, alcohol-based cosmetics, spices, or lime on your skin while using Renova. These items all have an additive drying effect, that can further irritate your skin.

5. Do not use if you're pregnant, or trying to become pregnant. Birth defects have been associated with the use of the oral form of tretinoin, known as Accutane, in laboratory animals.

6. Do not use if you're nursing, since it is not known whether tretinoin is excreted in breast milk.

7. Do not apply on diseased or sunburned skin until it is completely healed.

Renova alone isn't a magic potion, or a fountain of youth for your skin. Preventative measures are the best method to avoid the ravages of sun-damaged skin.

When considering the substantial cost of Renova (approximately $50 a tube), the absence of insurance reimbursement, and the number of drug interactions and cautions involved, a practical alternative may be sunscreen, moisturizers, and wearing protective clothing. In addition, follow the preventative measures recommended by the manufacturer so as to remain side effect free.

Varicose Veins

For most people the term varicose veins conjures up thoughts of blue, bulging, veins in the legs, running up and down and roundabout just under the skin's surface and, in general, creating visual havoc. Yet any true sufferer of varicose veins will tell you that appearance is the least of their problems!

Varicose veins develop when valves in the vein malfunction. These valves, when healthy, help the body return blood to the heart by opening and closing to keep blood flowing in the right direction. But the more we stand or sit, the harder our leg veins must work against the force of gravity to do this job. If you are female, eventually one or more of these valves will usually malfunction, allowing blood to flow in the wrong direction and pool below the valve. Over time, this pooling can cause distention or varicosities in the vein.

It's estimated that nearly 50 percent of all middle-aged Americans have varicose veins — and the majority of sufferers are female.

Symptoms of Varicose Veins

Achiness: This is usually experienced as a dull ache, or a feeling of heaviness. Affected legs may also feel tired and weak. Standing or sitting for long periods of time may bring on or worsen feelings of achiness. Night cramps or charley horses are also common. If you suspect you have varicose veins, and experience a sharp or sudden acute pain, it is wise to consult a doctor. This could be a symptom of a more serious vein problem.

Restlessness: Legs may become so uncomfortable that it is difficult to stand on both feet at once. Discomfort may include burning and itching.

Swelling: Legs and even ankles may become noticeably swollen. This can be accompanied by brownish pigmentation or other visual abnormalities. If you have swelling that has not been caused by special circumstances such as excessive standing, sitting with bent knees or socks or shoes that are too tight, consult your doctor. Swelling can also be a symptom of a blood clot, heart failure, and other serious conditions.

Enlarged veins: The unsightliness of varicose veins occurs when blood pools in the affected vein, causing it to become enlarged and distended. This is seen as twisted, bulging, rope-like blue lines just under the skin's surface. Affected areas may also be discolored (brownish, bluish, or whitish) or appear thin and shiny. *Spider veins are not varicose veins.* They can however, exist concurrently with varicose veins.

In general, a varicose vein continues to have its rope-like appearance even when the affected leg is elevated. If veins are very painful, and contain a red lump or lumps that don't decrease in size when the legs are elevated, you could have a thrombus or clot. This should be checked by a doctor. In addition, many varicose veins are not visible because they are hidden in the interior of the leg. Sometimes perfectly healthy veins are visible below the skin's surface if the skin is extra transparent.

The above symptoms in and of themselves are not life-threatening. The complications that can result, however, can be. In 1994, approximately 100,000 Americans died from varicose vein complications, while hundreds of thousands more became severely disabled. Complications that can arise from varicose veins include:

- phlebitis — an inflamed vein wall
- thrombophlebitis — in which a mass forms and sticks to the wall of an inflamed saphenous vein
- deep vein thrombosis — when a mass or blood clot forms in a deep vein
- post-thrombotic syndrome — a number of symptoms including leg ulcers
- hemorrhage — blood gushing from an erupted vein. (In the event this happens, put finger pressure on the open vein, using a gauze pad, washcloth, or other clean pad and go to your doctor right away.)
- pulmonary embolism — a blood clot that has traveled into the lung

What Causes Valve Malfunction in the First Place?

The number one cause appears to be sedentariness. Apparently, in less-developed countries where much higher activity levels are an everyday part of life, varicose veins are quite rare. This is because exercise from activity helps valves and veins stay strong and in good working order. It also provides important secondary support for our veins. Exercise helps you maintain a stronger heart — which produces a stronger pumping action to help circulate blood. Second, it helps maintain good muscle tone, and well-toned muscles provide more support for neighboring veins. Also the action of muscles flexing and relaxing helps push blood through the veins.

In addition, sitting in a chair (which happens less in less-developed countries) requires veins to work harder against the force of gravity to move blood back up to the heart. Sedentary standing, such as working on an assembly line or standing behind a counter also put extra stress on the veins.

The fact that varicose-vein incidence increases with age also suggests that we lose vein health slowly — over the course of many decades. This loss of tone might not be significant enough to cause problems for people in less-developed countries. Higher activity levels probably result in less loss of tone. But the loss of vein tone with age appears to be enough to cause problems for persons in sedentary societies such as ours.

Being female also puts a person at greater risk for developing varicose veins: four times as many women as men have them. Reproductive differences apparently make us more vulnerable — especially during pregnancy and menopause. Both of these conditions are characterized by significant hormone balance fluctuations. In addition, pregnancy is extra stressful for our veins (as well as the rest of our circulatory system) because of the tremendous increase in blood volume at this time.

Many experts believe that varicose veins can also be caused by weak vein walls, heredity, and a low-fiber diet. Howard C. Baron, MD, and author of *Varicose Veins a Guide to Prevention and Treatment*, also believes that hormone replacement therapy and birth control pills may contribute to varicose vein development.

Prevention

If you don't already have varicose veins, here are some suggestions to help you reduce your risk of ever getting them:

Maintain a healthy lifestyle.... This covers the basics with which you should already be familiar: a healthy diet, a well-balanced aerobic and weight-bearing exercise program, and no substance abuse (that includes cigarettes and alcohol). Smokers have a higher incidence of varicose veins.

Your diet should be high-fiber to prevent constipation, which can cause pressure that may contribute to varicose veins. And as always, it's advisable to keep the muscle and lose the fat. The more fat you have, the more blood your body has to circulate. Muscle movement, however, helps circulate blood. When you are leaner, you have less blood volume, and more muscle power to circulate the blood you have.

Dr. Julian Whitaker, of the Whitaker Wellness Center in Newport Beach, California, also recommends eating plenty of blackberries and cherries, which may help prevent varicose veins and ease symptoms in those who have them. These and other dark-colored berries contain anthocyanins and proanthocyanidins, which help tone and strengthen vein walls.

Here's another lifestyle tip from Mitchel P. Goldman, MD and assistant clinical professor of dermatology at the University of California, San Diego: Wear flat shoes. "When you wear high heels, you do not activate your calf muscles properly, which allows blood to collect in your vein," says Dr. Goldman.

Avoid sedentariness.... This takes a little more thought and creativity. The objective is to avoid inactive standing and sitting. This puts extra stress and pressure on the veins by making them work against the force of gravity — without the extra assistance that comes with muscle movement, such as walking. If you must stand for long periods of time, try to exercise your legs in place as much as possible. This might include shifting your weight from one foot to the other; doing repetitions of standing on your toes; and taking a short walk every 30 to 60 minutes. The idea is to work your leg muscles so they can help your veins push blood back up to your heart. Sitting on a stool can also be helpful because it at least takes pressure off your veins.

If you are sitting — at a desk, around your house, or somewhere else on a chair or sofa — there are creative ways to reduce stress and pressure on the veins as well. For starters, try flexing various leg muscles, wiggling your toes, and taking short walks periodically. (For example, when watching television, train yourself to get up and walk somewhere during each commercial break.) If you can sit with your legs in a more horizontal position, that will also help reduce the force of gravity against which your legs must work. If you sit at a desk a lot and can get away with resting your feet on the desk or other piece of nearby furniture, do that. I also keep a plastic milk carton under the desk so I can sit with my legs extended horizontally. A wonderful piece of furniture to help you do this at home is called an ottoman. A sturdy coffee table or recliner chair also makes it easy to sit with your legs extended in front of you. Or simply sit on the floor and use a chair or sofa as a back rest. The idea here is that the more horizontal your legs, the less your leg veins must work against the force of gravity to keep blood flowing in the right direction.

Finally, choose jobs that do not require prolonged sitting or standing. This, however, will be easier for some and more difficult for others.

Be extra prepared for high risk times.... Pregnancy and menopause are times when American women are especially vulnerable to developing varicose veins. Knowing this in advance and doing something about it can give you a big preventive advantage. If you are planning to become pregnant, get yourself in extra-good shape (nutrition and exercise-wise) before conception. You will lower your risk of pregnancy-related health problems, including varicose veins. Plus, you'll lower your unborn child's risk of birth defects. The same holds true for menopause. In general, the better all-around shape a woman is in before menopause, the easier the menopause transition will be for her including fewer health problems, such as varicose vein development, during that time. Then after menopause, stay in good shape to reduce your risk of developing varicose veins even further.

But What If You Already Have Varicose Veins?

Are you hopelessly destined for them to become worse, possibly bad enough to require surgery or develop one of the associated complications? Not necessarily! For millions, varicose veins never progress beyond minor discomfort. In addition, the above suggestions may provide relief. And you may be able to arrest varicose-vein development, and even improve your vein health with the following:

Exercise: The rule of thumb here is to do nothing that will overstress your already stressed varicose veins. Walking is a good choice because it is gentle, yet helps strengthen the entire circulatory system, plus builds calf muscles (which help pump blood back to your heart as you walk). Other forms of exercise that build up leg muscles are also beneficial. But don't over-exert yourself. Excessive stress and pressure on the circulatory system can cause varicose veins to bulge more, make symptoms worse, and/or cause a temporary flare-up (especially excessive weightlifting with the legs). As always, remember to consult your doctor before beginning a new exercise program. A quick phone call can usually get you an official "go-ahead."

Elevation: You don't have to wait for symptoms to flare to benefit from elevating your legs (above the level of your heart). Elevating your legs at least once a day for 20 minutes will give your circulation a boost, even when you are symptom-free.

Support stockings: Some women find that support hose, extra thick nylon stockings, help legs feel better. Others like supportive knee socks. And for more serious cases, a doctor can prescribe special elastic support stockings. They can all reduce edema, or swelling (and in turn relieve symptoms), by providing your veins extra support. At the same time, it's important to avoid constrictive clothing. This means knee socks should

Natural Solutions to Varicose Veins

Varicose veins affect almost 50 percent of middle-aged people, and four out of five of them are women. Pregnant women and obese adults put more pressure on their veins, accounting for some of this high female percentage. Compression stockings, followed by surgical stripping, are the most common treatments for varicose veins. Now, horse chestnut seed extract is being used.

In a recent clinical trial, horse chestnut seed extract containing 50 mg of aescin (a natural ingredient), was tested against compression stockings or a placebo for three months. Compression therapy reduced the varicosity by 56.5 ml, and horse chestnut seed extract reduced it by 53.6 ml. People on the placebo had a 9.8 ml increase. If you have varicose veins, you may find that taking horse chestnut seed extract works almost as well as compression stockings. And if it's working from the inside out, instead of just pressing the veins, the results may last even longer.

Diehm, C., et al. "Comparison of leg compression stocking and oral horse chestnut seed extract therapy in patients with chronic venous insufficiency," *Lancet*, 347:292-4-1996; *Amer J Natr Med*, July/Aug 1997.

not be extra tight at the top since this can have a tourniquet effect and restrict instead of promote blood flow. Girdles and other constrictive clothing can also have a similar effect.

Herbal remedies: Michael T. Murray, a naturopathic doctor and author of *The Healing Power of Herbs,* recommends triterpenic acid extract of gotu kola for varicose veins sufferers. Studies have found it effective in treating symptoms (including a reduction of edema, spider veins, leg ulcers, and vein distensibility), plus improving blood flow, in approximately 80 percent of patients. The extract can be difficult to find, so gotu kola leaves can be substituted. Dr. Murray recommends using two to four grams per day of the leaves, which can be made into a tea or tincture.

Other remedies that Dr. Murray recommends are:

Bilberry — To help stabilize altered veins, help restore the connective tissue sheath that surrounds the vein, and help reduce blood pooling.

Ginkgo biloba — For stimulating improvement in vein tone and normalizing circulation.

Bromelain — To reduce the risk of thrombus formation, which may result in thrombophlebitis, heart attack, pulmonary embolism, or stroke.

Butcher's broom (Ruscus aculeatus) — For improving tone of the vein walls.

Homeopathy — Andrew Lockie, MD, and author of *The Family Guide to Homeopathy* recommends the following homeopathic remedies, c30 every 12 hours for up to seven days:

- *Hamamelis* for veins that feel bruised and sore.
- *Pulsatilla* if you feel chilly, but warmth and letting the legs hang down makes veins feel worse.
- *Carbo vegetabilis* if the skin around the veins is mottled and marbled.
- *Ferrum metallicum* if legs are pale, but redden easily; walking slowly relieves feelings of weakness and achiness.

Hydrotherapy — Agatha Thrash, MD at the Uchee Pines Institute, a natural healing center in Seale, Alabama, suggests stimulating circulation by filling two tall buckets or wastebaskets with hot and cold water up to the level of your knees, then submerging your feet and lower legs in the hot water for three minutes followed by a 30-second cold water soak. She recommends doing this three times, once a day for a month to see results. *Note:* Diabetics should use warm water instead of hot.

On the other hand, Dr. Goldman advises against heating up the veins with hot baths, saunas, etc. Even a bout of hot weather is enough to make symptoms flare by dilating the veins. For some sufferers, ice packs or cold water, without heat from any source, might provide better relief although it won't stimulate circulation as effectively.

Massage — Circulation in the legs can be stimulated with gentle massage. But don't massage the veins directly. Instead massage the surrounding areas. If you'd like to use a massage oil, Judith Jackson, author of *Scentual Touch: A Personal Guide to Aromatherapy* recommends a varicose vein blend of 12 drops each of cypress and geranium essential oils in four ounces of a carrier oil such as sesame.

Reduce sodium intake — Lowering the amount of salt you consume may help relieve swelling.

Sclerotherapy — This procedure calls for an irritant to be injected into a varicose vein. Then an elastic bandage is worn for about two weeks. During this time the irritant causes a clot to form in the vein, blocking it, and causing blood to be rerouted to healthier veins. Clots are locked in place by scar tissue that forms around them. This procedure is repeated for every varicosity. If a bandage is removed too early, the clot can be dislodged — creating a potentially life-threatening situation. This may not be worth the trouble since problems reappear in approximately 65 percent of all patients within three to four years.

Vein stripping — This is another allopathic medicine treatment in which the saphenous vein is removed and connected perforator veins are tied off. This forces blood to be rerouted through the deep interior leg veins that already carry nearly 90 percent of venous blood. After this procedure, new varicose veins rarely develop, and if they do, they are usually tiny.

Micro-extraction — The medical term for this procedure is ambulatory phlebectomy. It is a procedure from Europe that is basically a kinder and gentler version of vein stripping. With micro-extraction, a local anesthesia, called tumescent technique, is used, allowing doctors to safely give patients higher volumes of local anesthetic in an office setting. This anesthesia is an important part of the procedure because it presses the vein up against the skin's surface, making it easier to grasp.

The procedure leaves scars no larger than a pin point, is virtually pain-free, and offers a recovery period of only one day. This, combined with the fact that it can be performed on an out-patient basis, makes the procedure much less painful and expensive than traditional vein stripping.

As with all surgeries, there are risks. In the case of micro-extraction, the risks are similar to those of vein stripping. These include hemorrhage, hematoma, lymphocele, and nerve damage. According to a report that appeared in the *Journal of Dermatological Surgery*, however, the incidence and severity of these complications is much lower than in traditional vein stripping.

Doctors who are experienced in micro-extraction, though, can be difficult to find. If you are interested, you might call the Skin and Vein Center in Detroit (248-689-1400), which is operated by Dr. Sandy Goldman and Dr. Eric Seiger. They are among the most experienced physicians in this country doing the procedure.

Valve repair — Some surgeons are beginning to perform a valve repair procedure in which the vein around a malfunctioning valve is wrapped with a synthetic material — restoring it to its previously healthy diameter. This restores normal valve functioning. This is a relatively new procedure, so if you are considering it, make sure your surgeon has a good track record for doing it.

One Final Word About Remedies

Oftentimes, the simplest and easiest ones work best, plus are safer and less expensive. That makes them a great place to start to finally get your varicose veins under control.

Chapter 12

Supplements, Herbs, and Oils

What You Need to Know About Vitamins

Vitamins and minerals are nutrients that feed all the cells in your body. Without them your cells would starve and you would die. When you have too few of one or more nutrients, you run the risk of not feeling completely well and energetic or eventually of having a nutrient-deficiency disease. Many of these diseases, like scurvy from a vitamin C deficiency, are no longer a health problem in developed countries. Others, like anemia, which can be caused by iron or B_{12} deficiencies, may result in fatigue. Sometimes nutrient deficiencies result in such discomfort as PMS (often caused by a lack of sufficient B_6 or magnesium) or skin problems and never lead to serious illness.

Your body uses extra amounts of nutrients when you're under stress, exercising, fighting off a cold or flu, smoking, exposed to environmental pollutants, or using medications. Can you get enough of the vitamins and minerals you need from your diet? And when you take vitamin or mineral supplements, how do you know they are getting into your cells and doing their job?

How Much Is Enough?

Many people believe that a healthy diet provides all the nutrients we need. At one time that may have been true. However, environmental toxins from smog, foods containing residues of antibiotics, pesticides and herbicides, and the additional stresses that come from living in the 20th century, all impact on our nutrient needs. A diet that once was enough may now be deficient. And many people are too busy to prepare and eat three balanced meals a day. They get their energy boosts from caffeine, alcohol, or sugar, all of which deplete the body of one or more nutrients. Sugar, for example, requires more B vitamins to be digested than you'll get in your regular diet. Whenever you eat foods high in sugar, you need extra B vitamins.

Supplements, Not Replacements

To evaluate your body's nutrient needs, first recognize that vitamins and minerals are supplements, not instead-ofs. They do not replace a healthy diet or a good night's sleep. If you want to be healthy, stay healthy, and be free from discomfort as well as disease, begin eating a diet low in fats (and very low in animal fats), low in refined sugar and high in whole grains, beans, and vegetables. Add a little fruit and small amounts of raw nuts and seeds. After you've been eating well for several months, consider taking vitamins and minerals.

Taking a multi-vitamin/mineral may be the least expensive health insurance you can find — or it may be a complete waste of money. You may be surprised to know that all vitamins and minerals do not necessarily have the ingredients their labels say they contain. Nor are these nutrients necessarily in a form your body can break down and use. There is no agency that monitors the content and bioavailability of vitamins, so you have to do a little of the research yourself.

Vitamin C and Older Women

Older women living in nursing homes were found to eat 25 percent lower amounts of vitamin C than women living independently. They ate less fresh fruit and fewer vegetables. While these women did not show signs of vitamin C deficiency, this vitamin is needed to help absorb iron and folic acid, prevent bed sores and leg ulcers, and protect against infections. Why not give your mother or friend in a nursing home the present of chewable vitamin C tablets for a tasty, helpful gift? Then follow up to make sure she is taking them, requesting help from the nursing staff if necessary.

Look for High Quality

Some vitamins and minerals are made from petroleum by-products. They are synthetic. Numerous doctors and scientists argue that these are as well-absorbed as the "natural" ones and that more expensive vitamins are a waste of money. You may choose to believe them. At one time, I did, too. Then, as a nutritionist, I started looking closely at my patients and their health concerns. I noticed over a period of 14 years that patients who used inexpensive vitamins and minerals from drug stores, discount stores, and even health food stores appeared to be taking sufficient amounts of vitamins and minerals, but still had signs of nutrient deficiencies. I had

---

RDA vs. DRI

The Recommended Daily Allowances for nutrients were designed to inform the public about the amount of vitamins and minerals necessary to prevent illnesses, like scurvy and kwashiorkor (uncommon to begin with in this country). They were not to give optimal levels for people to recover from illnesses, or to keep people healthy.

Now, the National Academy of Sciences, which helps set nutrient levels, has asked a nonprofit organization, the Institute of Medicine (IOM), to re-do nutrient levels for specific conditions. The first condition being addressed is osteoporosis. Sound good? Read further.

We believe there is a great deal of confusion about how much calcium a woman needs for healthy, strong bones. The ideal amount, 1,000-1,500 mg, suggested by most doctors will, unfortunately, not get into women's bones. Calcium absorption after age 25 (except during pregnancy), deteriorates. Unabsorbed calcium can lead to arthritis and heart disease. And heart disease is the number one killer of post-menopausal women.

We think the impartial IOM may not be so impartial after all. The current study was funded by the FDA, Health Canada, the National Institutes of Health, and the United States Dairy Association (USDA). With the USDA in the picture, how can we expect impartial information, which must include our body's ability to use various nutrients.

When you see DRI levels in the future, remember that they may or may not be truly optimal. Unfortunately, biased information like increasing calcium beyond the body's ability to utilize it can lead to pain and heart problems in thousands of women.

Granato, Heather. "What is the DRI?" *Natural Foods Merchandiser,* October 1997.

them take natural vitamins and their deficiencies and symptoms disappeared.

For 14 years, I have noticed the relationship between good quality, well-absorbed nutrients and those that do not appear to do anything. My patients often decide to continue taking multi-vitamin/minerals because they notice a difference when they stop taking them.

Match Your Needs With a Formula

Look for a complete formula rather than buying bottle after bottle and making your own mixture. Some formulas are put together in such a way that they break down and are absorbed without competing with one another.

Most multivitamin/mineral formulas are based on old information stating that women need twice as much calcium as magnesium. The truth is, excessive calcium without sufficient magnesium is not absorbed into the cells, but rather collects in the joints where it becomes arthritis or in the arteries where it contributes to atherosclerosis. No wonder so many women suffer from heart attacks and painful arthritis as they age!

If you have PMS or are postmenopausal and concerned about osteoporosis, contact Optimox, Inc. They are the only company that has done controlled double-blind studies showing the effectiveness of their ratio of calcium to magnesium on eliminating PMS (Optivite formula) and reversing osteoporosis (Gynovite formula). Their formulas contain more magnesium than calcium and are extremely well-absorbed. You can call them at 800-223-1601. Other similar formulas are based on Optimox research. They may or may not break down in your body as well.

Flax Seed

Flax seed is another recently discovered nutrient powerhouse that in my opinion is not just a fad but is here to stay. It's rich in essential fatty acids and has strong antioxidant properties. I have a special coffee grinder that I use to grind a tablespoon or two of flax seed daily, which I then sprinkle on a salad.

A Final Note

Most companies put together formulas based on research on individual nutrients. They do not run expensive studies based on their finished product. Therefore, since each of us is unique and requires more or less of a specific nutrient, and our bodies differ in their abilities to utilize them, a formula that works for one person may not work as well for another.

You may want to try a particular formula for three months, then stop for a week or two to see if you notice any difference. If not, perhaps there is a better formula for you. Is a less than ideal formula better than nothing? If you're stressed, have less energy than you think you should, and if you're living in the same polluted world as the rest of us, you'll probably benefit from a good multivitamin/mineral whether you experience the benefits now or in the future.

What to Look for in Supplements

Vitamins A & E: Studies have shown that water-soluble vitamins A and E are better absorbed than the more commonly found oil-soluble ones. Look for dry or water-soluble forms.

Natural vs. Synthetic Vitamins

Many people would like you to believe there is no difference between natural and synthetic vitamins. They are all chemicals our bodies can use. But to what degree? A recent study on women and vitamin E was published in the *American Journal of Clinical Nutrition*. Each of three types and strengths of vitamin E was used for one month, with three months on no vitamin E used in between.

It took 300 mg of synthetic vitamin E to equal the blood levels of 100 mg of the natural vitamin. If you're taking vitamins with synthetic vitamin E (the label will say dl-alpha tocopherols, rather than d-alpha tocopherols), you are probably getting one-third the amount you're taking. We look forward to seeing studies on other synthetic vitamins.

Kiyose C., et al. "Biodiscrimination of alpha-tocopherol sterioisomers in humans after oral administration," *Am J Clin Nutr 65*, 785-9(1997); *Intl Clin Nutr Rev*, July, 1997.

Calcium: The most easily absorbed calcium is calcium carbonate or citrate. But calcium needs acid in order to be absorbed, so calcium carbonate in an antacid is poorly absorbed.

Minerals: Minerals in citrate form usually are not irritating and are well-absorbed. If the name of a mineral is followed by the word "picolinate" such as chromium, iron, and zinc, the absorption rate into your body is very high. You get more of these nutrients into your cells than minerals in other forms.

Calcium & Magnesium: Choose a formula that has at least as much magnesium as calcium. Numerous recent studies indicate that 400 to 600 mg of calcium a day is sufficient, and you get some from the foods you eat. A formula with more than 600 mg of calcium may lead to more problems than solutions.

Iron: If you have had cancer, or if there is a high incidence of cancer in your family, you may want to take a formula without added iron. High iron has been found in women with cancer.

Selenium: Low selenium levels are associated with cancer, AIDS, and other immune problems. A protective amount is 200 mcg.

Chromium: Chromium helps the body utilize carbohydrates and is helpful in stabilizing blood sugar levels and reducing excess weight. You

---

Early-Onset Treatment for Alzheimer's

L-acetylcarnitine (LAC) is a molecule made from L-carnitine, an amino acid, and acetic acid, an organic acid found in vinegar. It is a combination that occurs naturally in our brains. Over the past 10 years, LAC has been studied in relationship to Alzheimer's, age-related memory loss, and depression in older people. LAC is related to an important neurotransmitter that is responsible for brain function, called acetylcholine. As we age, we utilize acetylcholine less well. This is where LAC comes in.

A recent study published in *Neurology Journal* (47:705-11, 1996) shows that LAC has a similar effect on the brain as acetylcholine, and was not only helpful for patients under age 65 with early stage Alzheimer's, it also benefitted people under 65 with memory loss and depression. Three grams of LAC were given to patients in this study for a year. People over 65 had less benefit than those who were younger.

Thal, L.J., et al. "A one-year multicenter placebo-controlled study of acetyl-L-carnitine in patients with Alzheimer's disease," *Neurology* 47:705-11, 1996.

need at least 200 mcg. of chromium — often more for weight control and excessive sugar cravings.

Women, Girls and Iron Deficiency

A recent article in the *Journal of the American Medical Association* has come out with startling statistics. Nearly 700,000 young children and 7.8 million women in this country have an iron deficiency. "Nine percent of toddlers aged one to two years and 9-11 percent of adolescent girls and women of child-bearing age were iron deficient," the article states.

Many young girls are iron-deficient without being anemic, so their problem is masked. Now, a study from Baltimore shows a correlation between this iron deficiency and cognitive functioning. The girls in this study were given 650 mg of oral ferrous sulfate twice a day for two months. They were not give any other vitamins or minerals. At the end of the program, their verbal learning and memory improved considerably. Their ability to pay attention in class, however, did not change. Since adolescent girls don't always eat properly, iron supplementation was used to correct the iron deficiency.

Iron is a mineral that is either deficient in our diets, or difficult to be absorbed. To absorb iron, you need acid in your stomach or in the iron-rich foods you eat. Two simple suggestions for food preparation can help you and your children replenish depleted iron stores. First, cook iron-rich green leafy vegetables, whole grains, and beans in cast-iron pots whenever possible, adding an acidic substance to it like lemon juice or tomatoes. This allows some of the iron to get into the foods and into you in a more absorbable form.

A Brazilian study indicated that iron increased at least six times when cast iron cookware was used. Always eat iron-rich foods with some form

If You're Anemic, Watch Your Calcium

Don't mix yogurt into your stewed prunes or eat a salad with cheese if you're anemic. Calcium (found in dairy products) inhibits the absorption of iron. If you've been eating these foods and your iron levels are fine, don't worry. But if you have low iron and have been combining dairy products with high-iron foods, you may want to eat them at separate times for maximum iron absorption. (Proceedings of the Nutrition Society, UK, 52, 1993) of acidic food. Even sipping lemon water helps the iron to be increased at least two or three times, and is more easily metabolized.

If you have a teenaged daughter who has heavy menstrual flow, or who is having difficulty remembering what she's learning in school, you may want to have her tested for a slight deficiency. Try adding iron-rich foods to her diet and see if this increase in dietary iron helps her school work improve.

The Healing Power of Essential Oils

Essential oils might be one of the most misunderstood remedies in the alternative medicine cabinet. In this country, they're most widely used for creating fragrances. But in Europe, essential oils are a first therapy of choice for many doctors and other healers. Why? Because they make up a virtual medicine cabinet of therapies, with effects ranging from analgesic to antidepressant to antiseptic to anti-inflammatory to antiviral and antibiotic. I'd like to share with you some powerful, but lesser-known uses of essential oils.

Essential oils are "oils" derived from various plant materials through a variety of distillation processes. Not all essential oils are oily, however. Some are extracted through a distillation process that uses alcohol. These oils tend to be more watery and can evaporate quickly, like alcohol. Proper extraction is critical to an oil's performance, and (in order to avoid a lengthy discussion of extraction methods, let me simply say that) a top-quality supplier is your best insurance that an oil has been properly extracted.

Oils are then put in dark-colored bottles, which should be stored in a cool, dark, dry place, such as a drawer. These precautions help guard against degradation from light and other types of exposure. Also, look for bottles that have an insert at the top to facilitates measuring drops. This helps preserve oils from oxygen degradation. Plus makes oils easier to use. For example, when making an essential oil bath or massage oil, it's necessary to measure a precise number of drops into an ounce or so of a carrier oil, such as almond or sesame oil. Carrier oils have their own beneficial properties, help balance and stabilize essential oils, plus are a convenient vehicle for diluting an oil(s), which may be too powerful to use neat (pure). Essential oil suppliers are also good sources for top quality carrier oils.

Healing Infections With Essential Oils

You can use essential oils as a first-line therapy against bacterial infections, and completely avoid the risks of antibiotic use. There is no risk of developing dangerous, antibiotic-resistant bacteria (sometimes called superbugs), because bacteria do not develop resistance to essential oils. Antibiotics also weaken the immune system, while many essential oils (such as lavender) actually strengthen it.

I gained a new respect for the healing power of essential oils on a cold night last December when my four-year-old began complaining of ear pain. Within an hour, he progressed from whining to wailing. Being an anti-antibiotic mom confronting an ear infection for the first time, I calmly explained that he should feel better in a few days.

After a few more hours, though, I realized my mental health was quickly being deteriorated by the non-stop crying and retreated to my office. There I reviewed several reference books, and found a discussion of how to use essential oils to treat ear infections. I didn't have the recommended oils, so I grabbed what I did have on hand and knew was both safe and antibacterial: lavender and tea tree oils. I rubbed a couple drops of each oil, neat (pure) around the outside of each ear. Then I mixed a few drops of each oil with a little carrier oil and put four drops of the solution inside each ear. In addition, I gave him Tylenol to relieve the pain, a decongestant to relieve the pressure, and triple doses of echinacea extract and a liquid multivitamin to boost immune response.

Within an hour he fell asleep, and I didn't hear another peep from him until the morning. But instead of more whining and crying, he was running around laughing and playing tricks on his brother. Although this report is anecdotal, I'm convinced the explanation for the dramatic recovery is that the oils cured the infection — faster than I could have gotten my boy to a doctor and started antibiotics, I might add.

Academic research has also discovered the superiority of essential oils for treating childhood ear infections. A study reported in the *Chinese Journal of Integrated Traditional and Western Medicine* in 1990, compared treatments of middle ear infections with pus: 170 children received eardrops of borneol oil (20 percent) and walnut oil, while 108 children received eardrops of the antibiotic neomycin. The oil proved 98 percent effective compared to 84 percent effectiveness for neomycin. The research report declared, "Due to its simple composition, significant therapeutic effects and nontoxic reactions, the borneol-walnut oil has been proven a promising external remedy for the treatment of purulent otitis media (infection of the inner ear)."

Another study, from India, showed lemongrass oil was more effective than the antibiotics penicillin and streptomycin against staphylococcus aureus (the bacteria that causes staph infections).

Yet another study tested the antiseptic phenol, found in Lysol, Pinesol, Chloraseptic throat spray, and other antimicrobial products. Phenol's antibacterial and antifungal activity was randomly assigned a reference value of 1.0. All essential oils that were tested received higher antimicrobial activity scores than phenol: lavender at 1.6, lemon at 2.2, citral at 5.0, clove at 8.0, thyme at 13, and oregano at a whopping 21.

Here are some other common infections that can be treated with essential oils:

Bladder Infections. Dr. Schnaubelt, a world-renown essential oil expert and author of *Advanced Aromatherapy*, reports relieving acute bladder infections (accompanied by painful urination) within hours of using tea tree oil. His protocol is to take one to three drops of the tea tree oil every 30 minutes with lots of water or herbal tea. The pain should clear within one to three days. For recurrence or persistent symptoms, though, consult your doctor to discover and treat the primary cause.

Cystitis. Maggie Tisserand, author of *Aromatherapy for Women*, recommends drinking two drops of juniper oil in honey water, twice daily until symptoms are relieved. Also avoid refined sugar and alcohol, which can contribute to cystitis.

Skin infections with pus. Dr. Schnaubelt recommends applying a small amount of neat (pure) tea tree oil up to five times daily.

Fungal infections. Same as above. For more stubborn toenail fungus, combine two parts thyme (thymol type) oil, one part oregano oil, one part cinnamon oil, and seven parts carrier oil, such as almond oil. Apply twice daily for up to two weeks.

Other Therapeutic Uses of Essential Oils

The usefulness of essential oils is not limited to treating infections, either. Here are some other simple treatments that are easy to use at home:

Arthritis pain. In her book, *Aromatherapy, a Lifetime Guide to Healing with Essential Oils*, author Valerie Gennari Cooksley, recommends her Easy Arthritis Rub: made of 14 drops lavender oil, 10 drops rosemary oil and six drops juniper oil mixed in two tablespoons of a carrier oil. This mixture should be stored in an amber glass bottle and massaged as needed into painful areas. For overall pain, add the mixture to a warm bath and soak in it for 20 to 30 minutes.

Digestive problems. A drop or two of peppermint oil mixed in a small glass of water with a little honey clears most digestive problems in minutes. If problems persist, you'll need to seek treatment for the underlying cause.

Heart attack. A couple drops of lavender augustifolia oil in the fold of the elbow will help prevent heart damage if applied during a heart attack, according to northern California lavender farmer Danielle Penzer.

High blood pressure. Lavender oil is also reputed to help control hypertension. Can be mixed with a carrier oil or cream and applied as needed. Also, if you feel a surge in blood pressure, inhale the vapors from a drop or two of lavender oil on a tissue for a few minutes until you feel the pressure subside (from Maggie Tisserand).

Varicose veins. Dr. Schnaubelt recommends mixing one part laurel oil, 30 parts calophyllum oil, and 30 parts rose hip seed oil. Apply three times a day for 7 to 14 days. For a cold compress, wet a washcloth in water that has a few drops of laurel oil mixed into it. Apply to irritated areas.

Weight loss. Juniper oil is a natural diuretic that also helps flush toxins from the body. Take a drop or two of neat oil in some honey daily for a 7 to 10 days to increase water elimination. Or use juniper in a bath or massage oil (also from Maggie Tisserand).

This is just a tiny sampling of essential oil therapies. Still, it illustrates the impressive range of applications. Other conditions that essential oils can be used to treat include acne, asthma, candida, herpes, shingles, and a wide range of mental conditions including depression, stress, anxiety, compulsive disorders, and addiction. Just as with other advanced therapies, it's advisable to work with a trained professional when pursuing advanced essential oil therapies.

How to Apply Essential Oils

When we think of essential oils, most of us think about inhaling vapors. This is just one of many ways in which oils can be used: the application depends on the treatment. For psychological and emotional healing, respiratory conditions, and immune system stimulation, inhalation is most common. For surface conditions, topical application to the skin (including being applied neat (pure), mixed with a carrier oil, or as a compress) is standard. Within five minutes, oils are absorbed through the skin and into the bloodstream. For internal healing, oils are often swallowed in capsules or after mixing with honey or water. *Some oils are toxic if used excessively, so don't automatically assume that more is better.* In general, more toxic oils are not widely marketed to the public. Also follow these preparation guidelines:

bath: up to 8-15 drops total (can be mixed in a carrier oil such as almond)

clothing, dressings (such as Band-Aids), pillows, handkerchiefs, tissues: 1-2 drops

diffuser: according to instructions

gargle: 1-2 drops/oz. water

massage oil: 10-30 drops total per one oz. carrier oil

creams and lotions: 5-10 drops total per ounce of cream or lotion.

vaporizer: 2-10 total drops

wet compress: 3-5 total drops in 1/2 cup of water or sprinkled on wet compress

The Right Oil for the Job

If you're a beginner at using essential oils, you don't need a huge selection to get started. Instead, just two or three oils from several categories can offer tremendous flexibility. The key to getting the most mileage from your oils is selecting a small, but versatile, assortment. Here are some of my favorites:

Tea Tree. This popular oil is antibacterial and antifungal. Uses include household cleaning solutions, and preventing and treating infections. Can be applied neat for treatment of cold sores, herpes lesions, and athlete's foot. Considered one of the safest oils for extended use.

Eucalyptus. Look for eucalyptus radiata. It is antiviral and antibacterial and especially effective as an expectorant in treating bronchitis, cold, flu, and sinusitis. Diffuse it, or mix with a carrier oil to make a chest rub.

Lavender. One of the most popular essential oils, lavender is antibacterial and boosts immunity, making it ideal for regular diffusing during the cold season. Lavender is also relaxing and sedative, making it a good choice for relaxing evening baths and as a fragrance for pillows. For cooking and other minor burns, apply neat (pure) lavender, then cool with ice. In a massage oil or cream, lavender can promote circulation and reduce inflammation of varicose veins. It's especially safe and gentle.

Basil. When unwanted mental fatigue sets in, a whiff of basil oil, or a quick bath with a drop or two of basil (in a carrier oil), can be especially stimulating. Other energy-boosting oils include rosemary, rosewood, lemongrass, lemon, orange, bergamot, and grapefruit. Don't use during pregnancy, otherwise it's safe.

Clary sage. Emotionally uplifting, especially for depression. A classic remedy for easing menstrual and menopause-related problems, as well as other hormone-related transitions such as childbirth, mild postpartum depression, and hormone-related headaches. Reported to be an aphrodisiac as well. Use during pregnancy only to promote onset and progression of labor, otherwise it's safe.

Is It Pure?

Before running out and buying any essential oils off a shelf, you should know that there is concern in the field about essential oil purity, as well as the practice of standardization. In a recent letter to the editor of *Aromatherapy Quarterly*, British aromatherapist Ian Smith summarized the issue by writing, "All I ask for is essential oil that comes from a single, identified botanical source, produced from a single batch of plant material and which has not been blended with anything else — natural or synthetic; i.e. nothing added and nothing taken away."

In other words, the essence of essential oils — for maximum therapeutic value — is purity. In fact, if you've been disappointed with the results of aromatherapy treatments in the past, the quality of the product you were using may well have been the reason. In researching information for this article, I asked one expert about an inexpensively priced leading brand and she simply replied, "don't expect results." Everyone else I spoke with shared this view as well. So where can you find pharmaceutical-grade essential oils? Two highly recommended sources are Simplers at 800-652-7646, and Original Swiss Aromatics at 415-479-3979. Both can send you product brochures and take orders by mail.

In the future, you will see an increasing number of alternative doctors and others using essential oils. For a long time, the healing power of essential oils was one of Europe's best-kept healing secrets. But now the secret's getting out.

Minimizing Colds and Flu

You might think you're helpless in the face of new, potent strains of flu that sweep the country every few years. Or the myriad of colds that your friends, family, and strangers in the movies and supermarket pass along from one person to another. But you can do a lot to strengthen your immune system and create an army inside your body that can stave off these germs — or minimize their effects.

The microorganisms that cause disease are all around us — in the air and water, in our food, and on everything we touch. It's our immune system that attacks these foreign invaders (pathogens) and protects us from getting mild or serious illnesses.

One of the problems we're facing today is that many of today's germs are stronger than those that were around decades ago. This is because we're using more antibiotics. Antibiotics have encouraged "survival of the fittest" for pathogenic bacteria by killing off the weak strains and allowing the strong ones to flourish. They also cause some bacteria to mutate into antibiotic-resistant forms. So the truth is, antibiotics are breeding stronger varieties of germs.

Our bodies fight off disease-causing bacteria with probiotic — or friendly — bacteria. These friendly "bugs," acidophilus, bifido, bulgaricum, and others, keep the bad "bugs" in check. But while stronger varieties of pathogenic bacteria appear, probiotics have not been getting stronger. And some of the friendly bacteria sold in health food stores is low in potency compared with these super strains of pathogens.

How We Get These Germs

Beef cattle and chicken are often given high amounts of antibiotics to keep them healthy or to increase their weight. These antibiotics are creating stronger forms of pathogenic bacteria in the animals, and they are being passed along to us when we eat them. The more antibiotics we have inside us, the stronger our own pathogenic bacteria becomes.

Germs are passed along from person to person, so when you or your family come in contact with people who are sick — through day-care centers, supermarkets, work, movies, etc. — you run a higher risk of getting sick. That is, unless you have a strong immune system.

We are coming into contact with new tropical viruses as more people clear-cut trees in previously uninhabited regions of the world. These are viruses that we have no immunity against, because our bodies haven't needed to develop a defense against them. All it takes for a tropical virus to reach you is for one person working in a jungle to get sick and pass it along from one person to another until it reaches this continent. As HIV has shown us, this is not an impossibility.

We all have pathogenic bacteria inside us, yet we're not constantly sick. Our immune system can fight these germs if it's strong. But nutrient deficiencies created by eating foods low in particular vitamins and minerals have reduced the ability of our immune systems to keep us healthy. And the overuse of pesticides on non-organic foods has lowered our immune systems as well.

A diet high in sugar suppresses your immune system and feeds the pathogenic bacteria at the same time. In fact, according to naturopathic doctor Joseph Pizzorno, N.D., in his excellent book *Total Wellness* (Prima Publishing, 1996), just three ounces of sugar — including honey, alcohol, and fruit juice — reduces your white blood cells (your body's defense against disease) by 50 percent for up to five hours! Stress has the same immune-lowering effect, which means you may want to find effective techniques to reduce the impact of stressors on your body. You're not likely to find a stress-free environment.

Medications suppress the immune system, as well. Aspirin, ibuprofen, and antibiotics all reduce your body's ability to fight colds and flu. Some antibiotics are more detrimental than others, like tetracycline and erythromycin, while penicillin has a lesser negative impact on immunity.

Creating a Strong Immune System

Begin with good personal hygiene. Wash your hands frequently, especially during cold and flu season. Don't touch your eyes, nose, or mouth with your hands. Teach your children to wash their hands frequently, as well. Even a moderate change in hand-washing could reduce the incidence and the severity of illness.

Practice good kitchen hygiene. When you buy raw meats, don't repackage them. The bacteria on them can easily spread to other foods and multiply. Instead, double-bag them in the grocery store, so none of their juices contaminate other foods. Wash your hands after you handle raw meat at home. Disinfect your cutting board, knives, and sponges after each use. A container with diluted Chlorox or other disinfectant can be kept under the sink for sponges.

Eat a nutrient-dense diet. Vitamins A, C, E, selenium, and zinc are all needed for a healthy immune system. Fresh, organic fruits and vegetables, along with whole grains and beans, have good amounts of these nutrients. Make sure that 80 percent of the foods you eat are high in vitamins and minerals. Avoid highly refined foods like white flour, sugar, and processed foods with a lot of chemical preservatives.

Avoid fried foods. Any oil that has been reheated is rancid (spoiled) and requires large amounts of vitamin E to keep this rancidity from reducing your immune system. Foods that have been deep-fried commercially are loaded with rancid oil. It doesn't matter whether or not this oil is lard or vegetable oil. If it's been reheated, it can lower your immune system.

Supplements That Boost Your Immune System

Probiotics. Since pathogens are kept in check with probiotics (friendly bacteria), we begin our list with acidophilus (for your small intestines), bifido factor (for your large intestines), and bulgaricum l.b. (a transient bacteria that needs to be replenished periodically). If you know your immune system is low (such as from recent or repeated antibiotic use, or radiation or chemotherapy), or if you've had intestinal problems like gas, diarrhea, or constipation, you will want to add these good bugs to your diet.

Probiotics don't live well with one another, so avoid those brands that put a number of them together. Instead, begin with a bottle of acidophilus, then follow with a bottle of bifido factor. We have found Natren brands to be strong and effective. Their Healthy Trinity is an exception to the "don't mix 'em" rule. Each probiotic in this formula has been surrounded in an oil base that prevents the bacteria from competing with one another.

Feed the probiotics. When you eat cultured foods containing other live bacteria, you feed the probiotics in your intestines. Miso soup, sauerkraut, and both yogurt and kefir (without sugar) all contain food for your good bugs. Refined sugar feeds the bad bugs, so replace it for now with foods containing fructose.

Take a good quality supplement. This is not instead of eating a good diet. It's additional protection. Find a good quality multi-vitamin/mineral with lots of vitamin E, A, C, zinc, and selenium. If it contains additional antioxidants like methionine and cysteine, all the better. If you are not low in iron, get a formula without it. More iron than you need can lower your immunity. Twin Lab is one of a number of brands found in health food stores with a good protective formula. AMNI (800-356-4791) has one (Added Protection) without iron and with added antioxidants and will ship them to you.

Vitamin C and Zinc. In combination, especially, these two nutrients offer powerful prevention and treatment for colds and flu. For prevention, take 500 to 1,000 mg of vitamin C, once or twice a day. Plus 30 mg a day of any form of zinc. If you still catch a cold or the flu, don't think your prevention efforts were to no avail. Your illness will be milder and of shorter duration. In addition, bump up your intake of these nutrients to treatment levels: 1,000 mg of vitamin C per hour (or as much as you can tolerate without developing diarrhea), and continue 30 mg daily of zinc. If you have a sore throat, use zinc gluconate lozenges.

Stress reduction. Worry and other stress, including physical stress such as lack of sleep, reduces your immune system as much as a poor diet. Daily meditation — just 10 minutes in the morning or evening — can go far to change your attitude and the way you handle stress. The simplest form of meditation is to simply close your eyes and watch your breath go in and out. When you forget, go back to watching your breath. Or get a relaxation tape and listen to it each evening.

Exercise and nature. Regular exercise, like a half-hour walk, housework, or gardening will reduce your stress as well. Do stretching or yoga on a regular basis. Connect with nature. Look at the sky. Watch the birds in your yard or a park. Hug a tree.

Herbs for Immunity

Garlic. The safest herb to use consistently is garlic, which has been used for over 5,000 years. It has a number of sulfur-containing chemicals that increase the immune system. But you need to eat a lot of it. Dr. Pizzorno suggests half a bulb of garlic three times a day. That's a lot, even if you're Italian! Instead, you can supplement your daily garlic intake with odorless garlic. Kwai brand has a lot of studies to back up the effectiveness of their garlic capsules. Use 1,800 mg of any aged, odorless garlic.

Most herbs that boost immunity are most effective when they're taken when needed, not all the time. Some of the best herbal boosters we've seen are:

Echinacea. An antiviral, antibacterial, immune-stimulating herb that should be taken at the first sign of a cold or flu. Of all the brands we've tested, Zand Echinacea worked the fastest. It comes in liquid or capsules (liquid is stronger) and can be taken every hour or two for the first day, then three times daily until your symptoms have lessened.

Goldenseal root, or Hydrastis canadensis. This bitter-tasting herb boosts the immune system and fights pathogenic bacteria. It directly affects the mucous membranes and is particularly good for colds and flu. You can take 500 mg three times a day, or get a combination of Echinacea and Golden Seal.

Shiitake mushroom. In Chinese medicine, shiitake mushroom has been used both to reduce tumors and increase immunity against infections. You can find them fresh in some supermarkets (although they're expensive) or get them in capsule form and take 500 mg three times a day.

Licorice root, or Glycyrrhiza glabra. Some chemicals in this naturally sweet root help the body make interferon, a potent antiviral. You can make a strong tea infusion of licorice root and add it to herb teas to sip throughout the day. Or you can take 1,500 mg capsules three times a day until your symptoms lessen. Do not take licorice root if you have high blood pressure. It can cause a rise in blood pressure if it's used daily for more than a month. But all immune-boosting herbs work best when they are taken infrequently.

Creating Your Immune-Boosting Program

Begin with a good diet. Add the appropriate nutrients to give your immune system extra support, like probiotics and a good multi-vitamin/mineral formula. Do some daily exercise and stress-reduction, like meditation. Watch your hygiene and that of your family. And laugh a lot. As Norman Cousins found in *Anatomy of an Illness*, it actually increases your resistance to disease!

When You Have a Confusing Array of Health Problems — Simplify!

Many people wait until their numerous health problems pile one on top of another before being willing to take their health into their own hands. By then their doctors often have them taking daily collections of pills, for symptoms as well as side effects.

In response, many people feel overwhelmed and immobile, unable to move in any direction. This is certainly understandable. It's frightening to realize your health is deteriorating and you may never be well again. But we've all heard of stories of people with seemingly insurmountable health problems who have spontaneous healings, or who find answers that doctors couldn't find.

When your health problems are complex and the people you have placed your faith and trust in don't seem to be helping you, it's difficult to believe you can unravel the problems yourself and find a better solution. Still, people do it every day.

The key is in simplifying and moving slowly one step at a time. Often taking small steps can make a significant difference. We'd like you to consider some simple steps that have helped a number of very sick people turn their health around. This is also an excellent plan for protecting good health.

Instinctively, You Know Best

Remember this: no one knows your body better than you. No one feels your feelings or is as able to tap into your body's innate intelligence to find answers better than you. Even without a medical degree, even without a thorough understanding of biochemistry, anatomy, and physiology, you can often find many of the answers you seek. One of the most profound statements on healing I ever heard was made by a world-renowned teacher in a graduate course for doctors. He told his class that if practitioners listened to what their patients said, they would be led by them to the correct course of treatment. So relax and listen for any intuitive advice from within.

Breathe

Don't underestimate the importance of breathing. I don't mean the shallow respiration that allows you to stay alive, but the deep breathing that brings oxygen to your brain and energy to your entire body. You need to breathe every day.

Begin now by taking a deep breath. Then another. Breathe deeply 10 times. Take in each breath to the count of eight. Hold it for a few seconds, then release it slowly to the count of 10. This deep breathing not only brings oxygen to your brain, it also brings a state of calmness and relaxation. And this is necessary for you to tune-in to your next step.

Exercise

Exercise means moving your body. You may be able to do a lot; you may be able to only raise and lower your arms. Whatever you can do, start moving. If you can, go for a walk, preferably in nature. A park in the middle of the city will do. If you can't walk, go for a drive and find a place that's as natural as possible where you can sit: a lake, a bench by the ocean, or even your backyard.

Take deep breaths and pay attention to the sound of birds, the flight of bees and insects, the shape of a leaf, or the color of a flower. Look around you and see that all of nature knows instinctively how to take care of itself, what nutrients are needed to repair itself and survive. You can too, but not if you're in a panic. Feel the increased energy that comes from moving, and from spending time with nature.

Trust — Your Next Step

Next, trust that you will be led to an answer or, at least, the first part of an answer. You don't have to believe this, but trust that it's possible. Enter into your healing process with a bit of faith. It's all right to be skeptical and to recognize how much you don't know. By the way, you'd be amazed at the number of excellent doctors and other health care practitioners who don't "know" what course of treatment to use for a patient. Often, they just know the next step. A person's response to one step can lead them to the next, and the next. So can yours. I'd much rather be in the care of someone who admits they don't know everything than someone who insists they do!

Talk to Your Doctor

All medications have some side effects. These side effects may lead a doctor to prescribe additional drugs which may have different side effects. I know many people whose health improved greatly when they lowered the amount and number of medications they were taking. Some of their symptoms disappeared completely. Even though this may be the case with you, don't attempt to stop or reduce your medications on your own.

You may be taking a drug that is crucial to your health, or you could harm yourself by reducing the dosage improperly and create other problems. The subject of drug interactions is a complicated one, as is knowing how to come off certain medications. Some are safe to stop completely, while others need to be tapered off over a period of time.

While there may be more natural substances than the medications you're now on that you'd like to try, the best approach is to have your doctor monitor you as you make changes in your medications. Contact your doctor or doctors and let them know what you'd like to do. Ask which medications you can reduce or eliminate temporarily. Explain that you want to simplify your treatment plan and you have not been getting the results all of you hoped for and expected. Let them know you'd like to consult with them if you have any questions or side effects that need to be considered. Make it clear that you want to take more responsibility for your health. If your doctor insists you stay on your present regime, find another health care professional who is willing to help you take a different approach and who will monitor your condition.

Improve Your Digestion

Help your diet by improving your digestion. This single step is responsible for more health improvements than any other one I know. I've said it before: You are not what you eat. You are what you eat, digest, and absorb.

If you are upset when you eat, you won't digest your food completely. Why? Because your stomach doesn't produce enough hydrochloric acid to break down foods into usable particles. The nutrients in your meals don't get small enough to get into your cells and help your body repair itself. If your digestion is not good (you get gassy, bloated, or sleepy after you eat), you may want to consider taking digestive enzymes with your meal. Papaya enzymes are not very strong. Instead, look for pancreatic enzymes or plant-based enzymes in a health food store and take one or two with each meal. Do not take enzymes if you know or suspect you have an ulcer.

Choose easy to digest meals that are low in fat, low in animal protein, high in fresh vegetables, fruits, grains, and legumes. If beans give you gas, use Beano, it works. Also remember that the first stage of digestion for all starches and sweets is in your mouth. Chew all your foods very, very well. Instead of stuffing yourself, stop eating when you feel satisfied. This will allow your body to better digest and utilize the foods you've eaten. Even though you may be tempted to eat junk foods, the time to eat the best is when you're the least healthy.

Many people who have been ill for a long time or have taken numerous medications have low levels of helpful bacteria in their digestive tracts. These friendly bacteria (acidophilus, bulgaricum, and bifido, among others) boost the immune system and support both good digestion and intestinal health. If your bowel movements are not regular, formed, and medium-to-dark in color, begin taking some friendly bacteria on a daily basis. There are many formulas in health food stores. The strongest, and the one we feel would work fastest for someone who has a myriad of problems is Healthy Trinity by Natren, Inc. (800-992-3323). Although it appears to be more expensive than other brands, we have found that one capsule a day is infinitely stronger than much larger doses of other brands taken two or three times daily. Plan on taking it for at least three months.

Watch Your Blood Sugar

When you skip a meal or eat a lot of sweets, you run the risk of having fluctuating blood-sugar levels. In plain language, this means you could feel strong and energetic for a while, then feel like the bottom has dropped out and you're suddenly exhausted.

If your energy fluctuates, especially if it's lower in the afternoon or when you haven't eaten for four to six hours, eat more frequently. Make sure you're getting a little protein for breakfast and lunch. Soy products like frozen Boca Burgers (veggie burgers with a meaty taste) or lentil soup are two kinds of vegetable proteins that will help keep your energy stable over a long period of time. If you don't have protein with a starchy meal, have a little fat with your starch. Putting a teaspoon of olive oil on your pasta will help slow down its conversion to sugar and give you longer-lasting energy than pasta with no oil.

Avoid alcohol and refined sugar. Instead, look for fruit-juice-sweetened desserts and treats like cookies or muffins, and try putting fruit-only jams on whole grain crackers for a mid-afternoon snack.

Be Patient

It is said that it takes twice as long to get well as it did to create any illness, so be patient with yourself. Chart any improvements so you don't lose sight of your progress. Focus on how much better you're getting, not on how bad you feel. Taking charge of a complicated medical condition may feel overwhelming if you look at the whole picture at once. But if you break it down into smaller steps it becomes more manageable. If you simplify your treatment and improve to any degree, your health provider may be able to help see other steps you can take. Don't be discouraged. Be in charge!

Consider Supplements

Once you've improved your diet, it might be smart to consider taking a good multivitamin/mineral. We like Added Protection III for women who are not menstruating, and Added Protection III with copper and iron for women who are (800-356-4791). Source Natural, found in many health food stores, and TwinLab, are two other companies that make good high-potency formulas that are well-absorbed. AMNI products have the advantage of being able to be returned if for any reason they don't agree with you.

Ginkgo biloba is an herb that has been found to increase the circulation and thus contribute to a better memory and clear thinking. Studies have shown that the amount necessary to do the job is 40 mg taken three times a day. After taking a multi, this may be an herb to consider.

Don't think of replacing the number of medications you've been on with a similar number of natural products. Try one or two supplements for a few months. You may find that's all you need.

Most of all, be persistent and find something each day to bring joy to your life. It may be watching a flower open or talking to a youngster in your family. It can be anything at all, so long as it's enjoyable. Life is not to be tolerated, it's to be lived.

When You Need to Call a Doctor

After trying many of the methods mentioned in this book, you may find that you need the assistance of a medically trained professional. If this is your situation, here is some information on how to find a doctor that can help with your particular ailment:

Alternative MD: As consumers become increasingly interested in alternative healing, so are doctors. And many allopathic doctors now offer various alternative treatments. In addition to alternative, some of these MD also call their practices holistic, complementary, and integrative. The common link is that these are conventionally trained MDs who have expanded their practices beyond conventional medicine to incorporate any number of a wide array of alternative healing methods. Therefore, when shopping for an alternative doctor, it's important to find out which alternative treatments are offered. Some have a holistic mind/body treatment approach. Some are highly specialized, such as a chelation specialist. Some combine allopathic with other healing approaches, perhaps nutrition. Others have abandoned allopathic medicine entirely.

If this sounds a bit confusing, bear with me. A little bit of investigative know-how can usually help you find the type of doctor you're looking for. Start by calling the American Holistic Health Association at 714-779-6152. (This organization also serves as a general clearinghouse to help you find pretty much any type of alternative practitioner, plus evaluate the effectiveness of various alternative treatments for specific health problems.) Or the American College for Advancement in Medicine at 949-583-7666. You might even call both. Ask for the names and numbers of alternative MDs in your area. Then call their offices and query the receptionist about the doctor's training, experience in treating conditions like yours, and types of treatments used. Always do this when considering any health care service provider. Another good general rule of thumb when considering various alternative treatment options, is to try the ones that you think might be best-suited to you first.

Chiropractor: Chiropractic medicine is based on the idea that joint dysfunction and misalignment (especially of the spine) may impair function of the neuromusculoskeletal system, leading to or causing disease. The objective of treatment is to restore proper alignment and balance to the body for improved functioning. Many people think of chiropractors as mainly back doctors, and they do excel at treating lower back pain. Studies have even found chiropractic treatment to be more effective (and less expensive) than allopathic treatment for acute and chronic lower back pain. Chiropractic medicine is also effective in boosting immune system strength (even for children with recurring ear infections), alleviating or eliminating migraines and other headaches, and much more.

Anyone interested in chiropractic care should know there are two main schools of doctors: straights and mixers. The mixers go beyond traditional chiropractic medicine to offer other treatments which may include hydrotherapy, electrotherapy, ultrasound, vitamin and mineral supplements, nutrition and diet, physical therapy, sacro-occipital technique, craniopathy, activator technique, and applied kinesiology.

To find a chiropractor in your area, call the International Chiropractor's Association (most members are straights) at 703-528-5000. Or call the American Chiropractic Association (most members are mixers) at 703-276-8800.

Homeopath: These doctors practice a system of medicine that's nearly 300 years old and is based on the principle that "like cures like". Here's an example. A minute dose of the poison belladonna may be prescribed for symptoms similar to those of belladonna poisoning. How such homeopathic remedies actually work has yet to be scientifically understood, but it's believed that they stimulate a healing response in the body. Even if you've tried over-the-counter homeopathic remedies without success, don't think they won't work for you. As my homeopath explained to me on my first skeptical visit, "there are thousands of homeopathic remedies and when one is correctly prescribed for you specifically, it can work like gangbusters." He was right and I was very pleasantly surprised. To find a trained doctor in your area that practices homeopathy, call the National Center for Homeopathy at 703-548-7790.

Naturopath: These doctors use natural therapies to stimulate the body's own innate power to heal itself. This system aims to treat the whole person as well as the cause, and incorporates many ancient healing arts from a variety of cultures. While practices vary from doctor to doctor, a typical naturopath might combine homeopathy, nutrition, herbs, hydrotherapy and Chinese medicine, and even soft tissue and skeletal manipulation. Naturopaths are also trained in minor surgery, prenatal care, and natural childbirth. To find a naturopath in your area, call the American Association of Naturopathic Physicians at 206-298-0125.

Nutritionist: WHL readers have the advantage receiving advice each month from their very own nutritionist, Dr. Fuchs. If you've been following her counsel, you're already enjoying the general health benefits of outstanding nutrition. You've probably also gotten some helpful tips for more specific problems. Still, few of us think of nutrition first when we have a health problem. Maybe we should. Good nutrition can prevent most birth defects. Nutrition has recently been discovered to be highly effective in treating and even reversing Down's Syndrome. In fact, the applications for therapeutic nutrition are so extensive that the Center For Science in the Public Interest estimates that poor nutrition is the cause of most deaths. I myself continue to be amazed by Dr. Fuchs' success stories. She has even helped diabetics get off of insulin using nutritional therapy alone. And she has patients all over the country with whom she consults. That means you have no further to look for a nutritionist than this article. You can call Dr. Fuchs' office directly at 707-824-1123.

If you prefer to work with a local nutritionist, they can be hard to find but well worth the effort. In looking for one, Dr. Fuchs advises avoiding anyone who says you have to buy supplements from him or her. Also, most well-trained nutritionists do not consider hair analysis or live-cell analysis to be reliable tests to show nutrient deficiencies, and don't use the same dietary program for everyone. Instead, a top notch nutritionist will custom tailor a nutritional program for you based on your lifestyle and food preferences and can be expected to explain everything to your satisfaction.

To locate a good nutritionist, ask for referrals from friends, from your medical doctor, or another health-care professional whose opinions you value. The nutritionist you end up working with may be a medical doctor with a strong emphasis on nutrition, a credentialed nutritional counselor

(MS, or PhD), or a registered dietitian (RD). You can also call the Price-Pottenger Nutrition Foundation at 800-FOODS-4-U to find a nutritionist in your area.

Osteopath: With an osteopath, you get a super-MD, of sorts. These physicians are licensed to perform all aspects of medicine including surgery, emergency medicine, and prescribing drugs. Some osteopaths offer prenatal care and natural childbirth. Osteopaths also use a variety of manual treatments including cranial manipulation, thrust technique, muscle energy, counter-strain, and myo-facial release. These are all aimed at making changes in the musculoskeletal system, and thus stimulate the body's own healing ability. This use of manipulative techniques has led the general public to frequently confuse osteopaths with chiropractors. Although this is a similarity, osteopaths receive much more extensive training that goes well beyond chiropractic training. Osteopathy was first developed by Dr. Still, a medical surgeon during the Civil War, who was dissatisfied with the effectiveness of prevailing medical practices of the day. Not all osteopaths today practice manipulative therapies, so if you are interested in these, confirm whether the osteopath you are considering seeing uses them. To find an osteopath in your area, call the American Osteopathic Association at 312-202-8000.

Doctor of Oriental Medicine: These doctors practice a tradition of medicine that dates back to ancient China, over four thousand years ago. It is also known as traditional Chinese medicine. Health is restored by rebalancing yin and yang, and unblocking trapped chi (vital energy). Therapies include acupuncture, acupressure, cupping, moxibustion, herbs, food, massage, and exercise. Although this might sound like fancy hocus-pocus to many, the World Health Organization recommends Chinese medicine for over 100 illnesses including migraines, sinusitis, asthma, brain damage, sciatica, and disorders of the eyes, ears and throat. Those who are intimidated by the thought of being stuck with lots of acupuncture needles, should simply put their preconceptions aside. There is minimal, if any, discomfort and the results can be very impressive. So impressive that one of my favorite places is the acupuncture table of Dr. Nic Mainferme in Pasadena, CA. To find a doctor of oriental medicine in your area, call the American Association of Oriental Medicine at 610-266-1433.

Take Matters Into Your Hands*

After you've gone to the doctor, if you're waiting by the phone to hear the results of your recent medical test, don't wait too long before taking matters into your own hands. A recent study shows that 36 percent of physicians do not always notify their patients of abnormal test results. And only 28 percent notify patients about normal test results, while the other 72 percent leave patients to assume "no news is good news."

The study of 207 physicians in Michigan, reported in the February 12, 1996 issue of *Archives of Internal Medicine*, showed that physicians are often lax in contacting patients, especially when the individual is due back for a follow-up visit. It also found that physicians often lack methods to ensure that they receive the results of tests ordered for their patients and that many don't document telling patients their results.

The reasons doctors gave for not getting in touch with their patients included unimportant results, an upcoming office visit, inability to contact the patient easily, lack of time, and forgetfulness. In addition, the sheer number of people that doctors and testing laboratories deal with can lead to delays and mix-ups when reporting test results.

Not only does poor follow-up from your doctor mean more worry for you, it can also endanger your health and cost time and money. To make sure you don't get lost in the shuffle:

● Let your doctor know you're waiting to hear your results, even if you have a follow-up appointment. Some doctors plan to tell patients their results at the next meeting.

● Know when to expect your results. Some tests may take longer than others to interpret, so find out when the results are due. If you don't hear from your doctor, call.

● Make yourself available. If you're hard to reach, give your doctor your home, work, and cellular phone numbers, or make arrangements to call the office yourself at a time when the doctor is available.

● Request that you be notified of test results even if they are normal. Don't assume that "no news is good news" — your doctor's silence may mean your results have been misplaced or forgotten.

● Find out what's being done where. Many tests ordered by physicians are performed at outside clinics or laboratories, and even tests

---

* Ref: *People's Medical Society*

performed in the office are often sent out for interpretation. Ask your doctor about how she keeps track of test results coming in and what her procedure is for notifying patients. This information can also help if tests are misplaced and need to be tracked down.

● Keep your own medical records. Documentation of tests and results can help you keep track of your health and medical history and can alert you when test results aren't received. A good record can also tell you when you're due for routine tests, such as Pap tests.

● Don't hesitate to double-check. Mixed-up test results are more common than you think, especially with all of the traffic to and from high-volume laboratories that interpret results. If you suspect a mistake or simply want to be sure, request a second opinion or have the test done again.

Resolve to Take Greater Control of Your Health!

Are you taking medications to correct or suppress the symptoms of a health problem? They may be the best solution — or there may be a more natural alternative that works just as well. Perhaps it's time to talk with your doctor about what you're putting into your body and why. Find out what each of your medications does and what nutritional or lifestyle changes you could make that would effect a similar reaction. Resolve this year to take more control of your health.

The problem with all medications is that they have side effects. Just go into a book store and pick up a copy of the *Physician's Desk Reference*. Then look up the prescription and over-the-counter drugs you're taking. What you read there may surprise and horrify you. While the odds may be in your favor, many thousands of people every year have significant side effects from drug therapy.

Some side effects are only irritating: fatigue, weight gain, or headaches. Still, a change in your diet, an herbal formula, or specific nutritional supplements might give you similar results without any side effects now or in the future.

Here's another reason to opt for natural alternatives when possible: You could experience an unpublished side effect! One reader recently wrote that a commonly prescribed sleeping medication has had the side effect of putting her in a state of constant sexual arousal — and stopping the medication and other efforts have failed to help her return to normal. Many people might consider such a side effect desirable. But the experience has been very disruptive and difficult for her. Even wearing pants can be extremely painful. And she has been unable to find other women who have gone through the same experience and might know of a solution for her. This particular side effect is unpublished. To date, the side effect of constant sexual arousal with this drug has only been acknowledged by the manufacturer and reported in men.

We're not suggesting you stop taking your medications. That's not smart. Some may be your best option, while others may need to be reduced slowly before they're stopped. Still, you can learn more about your condition and more natural options. Then make a well-informed decision about what solution is truly best for you.

Most doctors are trained in the use of medications, so that's usually what they suggest. Had they been trained in nutrition or herbs, they might suggest alternatives to drug therapy.

Start by asking your doctor to explain your condition. Or, if it's a common complaint like menstrual cramps, pregnancy-associated nausea, menopausal symptoms, anxiety, or depression, look them up in reference books that offer nutritional and herbal solutions. Two of the most valuable books we've seen on natural healing and recommend for your personal home reference library were written by doctors. They are *Healing with Foods* by Melvyn Werbach, MD (Harper Collins, 1994) and *The Healing Power of Herbs* by Michael T. Murray, ND (Prima Publishing, 1995). These authors, who have written nutritional and herbal textbooks for doctors as well as lay persons, base their information on good, sound scientific studies, not just personal experience or hearsay.

Let me walk you through this concept of taking more control of your health. Let's say you are anxious and your anxiety has bothered you enough for you to consult with a doctor. Your doctor gave you a prescription that you take and now you're not as anxious — so long as you continue taking your medication.

First, look to the cause of your anxiety. All of us are anxious at times, sometimes appropriately. But if you're frequently anxious and it's interfering with your life, you obviously have to do something. You may understand why you're anxious and feel stuck, even if you're in therapy. But does this mean that medications are the next step? Not necessarily. Most conditions have both emotional and physiological components. When you remove the physiological imbalances it's much easier to deal with your emotions. With this in mind, let's look at what Dr. Werbach and Dr. Murray say about more natural answers to anxiety.

Dr. Werbach explains the association between anxiety and refined sugar, caffeine, and food allergies. If you eat a lot of candy, cookies, or ice cream it would be smart to eliminate sugar entirely from your diet for two weeks. This is all many people need to do to reduce their anxiety or depression. Since natural sugars don't cause the same effect, you can substitute fruit-juice sweetened desserts and not feel deprived. If sugar is not the answer, try eliminating caffeine or look for a source of food sensitivity. Dr. Werbach tells you just how to find out which foods you react to that may be contributing to anxiety.

He continues by explaining the association between anxiety and a number of B vitamins, calcium, and magnesium, and a fatty-acid deficiency. And he tells how much of each nutrient to take as well as when you need medical supervision. If you read his clear analysis and follow his program step-by-step, you will find out how much of your anxiety is caused by nutritional excesses or deficiencies.

Dr. Murray adds to this information by naming two herbs that reduce anxiety: kava and valerian. He suggests beginning with kava for one month and, if you're still feeling anxious, trying valerian. Valerian root is one of a number of relaxing herbs used in Celestial Seasoning's Sleepytime Tea. Other herb tea companies also make relaxing teas with valerian that you can safely drink during the day or before going to sleep.

Here are a few suggestions for drug-free approaches to other common complaints:

For hot flashes associated with menopause: reduce the amount of spicy foods, fats, and sugars in your diet. They create heat. Add more foods that cool you from the inside out like fruits and vegetables. Add lemon to your water and sip it frequently throughout the day. Remember, water puts out fire. If your problem persists, consider a natural substance found in citrus fruits, a flavonoid called hesperidin. I have given many of my menopausal patients two capsules of hesperidin in the morning and evening and find it eliminates their hot flashes within a week or two. Dr. Murray also lists a number of herbs that have been used success- fully to eliminate hot flashes including dong quai, licorice root, chaste berry, and black cohosh.

For nausea associated with pregnancy, you want to avoid medications as much as possible since they can affect the fetus as well as you. Begin by trying a light abdominal massage — or increase your intake of vitamin B_6. If these don't work, have some ginger, an herb used for motion sickness and morning sickness. The ginger can be taken in capsules or grated into a cup and made into ginger tea. Traditional Medicinals herb tea company has a delicious tea called Ginger Aid found in most health food stores and some super- markets. (Note: Some nutritional supplements and herbs are not recommended during pregnancy, so as always, check with your health care provider about the safety of any treatment you are considering.)

For menstrual cramps, Dr. Werbach suggests a program of 100 IU of vitamin E three times a day for two weeks beginning 10 days before your menses. He also points out a frequent need to increase your magnesium intake, a mineral that causes muscles to relax. Calcium has the opposite effect and causes muscle contractions, so you may want to reduce your calcium intake, including all dairy products, and eat more whole grains and beans, which are higher in magnesium. Check your vitamins to make sure you're taking more magnesium than calcium if you have menstrual cramps. Bilberry is an herb you may want to try that contains a flavonoid that relaxes smooth muscles. Common over-the-counter drugs like ibuprofen cause the cycle of menstrual cramps to· continue by destroying anti-cramping substances called prostaglandins along with the prostaglandins that cause cramping. Although they may take away your pain this month, they will guarantee you have them again next month — a good solution only for the manufacturer, which is interested in selling as much product as possible.

For most common and even serious health conditions, there are safe and simple nutritional and herbal solutions. Instead of listening only to one authority who may represent the medical establishment and is trained to dispense medications, consult also with authorities who have studied other approaches and choose the path with which you feel most comfortable and works best for you. It may be traditional medicine, traditional Chinese medicine, naturopathy, nutrition, or a combination of any of these. This is your body and you should decide. Resolve to do so today!

Bibliography

Abraham, Guy E., MD. "Nutrition and the premenstrual tension syndrome," *Journal of Applied Nutrition*, September 1984.

Abraham, Guy E., MD and Harinder Grewal, MD. "A total dietary program emphasizing magnesium instead of calcium: effect on the mineral density of calcaneous bone in postmenopausal women on hormonal therapy," *Journ of Repro Med*, Vol. 35, No. 5, May 1990.

Ackerson, Amber, ND & Corey Resnick, ND. "The effects of l-glutamine, n-acetyl-d-glucosamine, gamma-linolenic acid, and gamma-oryzanol on intestinal permeability," Tyler Encapsulations, *Townsend Letter for Doctors*, January 1993.

Aldercreutz, Herman, et al. "Dietary phytoestrogens and the menopause in Japan," *Lancet*, May 16, 1992, 339:1233.

Am J Clin Nutr, 27(1):59-79, 1974; 60, 1994;129-135.

Am Journ of Nat Med, July/August 1997.

"Angioplasty Risks Found for Women," *Boston Globe*, 9 March 1993, p 1.

Angus, Rosalind, et al. "Dietary intake and bone mineral density," *Bone Min*, 88.

Arjmandi, BH, et al. "Dietary soybean protein prevents bone loss in an ovariectomized rat model of osteoporosis," *J Nutr* 126, 161-167 (1996).

Ault, Alicia. "FDA warns on calcium-channel blocker," *Lancet*, January 3, 1998.

Beattie, J.H., and H.S. Peace. "The influence of a low-boron diet and boron supplementation on bone major mineral and sex steroid metabolism in postmenopausal women," *Brit Journ Nutr*, 871-84 (1993).

Bland, Jeffrey, PhD. *Nutraerobics: The Complete Individualized Nutrition and Fitness Program for Life After 30*, Harper & Row Publishing, 1983.

Brandi, Maria Luisa, MD, PhD. "New Treatment Strategies: Ipriflavone, Strontium, Vitamin D Metabolities and Analogs," *The Amer Journ of Medicine*, Nov 30, 1993; 95 (Suppl. 5A):5A-74S.

Braverman, Eric R., MD, Carl C. Pfeiffer, MD, PhD. *The Healing Nutrients Within*, Keats Publishing, 1987.

Brown, Susan E. "Osteoporosis: Sorting fact from fallacy," *Network News*, Nat'l Women's Health Network, July/August 1988.

Bruner, Ann B., et al. "Randomised study of cognitive effects of iron supplementation in non-anaemic iron-deficient adolescent girls," *Lancet*, vol 348, October 12, 1996.

Caldu, P., et al. "White Wine Reduces the Susceptibility of Low-Density Lipoprotein to Oxidation," *Am J Clin Nutr* 62, 403, 1996.

Cass, Hyla, MD. *St. John's Wort: Nature's Blues Buster*, Avery Publishing, $9.95, 1998.

Chenoy R., Hussain S., et al. "Effect of oral gamolenic acid from evening primrose oil on menopausal flushing," *BMI* 308, 1994.

Classen, D.C., et al. "Adverse Drug Events in Hospitalized Patients," *JAMA*, 277 (1997):301-6.

Collin, Jonathan, MD. "Treating candidiasis without nystatin, ketoconazole, or diflucan," *Townsend Letter for Doctors*, #161, December 1996.

Collins, Peter, et al. "Cardiovascular Protection by Oestrogen — A Calcium Antagonist Effect?" *Lancet*, May 15, 1993.

Cowley, Geoffrey. "The Heart Attackers," *Newsweek*, August 11, 1997.

Cox, Cat. "Chocolate Unwrapped: The Politics of Pleasure," The Women's Environmental Network, London, 1993.

Criqui, M.H., and B.L. Ringel. "Dies Diet or Alcohol Explain the French Paradox?" *Lancet*, 1719-1723, 1994.

Crouse, John R., III. "Gender, Lipoproteins, Diet, and Cardiovascular Risk," *Lancet*, February 11, 1989.

D'Adamo, Dr. Peter J. and Catherine Whitney. *Eat Right 4 Your Type*, G.P. Putnam's Sons, 1996.

Deadly Medicine, by Thomas J. Moore, Simon & Schuster, 1995.

Dept of Agriculture, Agricultural Marketing Service, "Pesticide Data Program: Annual Summary Calendar Year 1993," June 1995.

"Dietary calcium and the prevention of postmenopausal osteoporosis," review from the Nat'l Nutr Institute, Canada, *Nutrition Today*, May/June 1988.

Diethrich, Edward B., MD, and Carol Cohan. *Women and Heart Disease*, Times Books, 1992.

Dreher, Henry. *The Immune Power Personality*, Penguin Books, 1995.

"Drinking Green Tea Every Day May Keep Cancer at Bay," *Healthy Cell News*, Fall/Winter 1997.

Falck, Jr, Frank, et al. "Pesticides and polychlorinated biphenyl residues in human breast lipids and their relation to breast cancer," Archives of Environ. Health, March/April 1992 (vol 47, no. 2).

Fitzpatrick, Annette. "Calcium-channel blockers may increase breast-cancer risk," *Cancer*, 1997;80.

"Folic acid facts," Wheat Foods Council, 5500 S Quebec, Suite 111, Englewood, CO 80111.

Fuhrman, B., et al. "Consumption of Red Wine With Meals Reduces the Susceptibility of Human Plasma and Low-Density Lipoprotein to Lipid Preoxidation," *Am J Clin Nutr* 61(3), 549-554, 1995.

Gaby, Alan R., MD. *The Townsend Letter*, Aug/Sept 1995.

Ginsberg, Jean. "Environmental oestrogens," *Lancet*, January 29, 1994.

Gordan and Genant. "The aging skeleton," *Chrons Geriatr Med*, 1985.

Haris, Susan S. and Bess Dawson-Hughes. "Caffeine and bone loss in healthy postmenopausl women," *Amer Journ Clin Nutr*, 1994; 60:573-8.

Hegerfeld, Constance. "Osteoporosis: The pain facts," *Women's Health Connections*, Aug/Sept 1993.

Hernandez, Katie. "The Leaky Gut Syndrome," unpublished paper.

Hobbs, Larry S. *The New Diet Pills*, Pragmatic Press, Irvine, CA, 1995.

Hopper, John Llewelyn, PhD, and Ego Seeman, MD. "The bone density of female twins discordant for tobacco use," *New England J Med*, 2/10/94.

Horton, Richard. "Trials of Women," *Lancet*, March 26, 1994.

Horton, Richard. "Attacking Heart Disease Among U.S. Women," *Lancet*, August 27, 1994.

"House Approves Bill to Speed Federal Review of Medicines," *New York Times*, October 8, 1997.

HSR's Annual Guide to Herbs: St. John's Wort, Health Supplement Retailer, December 1977.

Imai, K. and K. Nakachi. "Cross Sectional Study of Effects of Drinking Green Tea on Cardiovascular and Liver Diseases," *British Medical Journal* 1995;310:693-696.

Immaculate Deception II, Suzanne Arms, Celestial Arts, 1994.

Ji H.T., et al. "Green tea consumption and the risk of pancreatic and colorectal cancer," *Int J Can*, 7;253-8, 1997.

Joo, S.J. and N.M. Betts. "Copper intakes and consumption patterns of chocolate foods as sources of copper for individuals in the 1987-88 nationwide food consumption survey," *Nutr Res*, 16(1), 41-49(1995). (*Intl Clin Nutr*, July 1996, 164-165).

Kamen, Betty, PhD. *Hormone Replacement Therapy Yes or No?* Nutrition Encounter Inc. 1993.

Katzin, Carolyn, MS, CNS. *Good Eating Guide & Cookbook*, Herbalife, 1996.

Keshgegian, A.A. and A. Cnaan. "Estrogen receptor-negative, progesterone receptor-positive breast carcinoma," *Arch Pathol Lab Med* 120:970-3, 1966.

Kilbourn, J.P., PhD. "Not all colloidal silver products are created equal!" *Townsend Letter for Doctors & Patients*, October 1996.

Klotter, Jule. "The Individualized Diet Solution," *Townsend Letter for Doctors & Patients*, June 1997.

Knekt P., et al. "Antioxidant Vitamin Intake and Coronary Mortality in a Longitudinal Population Study," *Am J Epidemiol* 139, 1180-9, 1994.

Kritz H., et al. "Passive Smoking and Cardiovascular Risk," *Arch Intern Med* 155:1942-8, 1995.

Lahorz, S. Colet, RN. *Conquering Yeast Infections: the Non-Drug solution*, Pentland Press, Inc., 1996.

Larkin, Marilynn. "Risk of age-related vision loss wanes with wine," *Lancet*, January 10, 1998.

LeShan, Lawrence and R.E. Worthington. "Personality as a factor in the pathogenesis of cancer: A review of the literature," *Brit J Med Psychol*, 29, 1956.

Lock, Margaret. "Contested meanings of the menopause," *Lancet*, 5/25/91.

Lukaczer, Dan, ND. "Antioxidants Offer Balance and Protection," *NFM's Nutrition Science News*, August 1996.

Martin, Jeanne Marie, Zoltan P. Rona, MD. *Complete Candida Yeast Guidebook*, Prima Publishing, 1996.

Matkovic, Velimer, et al. "Urinary calcium, sodium and bone mass of young females," *Amer Journ Clin Nutr*, 1995; 62:417-425.

Matthews, Karan A., PhD, et al. "Menopause and risk factors for coronary heart disease," *New Engl J Med*, Vol. 321, No. 10, Sept 7, 1989.

McCarthy, Michael. "Conflict of interest highlighted in debate on calcium-channel blockers," *Lancet*, January 17, 1998.

McCully, Kilmer S., MD. *The Homocysteine Revolution*, Keats Publishing, 1997.

McNulty, H. "Folate requirements for health in women," *Proc Nutr Soc* 56, 1977. *Int Clin Nutr Rev*, October 1997, pg 223.

Melina, Vesanto, RD, et al. *Becoming Vegetarian*, Book Publishing Company, 1995.

MenoTimes newsletter, Spring 1996

Miller, Alan L., ND, and Gregory S. Kelly, ND. "Methionine and homocysteine metabolism and the nutritional prevention of certain birth defects and complications of pregnancy," *Alt Med Review*, Vol 1, No 4, 1996.

Miller, Alan L., ND. "Cardiovascular disease — toward a unified approach," *Alternative Medicine Review*, September 1996.

Miller, Alan, L., ND, and Gregory S. Kelly, ND. "Homocysteine metabolism: nutritional modulation and impact on health and disease," *Alternative Medicine Review*, July 1997.

Moore, Thomas J. *Prescription for Disaster*, Simon & Schuster, 1998.

Mother-Friendly Childbirth Initiative, Coalition for Improving Maternity Services, 1996.

Murch, Susan J., et al. "Melatonin in feverfew and other medicinal plants," *Lancet*, November 29, 1997.

Murray, Michael T., ND. "Menopause: Is Estrogen Necessary?," *Amer Journal of Natural Medicine*, Vol. 2, No. 9, November 1995.

Murray, Michael T., ND. "Common Questions about St. John's wort extract," *Amer. Journ of Natural Med*, September 1997.

Murray, Michael T., ND. "St. John's wort extract in depression: Over three million prescriptions per year in Germany," *Amer Journ of Natural Med*, December 1996.

Ness, Roberta B., MD, MPH, et al. "Number of Pregnancies and the Subsequent Risk of Cardiovascular Disease," *NEJM*, May 27, 1993.

Nielsen, Forrest H. et al. "effect of dietary boron on mineral, estrogen, and testosterone metabolism in postmenopausal women," *FASEB Journ*, 1987.

Padus, Emrika. *The Complete Guide to Your Emotions & Your Health*, Rodale Press, 1986.

Pahor, Marco, et al. "Calcium-channel blockade and incidence of cancer in aged populations," *Lancet*, August 24, 1996. "Calcium-channel blockers: managing uncertainty," editorial *Lancet*, August 24, 1996.

Palmer, Julie R., et al. "Coffee Consumption and Myocardial Infarction in Women," *American Journal of Epidemiology*, 1995;141(8)724-31.

Pelletier, Kenneth R. *Mind as Healer, Mind as Slayer*, Delacorte Press, 1977.

Pini, Pia. "New candidaemia patterns emerge in the U.S.A.," *Lancet*, vol 348, August 10, 1996, p 395.

Pizzorno, Joseph, ND. *Total Wellness*, Prima Publishing, 1996.

Press Release, Sept. 10, 1996, The American Society for Bone and Mineral Research.

Quincy, Cheri, DO. "Issues regarding menopause ... the politics of estrogen?" privately published (707) 539-3511.

Revised 1990 Estimates of Maternal Mortality, A New Approach by WHO and UNICEF, April 1996.

Ricketts, C.D., et al. "Effect ot Dietary Caffeine Intake on Serum Lipid Levels in Healthy Adults," *Nutrition Research* 13, 639-647 (1993).

Rogers, Sherry A., MD. *Wellness Against All Odds*, Prestige Publishing, Syracuse, NY, 1994.

Rosenbaum, Michael, MD, and Murray Susser, MD. *Solving the Puzzle of Chronic Fatigue Syndrome*, 1992, Life Sciences Press, P.O. Box 1174, Tacoma, WA 98401.

Ross, Ronald K., et al. "Stroke Prevention and Oestrogen Replacement Therapy," *Lancet*, March 4, 1989.

Rowe, Paul M. "Housework Recommended for Cardio-vascular Health," *Lancet*, vol 347, January 13, 1996.

Sack, Michael N., et al. "Estrogen and Inhibition of Oxidation of Low-Density Lipoproteins in Postmenopausal Women," *Lancet*, January 29, 1994.

Sahelian, Ray, MD. "Author urges caution in DHEA sales," *Nat Foods Merchandiser*, January 1998.

Samuels, Adrienne, PhD. Correspondence, Truth in Labeling Campaign, PO Box 2532, Darien, IL 60561, 1997.

Sanchez-Guerrero J, et al. "Postmenopausal estrogen therapy and the risk for developing systemic lupus erythermatosus," *Ann Intern Med* 1995:122:430-433.

Santosh-Kumar C.R., et al. "Unpredictable intra-individual variations in serum homocysteine levels on folic acid supplementation," *Eur J Clin Nutr 51*, 188-192 (1977). From *Int Clin Nutr Rev*, October 1997, p 213.

Schauss, Alexander G., PhD. "Colloidal minerals: clinical implications of clay suspension products sold as dietary supplements," *Amer Journ Natural Med*, January/February 1997.

Schwartz, G.E. "Psychobiology of repression and health: a systems approach," 1990.

Schwartz, G.E. "Disregulation theory and disease: Applications to the repression/cerebral disconnection/cardiovascular disorder hypothesis," *International Review of Applied Psychology*, 32, pp 95-118, 1983.

Seelig, Mildred, MD and Ronald J. Elin, MD, PhD. "Myocardial Infarction and Magnesium," *Clinical Pearls News*, January 1996.

Seidler, Susan. "ERT: Drug company sales vs.women's health," *Nat'l Women's Health Network*, Mar/Apr 1994.

Selye, Hans. *The Physiology and Pathology of Exposure to Stress*, Montreal:Acta, 1950.

Shields, P.G., et al. "Mutagens from heated Chinese and U.S. cooking oils," *J Natl Cancer Inst*, 1995;87:836-841.

Shrive, E, et al. "Glutamine in treatment of peptic ulcer," *Tex. J. Med.*, 53:840-843, 1957.

Sibbison, J.B. "USA: Women's Health, Women's Rights," *Lancet*, July 21, 1990.

Stampfer, Meir J., MD, et al. "Postmenopausal Estrogen Therapy and Cardiovascular Disease: 10-Year Follow-Up From the Nurse's Health Study," *NEJM*, September 12, 1991.

Stampfer, Meir J., MD, et al. "A Prospective Study of Moderate Alcohol Consumption and the Risk of Coronary Disease and Stroke in Women," *NEJM*, August 4, 1988.

"Study Finds Bias in Way Women Are Evaluated for Heart Bypass," *New York Times*, 16 April 1990, p. A15.

Talley, R.B. "Drug-Induced Illness," *JAMA*, 229 (1974):1043.

te Velde, Egbert R., Huub A.I.M. van Leusden. "Hormonal Treatment for the Climacteric: Alleviation of Symptoms and Prevention of Postmenopausal Disease," *Lancet*, March 12, 1994.

Teo, Koon K., and Salam Yuuf. "Role of magnesium in reducing mortality in acute myocardial infarction: A review of the evidence," *Drugs*, 1993; 46(3).

"The Best & Worst Dressed List," *Nutrition Action Healthletter*, CSPI, June 1997.

"The FDA Approved a Drug. Then What?" *New York Times*, October 7, 1997.

"The PDR Family Guide to Women's Health and Prescription Drugs," *Medical Economics*, Montvale, NJ, 1994.

Troisi, R.J., Willett, W.C., et al. "Evidence for an oestrogen contribution to the pathogenesis of adult-onset asthma," *Am J Epidemiol* 139 (11), 7S21 (1994).

Truss, C. Orian. *The Missing Diagnosis*, Birmingham, AL, 1983.

"U.S. iron deficiency," *Lancet*, April 5, 1997, p. 1002.

Vakkanski, L. "Magnesium may slow bone loss," *Med Tribune*, July 22, 1993.

van Papendorp, DH, et al. "Biochemical profile or osteoporotic patients on essential fatty acid supplementation," *Nutr Res* 15(3), 325-334 (1995).

Verhoef, P., et al. "Homocysteine metabolism and risk of myocardial infarction: relation with vitamins B_6, B_{12} and folate," *Am J Epidemiol* 143,1966. From *Amer Journ of Clin Nutr*, April 1997, vol 17, No 2.

VERIS, Hammond B.R., et al. "Dietary modification of human macular pigment density," *Investigative Opthamol & Visual Science*, 1997;38:1795-1801.

Vrazo, Fawn. "FDA Panel Notes Heart Benefits of Postmenopausal Estrogen Drug," *Philadelphia Inquirer*, June 16, 1990.

Walsch, Neale Donald. *Conversations With God*, Hampton Roads Publishing, 1995.

Watts, David L. "Calcium and virus activation," *Trace Elements, Inc. Newsletter*, Vol. 3, No. 5, 1989. (P.O. Box 514, Addison, TX 75001).

Weaver, Connie M., et al. "Human calcium absorption from whole-wheat products," *Amer Inst of Nutr*, 3 May 1991.

Wei M., et al. "The Impact of Changes in Coffee Consumption on Serum Cholesterol," *J Clin Epidemiol* 48(10), 1189-1196 (1995).

Wenger, Nanette K., MD, et al. "Cardiovascular Health and Disease in Women," *NEJM*, vol 329, no. 4, July 22, 1993.

Werbach, Melvyn R., MD. *Nutritional Influences on Illness*, Second Edition, Third Line Press, 1996.

Whitaker, Julian, MD. *Is Heart Surgery Necessary?* Regnery Pub., 1995.

Whitehead, et al. "Effect of Red Wine Ingestion on the Antioxidant Capacity of Serum." *Clin Chem* 41:32-5, 1995.

Willett, W.C., et al. "Weight, Weight Change, and Coronary Heart Disease in Women," *JAMA* 273, 461-465, 1995.

Willett, Walter C., et al. "Intake of Trans Fatty Acids and Risk of Coronary Heart Disease Among Women," *Lancet*, March 6, 1993.

Wilson, Peter W.F., et al. "Postmenopausal Estrogen Use, Cigarette Smoking, and Cardiovascular Morbidity in Women Over 50," *NEJM*, October 24, 1985.

Wolff, Mary. "Blood Levels of Organochlorine Residues and Risk of Breast Cancer," *Journal of the Nat'l Cancer Institute*, 85, 8 (April 21, 1993):648-52.

Zang, E.A. and E.L. Wynder. "Differences in lung cancer risk between men and women: Examination of the Evidence." *J Natl Can Inst* 1996;88:183-91.

Index